INFLAMMATION AND OBESITY

INFLAMMATION AND OBESITY

A New and Novel Approach to Manage Obesity and its Consequences

Edited by

RAMAN MEHRZAD

Division of Plastic and Reconstructive Surgery, Rhode Island Hospital, The Warren Alpert School of Brown University, Providence, RI, United States

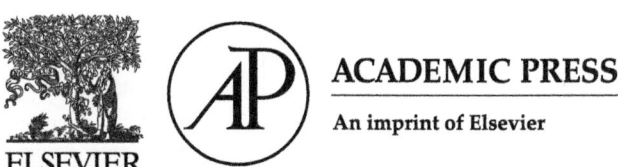

Academic Press is an imprint of Elsevier
125 London Wall, London EC2Y 5AS, United Kingdom
525 B Street, Suite 1650, San Diego, CA 92101, United States
50 Hampshire Street, 5th Floor, Cambridge, MA 02139, United States
The Boulevard, Langford Lane, Kidlington, Oxford OX5 1GB, United Kingdom

Copyright © 2023 Elsevier Inc. All rights reserved.

No part of this publication may be reproduced or transmitted in any form or by any means, electronic or mechanical, including photocopying, recording, or any information storage and retrieval system, without permission in writing from the publisher. Details on how to seek permission, further information about the Publisher's permissions policies and our arrangements with organizations such as the Copyright Clearance Center and the Copyright Licensing Agency, can be found at our website: www.elsevier.com/permissions.

This book and the individual contributions contained in it are protected under copyright by the Publisher (other than as may be noted herein).

Notices

Knowledge and best practice in this field are constantly changing. As new research and experience broaden our understanding, changes in research methods, professional practices, or medical treatment may become necessary.

Practitioners and researchers must always rely on their own experience and knowledge in evaluating and using any information, methods, compounds, or experiments described herein. In using such information or methods they should be mindful of their own safety and the safety of others, including parties for whom they have a professional responsibility.

To the fullest extent of the law, neither the Publisher nor the authors, contributors, or editors, assume any liability for any injury and/or damage to persons or property as a matter of products liability, negligence or otherwise, or from any use or operation of any methods, products, instructions, or ideas contained in the material herein.

ISBN 978-0-323-90960-0

For information on all Academic Press publications
visit our website at https://www.elsevier.com/books-and-journals

Publisher: Stacy Masucci
Acquisitions Editor: Katie Chan
Editorial Project Manager: Tracy I. Tufaga
Production Project Manager: Stalin Viswanathan
Cover Designer: Greg Harris

Typeset by STRAIVE, India

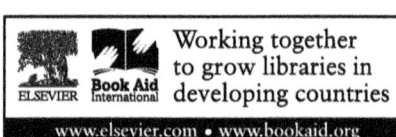

Dedication

To my mother, Shifteh Shahriari, who always inspired me to believe in myself; and to my sister Dr. Melorin Mehrzad, who always supported me in every aspect of my life. I love you both dearly, and I am proud that you have won the war against obesity.

Contents

Contributors   xiii

1. **Introduction to obesity and inflammation**   1
   Raman Mehrzad

2. **The obesity pandemic: How we are failing our patients**   5
   Ronald Tyszkowski and Raman Mehrzad

   Obesity as a disease   5
   Epidemiology   7
   Global impact of obesity   7
   Impact of increased incidence of obesity   8
   Origins of the obesity epidemic   8
   Sociodemographic factors associated with obesity   8
   Behavioral factors associated with obesity   10
   Obesity and disease   13
   Type 2 diabetes   13
   Failures in management of obesity   14
   References   16

3. **Inflammation: A multifaceted and omnipresent phenomenon**   19
   Ronald Tyszkowski and Raman Mehrzad

   Inflammation   19
   Allostasis and allostatic load   20
   Inflammation triggers   20
   Obesity   20
   Physical activity   22
   Dysbiosis   22
   Diet   24
   Chronic stress   25
   Disturbed sleep   25
   Chronic infections   26
   Xenobiotics   26
   References   28

4. Pathophysiology of obesity — 31
Jacqueline J. Chu and Raman Mehrzad

Structure of adipose tissue — 31
Phenotype of obesity — 32
Endocrine action of adipocytes in lean and obese states — 37
Putting it together: Treatment for obesity and metabolic syndrome — 39
Conclusion — 41
References — 42

5. Consequences of inflammation in obesity — 49
Mercy Adewale, Danielle Ruediger, and Jessica A. Zaman

Introduction — 49
Mechanism of inflammation — 53
Inflammatory processes in cardiovascular diseases and its relation to obesity — 55
Inflammatory processes in endocrine diseases and its relation to obesity — 57
Inflammatory processes in gastrointestinal diseases and its relation to obesity — 59
Inflammatory processes in musculoskeletal diseases and its relation to obesity — 62
Inflammatory processes in the central nervous system and their relation to obesity — 63
Conclusion — 65
References — 67

6. Inflammation and obesity — 71
Ronald Tyszkowski and Raman Mehrzad

Obesity and inflammation — 71
Changes in adipose tissue — 72
Adipokines: Origins and effects — 72
Tumor necrosis factor alpha — 73
Interleukin 6 — 73
Adiponectin — 74
Promotion of inflammation in obesity — 74
Insulin resistance — 75
microRNA — 76
Endothelial and microvascular dysfunction — 76
Obesity, inflammation, and cancer — 77
References — 80

7. Obesity, inflammation, and aging — 83
Jacqueline J. Chu and Raman Mehrzad

- Inflammation and aging — 83
- Inflammation and obesity — 87
- Connecting inflammation, obesity, and aging — 88
- Antiinflammatory intervention for aging-related illnesses — 92
- Conclusions — 93
- References — 94

8. Obesity, inflammation, and diseases of the gastrointestinal tract — 101
Anastasia C. Tillman and Marcoandrea Giorgi

- Introduction and epidemiology — 101
- Obesity incidence in certain groups — 102
- Etiology — 104
- The connection between obesity and inflammation — 105
- Obesity and gastrointestinal diseases — 108
- Interventions — 112
- References — 114

9. Obesity, inflammation, and cardiovascular disorders — 119
Afshin Ehsan

- Introduction — 119
- Atherosclerosis and coronary artery disease — 119
- Heart failure — 120
- Arrhythmias — 122
- Aortic stenosis — 123
- Aneurysmal disease — 124
- The obesity paradox — 126
- References — 126

10. Obesity, inflammation, and CNS disorders — 131
Sheel Shah, Justin Lee, and Michael Gong-Ruey Ho

- Introduction — 131
- CNS disorders associated with obesity — 132
- Conclusions — 144
- References — 145

11. Obesity, inflammation and muscle weakness   153
Per-Olof Hasselgren

Introduction	153
Obesity and relative muscle weakness	153
Sarcopenic obesity	156
Summary and conclusions	167
References	168

12. Resolution of inflammation   175
Ronald Tyszkowski and Raman Mehrzad

Resolution of inflammation	175
Cyclopentenone prostaglandins	176
Apoptotic cells and their clearance	180
microRNA	181
Resolution-directed lipid mediators of inflammation	182
Lipoxins	183
Resolvins	183
Maresins	185
Protectins	185
References	186

13. Physical activity in obesity and inflammation prevention and management   189
Ollin Venegas and Raman Mehrzad

Introduction	189
Obesity-related inflammation	190
Physical activity and obesity-related inflammation	193
Weight loss and maintenance	203
Conclusion	205
References	205

14. Diet and inflammation in obesity: Prevention and management   213
Kathryn Ottaviano and Jessica A. Zaman

The obesity epidemic	213
Pathophysiology of obesity	213
Leptin and inflammation	214
Obesity and markers of inflammation—Are they adequate?	215
Diet and obesity	216
Sugar and obesity	216

Sugar and inflammation	218
High fat	219
Essential fatty acids	219
Saturated and unsaturated fat	220
Trans fats	221
What is an antiinflammatory diet	222
Antiinflammatory diet and weight loss	224
Antiinflammatory benefits of popular diets	224
The long-term outlook	227
References	227

15. Management of obesity and related inflammatory disorders — 233
Nisrine I. Kawa and Souheil W. Adra

Introduction	233
Behavioral weight management strategies and inflammation	233
The role of the microbiome in treatment of obesity and inflammation	237
Role of weight loss medications	242
Bariatric interventions endoscopic/surgical and inflammation	248
A standardized evaluation of inflammation in patients with obesity	252
A stepwise approach for managing inflammation and weight in the obese patients	253
References	255

16. New therapeutic strategies in the management of obesity-modulated inflammation — 263
Ronald Tyszkowski and Raman Mehrzad

Staging obesity-related inflammation	263
Glucose-insulin homeostasis biomarkers	265
Adipose tissue biomarkers	266
Inflammatory biomarkers	266
Omic-based biomarkers	267
The microbiome and obesity	267
Alternative treatments for obesity	269
Artificial intelligence and management of obesity	271
Botanicals in the treatment of obesity and obesity-related inflammation	272
Sleep and obesity	273
References	274

Index — 277

Contributors

Mercy Adewale
Albany Medical College, Albany, NY, United States

Souheil W. Adra
Department of Surgery, Beth Israel Deaconess Medical Center, Harvard Medical School, Boston, MA, United States

Jacqueline J. Chu
College of Medicine, The Ohio State University, Columbus, OH, United States

Afshin Ehsan
Division of Cardiothoracic Surgery, Rhode Island Hospital, Brown University, Providence, RI, United States

Marcoandrea Giorgi
Surgery, Brown University, Providence, RI, United States

Per-Olof Hasselgren
Department of Surgery, Beth Israel Deaconess Medical Center; George H.A. Clowes Distinguished Professor of Surgery, Harvard Medical School, Boston, MA, United States

Michael Gong-Ruey Ho
Department of Neurology, David Geffen School of Medicine at UCLA, Los Angeles, CA, United States

Nisrine I. Kawa
Department of Internal Medicine, Waterbury Hospital, Yale School of Medicine, Waterbury, CT, United States

Justin Lee
Department of Neurosurgery, David Geffen School of Medicine at UCLA, Los Angeles, CA, United States

Raman Mehrzad
Division of Plastic and Reconstructive Surgery, Rhode Island Hospital, The Warren Alpert School of Brown University, Providence, RI, United States

Kathryn Ottaviano
Department of Surgery, Albany Medical Center, Albany, NY, United States

Danielle Ruediger
Albany Medical College, Albany, NY, United States

Sheel Shah
Department of Neurosurgery, David Geffen School of Medicine at UCLA, Los Angeles, CA, United States

Anastasia C. Tillman
Warren Alpert Medical School, Brown University, Providence, RI, United States

Ronald Tyszkowski
Private Practice, Allied Health, Women and Infants Hospital, Providence, RI, United States

Ollin Venegas
Department of Surgery, Rhode Island Hospital, Brown University, Providence, RI, United States

Jessica A. Zaman
Department of Surgery, Albany Medical Center, Albany, NY, United States

CHAPTER 1

Introduction to obesity and inflammation

Raman Mehrzad
Division of Plastic and Reconstructive Surgery, Rhode Island Hospital, The Warren Alpert School of Brown University, Providence, RI, United States

Obesity is a global, complex, multifactorial, and generally preventable disease. The global prevalence of obesity has doubled in the past 40 years regardless of sex, age, ethnicity, or socioeconomic status. Today, more than one-third of the world's population is classified as obese or overweight. If this trend continues, researchers estimate that by 2030, this number will hit over 50%. Based on this, there is continuous research being pursued each year with new scientific articles, evidence, guidelines, and management coming out on this topic.

Inflammation is a biologic sequence of events evolutionary designed to maintain tissue and organ homeostasis. Different mediators and expression of receptors are timely released to restore tissues to their original condition [1]. Additionally, inflammation is a protective tissue response to injury or destruction of tissues that serves to destroy or dilute both the injurious agent and the injured tissues [2].

Two main types of inflammation exist: acute and chronic inflammation. Acute inflammation lasts for a brief period and is characterized by edema and migration of leukocytes. Chronic inflammation lasts for a long time and is characterized by the presence of lymphocytes and macrophages and the proliferation of blood vessels and connective tissue [3].

Obesity, a feature of metabolic syndrome, is associated with chronic with secretion of inflammatory adipokines usually from adipose tissue, such as leptin, interleukin (IL-6), tumor necrosis factor-α (TNF-α), monocyte chemoattractant protein-1 (MCP-1), C-reactive protein (CRP), and resistin [4,5]. In recent years, it has been proven that obesity is associated with a low-grade inflammatory state and process with increase in circulating levels of the above proinflammatory cytokines in healthy obese subjects [6]. The same phenomenon is also seen in obese children who have higher CRP levels than normal-weight children [6]. Weight loss, mainly through diet, has been demonstrated in some studies to be associated with reduction in circulating levels of IL-6, TNF-alpha, CRP, and other markers of inflammation, independently of age, sex, and BMI. Similarly, subjects who lose weight after gastric bypass show decrease of CRP and IL-6 levels [6]. Sustained inflammation is considered a strong risk factor for developing many diseases including metabolic syndrome, cancer, diabetes, and cardiovascular disease.

Consequently, obesity and metabolic disorder are accompanied by chronic low-grade inflammation, which could have fundamentally consequences to our health. Thus, this foundation has changed our view of the underlying causes and progression of obesity. Inflammatory cascades are activated early in adipose expansion and during obesity, lastingly skewing the immune system to a proinflammatory state. Moreover, numerous studies have demonstrated that one of the major consequences of obesity is not only the initiation of inflammation, but its relevant role in causing insulin resistance, impaired insulin secretion, and disruption of other aspects of energy homeostasis [5].

Importantly, obesity-induced inflammation is different from other inflammatory types in that it involves stimulatory activation of the innate immune system that impacts metabolic homeostasis, that in many cases last for many years, if not a lifetime. Obesity-related inflammation also results in inadequate responses such as necrosis and fibrosis that can lead to significant tissue damage. Furthermore, this type of inflammation is unique in that it encompasses multiple organs, including the skeletal muscle, brain, adipose, pancreas, liver, and heart [5].

Therefore, outlining the reciprocal influence of obesity and inflammation is of crucial importance to not only find new therapeutic strategies to fight this pandemic but also to manage its complications. With this foundation, this book gathered a group of experts that has provided reviews that dive deeply into the mechanisms and links between obesity and inflammation, and furthermore, its consequences within different organ systems and our biology.

References

[1] Romano M. Inflammation resolution: does the bone marrow have a say? Am J Hematol 2008;83(6):435–6.
[2] Feuerstein GZ, Libby P, Mann DL. Inflammation—a new frontier in cardiac disease and therapeutics. In: Feuerstein GZ, Libby P, Mann DL, editors. Inflammation and cardiac diseases. Birkhäuser Basel; 2003. p. 1–5.

[3] Seki H, Tani Y, Arita M. Omega-3 PUFA derived anti-inflammatory lipid mediator resolvin E1. Prostaglandins Other Lipid Mediat 2009;89(3–4):126–30.
[4] Stępień M, Stępień A, Wlazeł RN, Paradowski M, Banach M, Rysz J. Obesity indices and inflammatory markers in obese non-diabetic normo- and hypertensive patients: a comparative pilot study. J Lipids Health Dis 2014;13:29.
[5] Ellulu MS, Patimah I, Khaza'ai H, Rahmat A, Abed Y. Obesity and inflammation: the linking mechanism and the complications. Arch Med Sci 2017;13(4):851–63. https://doi.org/10.5114/aoms.2016.58928. Epub 2016 Mar 31 28721154. PMC5507106.
[6] Rodríguez-Hernández H, Simental-Mendía LE, Rodríguez-Ramírez G, Reyes-Romero MA. Obesity and inflammation: epidemiology, risk factors, and markers of inflammation. Int J Endocrinol 2013;2013:678159. https://doi.org/10.1155/2013/678159. Epub 2013 Apr 17 23690772. PMC3652163.

CHAPTER 2

The obesity pandemic: How we are failing our patients

Ronald Tyszkowski[a] and Raman Mehrzad[b]
[a]Private Practice, Allied Health, Women and Infants Hospital, Providence, RI, United States
[b]Division of Plastic and Reconstructive Surgery, Rhode Island Hospital, The Warren Alpert School of Brown University, Providence, RI, United States

Obesity as a disease

Obesity is defined by the World Health Organization (WHO) as excessive fat accumulation that might impair health and is diagnosed at a BMI of $\geq 30\,\text{kg/m}^2$ [1]. The 2017 Global Nutrition Reports showed that 2 billion adults and 40 million children are overweight, worldwide [2].

The US Department of Health and Human Services called obesity "the single greatest threat to public health for this century [3]." It is universally recognized as a significant health hazard and is associated with a decreased life expectancy of from 5 to 20 years, depending on the severity of the condition and the presence of associated comorbidities including cancer, cardiovascular disease, diabetes mellitus [4], and poor mental health; all of which have a negative effect on quality of life, work productivity, and healthcare costs. In 2005, the Center for Disease Control estimated that 365,000 people die annually from obesity [5]. And some studies predict that life expectancy will level off or decline by 2050 due to childhood obesity [6]. In the United States, it has been estimated that the health cost incurred by a single obese individual was $1901 per year in 2014, extrapolating to $149.4 billion at the national level [7]. In England, the total direct and indirect costs attributable to overweight and obese individuals were equivalent to 0.47%–0.61% of the GDP [8].

This worldwide epidemic of obesity is not a new phenomenon. The International Obesity Task Force was formed in the mid-1990s with the aim of expanding awareness of this growing problem. The WHO in 1997 convened the Expert Technical Consultation on Obesity and published its findings in 2000. Obesity was officially classified as a disease in 1990 (ICD-10 E66.0) [9]. In 2013, the American Medical Association recognized obesity as a disease, of growing scientific, social, and political interest [10].

It stated that "recognizing obesity as a disease will help change the way the medical community tackles this complex issue."

Classifying obesity as a disease also produced a significant amount of criticism as well. It has historically been a "highly stigmatized condition that has long been generally regarded by the public as a reversible consequence of personal choices" [3]. Michael Tanner wrote in The National Review in 2015 that this move was a symptom of another disease, "the abdication of personal responsibility and an invitation to government meddling." [11]. Many other organizations have also adopted this terminology (Fig. 1)

Randolph Nesse wrote about disease classification: "Our social definition of disease will remain contentious, however, because values vary, and because the label 'disease' changes the moral status of people with various conditions, and their rights to medical and social resources." [12].

Box 1
Associations or organizations that have declared obesity is a disease

- National Institutes of Health
- US Food and Drug Administration
- Federal Trade Commission
- American Medical Association
- World Health Organization
- American College of Physicians
- American Association of Clinical Endocrinologists
- American College of Cardiology
- The Endocrine Society
- American Academy of Family Physicians
- Institute of Medicine
- The Obesity Society
- World Obesity Federation
- American Heart Association
- American Diabetes Association
- American Academy of Family Physicians
- American Society for Reproductive Medicine
- American Urologic Association
- American College of Surgeons

Data from Kahan S, Zvenyach T. Obesity as a disease: current policies and implications for the future. Curr Obes Rep 2016;5(2):291-7; and Bray GA, Kim KK, Widling JPH. Obesity: a chronic relapsing progressive disease process. A position statement of the World Obesity Federation. Obes Rev 2017;18(7):715-23.

Fig. 1 Associations that have declared obesity as a disease [13].

Epidemiology

Despite the universally accepted premise that it needs to be addressed as an urgent public health issue, incidence continues to rise in the United States and globally. No country or subpopulation within a country has achieved a decrease in obesity, representing one of the biggest population health failures of our time [14]. Trends in obesity, which had leveled off briefly in 2009–12, project to 50% of adults by 2030. In the United States, rates of obesity will surpass 50% by 2030 in 29 states and not below 35% in any state [15]. Additionally, severe obesity (BMI ≥ 35) will affect one in four and become the most common BMI category in women, black non-Hispanic adults, and low-income adults.

Extrapolating trends out to 2050 paints an even worse picture. Men in age group 31–40 (Fig. 2) project to an almost 70% rate of obesity by 2050. Interestingly, women also project to a slightly less percentage of obesity of 60%, but at a later age range of 61–70, possibly related to the hormonal variability of menopause (Fig. 3).

Global impact of obesity
Obesity worldwide

- In a majority of European countries, the prevalence of obesity has increased from 10% to 40% in the last 10 years [9].
- In England, prevalence has tripled in the last 10 years [9].

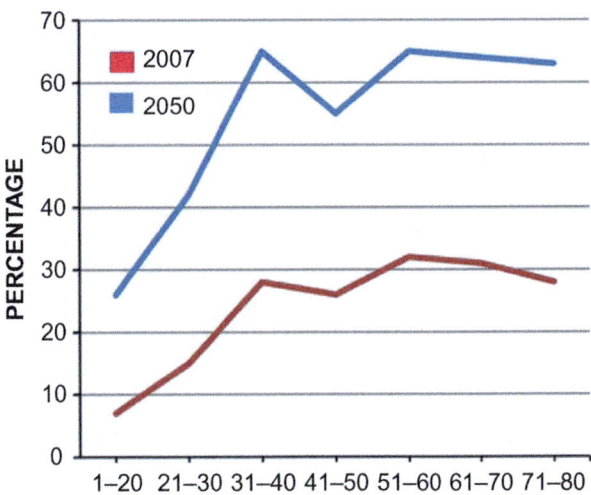

Fig. 2 Estimated percentage of males who are obese at 2007 and 2050 [9].

8   Inflammation and obesity

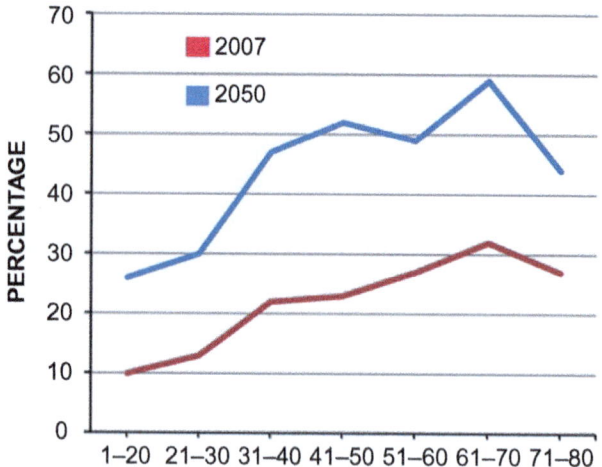

Fig. 3 Estimated percentage of women who are obese at 2007 and 2050 [9].

- In 2009, one in five Americans were morbidly obese [9]
- As the Western diet combined with modern food preparation techniques moves across the world, projected rates of obesity in Africa increase by 162%, in India by 150%, and in China by 104% by 2030 (Fig. 4) [16]. Fig. 5 shows the expected increase in rate of obesity as broken down by ethnic group.

Impact of increased incidence of obesity

In Fig. 6, the effect of obesity on quality of life is demonstrated over a 20-year period. Unhealthy obese patients show the greatest decrease in physical function and overall body pain.

This increase will inevitably coincide with an increase in medical costs and percentage of GDP directed to obesity-related costs.

Origins of the obesity epidemic

Studies into the origins of obesity can guide the clinician to target those with higher risk factors inherently and modify behavior strategically. Multiple literature reviews list those factors, which are summarized below.

Sociodemographic factors associated with obesity [18]

- Older age
- Married

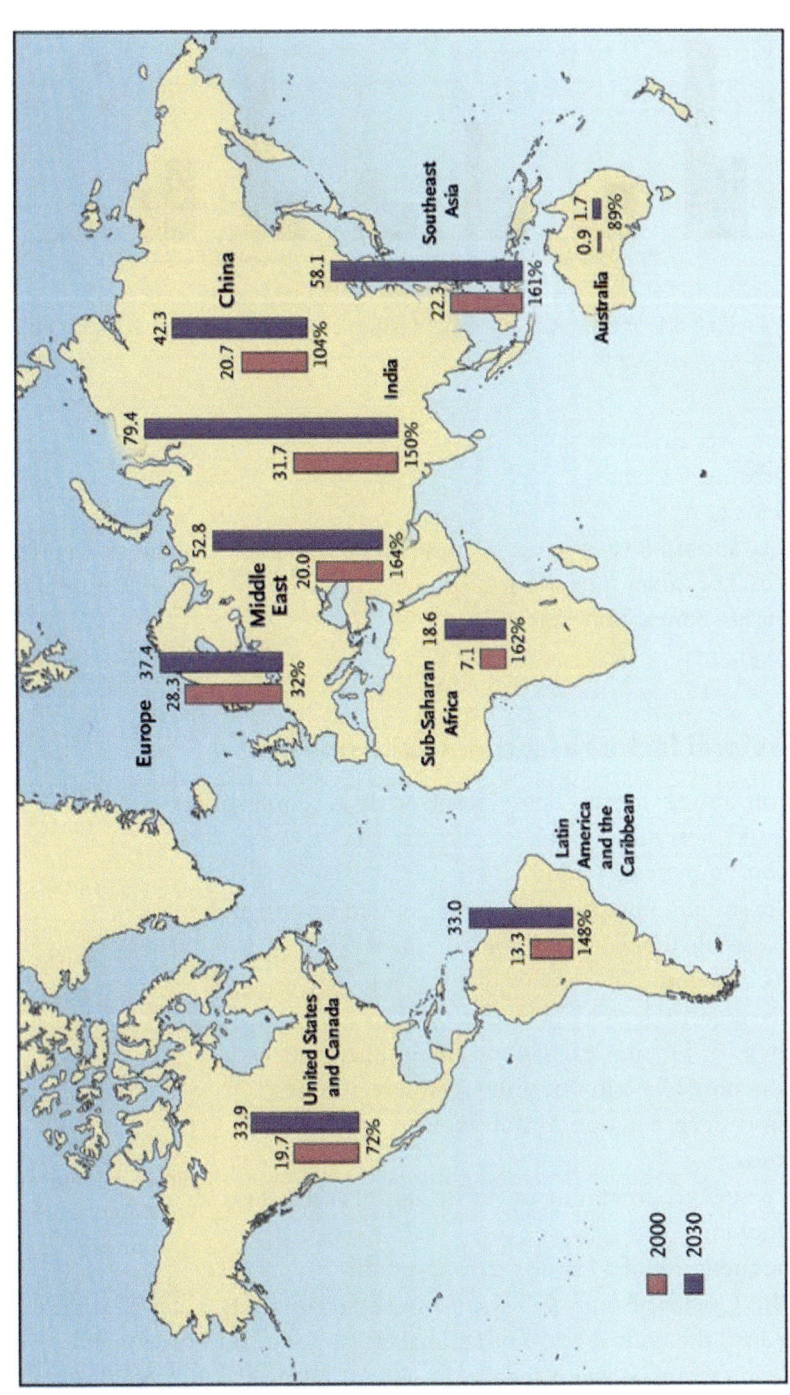

Fig. 4 The percentage obese in 2000 vs 2030, with the percent increase. [16].

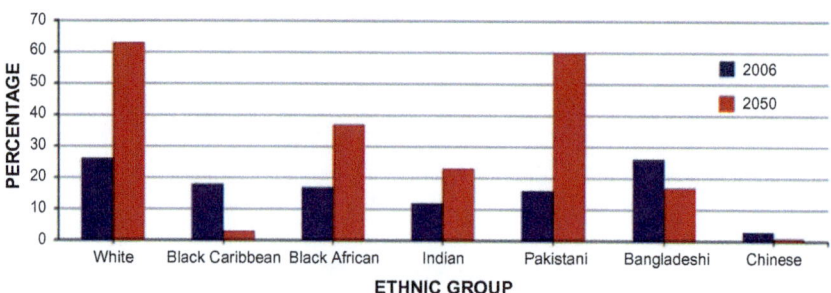

Fig. 5 Predicted percentage of male population obese at 2006 and 2050 by ethnic group [9].

- Low wealth index
- Urban residency
- Female
- Easy accessibility of nutrient dense foods secondary to a free trade policy
- Rural to urban migration
- Higher education levels
- Pregnancy

Behavioral factors associated with obesity

- Consuming energy-dense food, such as confectionaries, sugars, soft drinks, fats, and alcohol
- Consuming pastry foods
- Consuming ultraprocessed food (refined carbohydrates)
- Excess alcohol consumption
- Monotonous diet or poor diet quality
- Evening snack induces obesity
- Irregular physical exercise or physical inactiveness
- Watching television or prolonged screen time
- Short sleep duration or shift work
- Stress
- Obesogenic environment (urbanization and industrialization)
- Smoking
- Frequent use of a taxi for transportation

The Quebec Family Study, an observational study published in 2014, looked at "the contribution of familial resemblance and genetic effects on body fatness and behaviors related to energy balance" [19]. Fig. 7 shows the

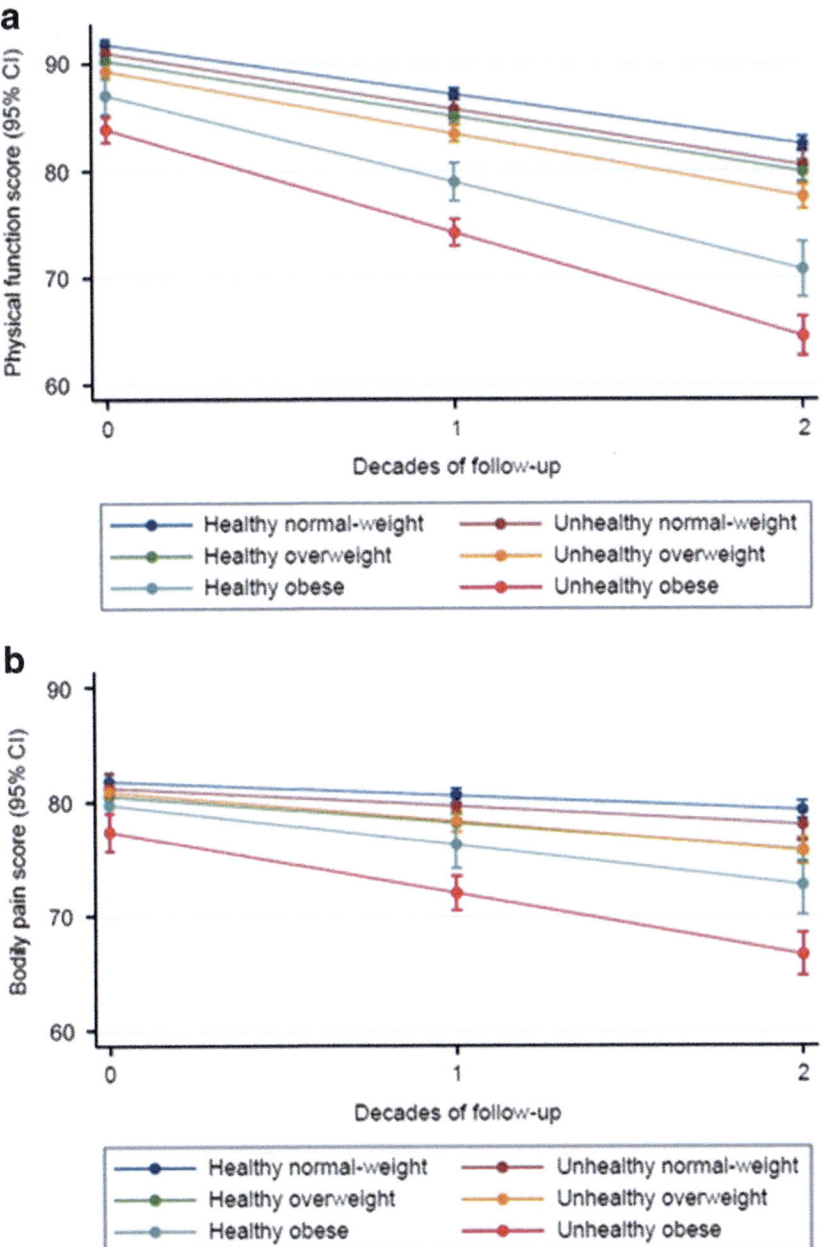

Fig. 6 Decline in physical function (A) and worsening of bodily pain (B) over two decades by initial metabolic and obesity status. Models include adjustment for 1991/1994 values of age, sex, ethnicity, occupational position, moderate-to-vigorous physical activity, smoking, alcohol, and fruit and vegetable consumption. [17].

Common risk factors
High lipid intake
≥40% fat/day (vs. <30 % fat/day)
Nonparticipation in hight-intensity physical activity
0 min/day (vs. ≥30 min/day)
Two risk factors combined
≥40% fat/day + 0 min/day
Emerging risk factors
Low calcium intake
<600 mg/day (vs. ≥1,000 mg/day)
High disinhibition eating behavior
≥6 disinhibition score (vs. ≤3 disinhibition score)
Short sleep duration
<6 h/day (vs. 7-8 h/day)
Low calcium intake and high disinhibition eating behavior
<600 mg/day + ≥6 disinhibition score
Low calcium intake and short sleep duration
<600 mg/day + <6 h/day
High disinhibition eating behavior and short sleep duration
≥6 disinhibition score + <6 h/day
Three risk factores combined
<600 mg of calcium/day + ≥6 disinhibition score + <6 h of sleep/day

Fig. 7 Common and emerging risk factors for obesity from the 2014 Quebec Study [19].

common risk factors, high-fat diet, and lack of physical activity. But it also shows newer emerging risk factors of:
- low calcium intake,
- binge eating,
- lack of sleep,
- various combinations of the three.

Since obesity has been so resistant to treatment, in that rates continue to rise, these risk factors can help us to identify vulnerable populations and dangerous behavior so that interventions can happen earlier before the disease sets in.

Obesity and disease

Obesity and its myriad of physiologic sequelae are a significant health issue. However, the problem does not stop there. It predisposes the affected individual to increased risk of a multitude of chronic, life-threatening illnesses. Type 2 diabetes and cancer are two disease states inexorably linked to obesity (Fig. 8).

Type 2 diabetes

In total, 90% of type 2 diabetes is attributable to obesity, and obesity-related metabolic syndrome causes impaired glucose tolerance in 197 million people worldwide. The prevalence of type 2 diabetes is expected to increase to 366 million by 2033, with the most prominent increase in developing countries [16].

Type 2 diabetes mellitus (T2D) is one of the defining medical challenges of the 21st century [21]. Overconsumption of relatively inexpensive, calorically dense, inadequately satiating, highly palatable food in industrialized nations has led to unprecedented increases in obesity [21]. In the United

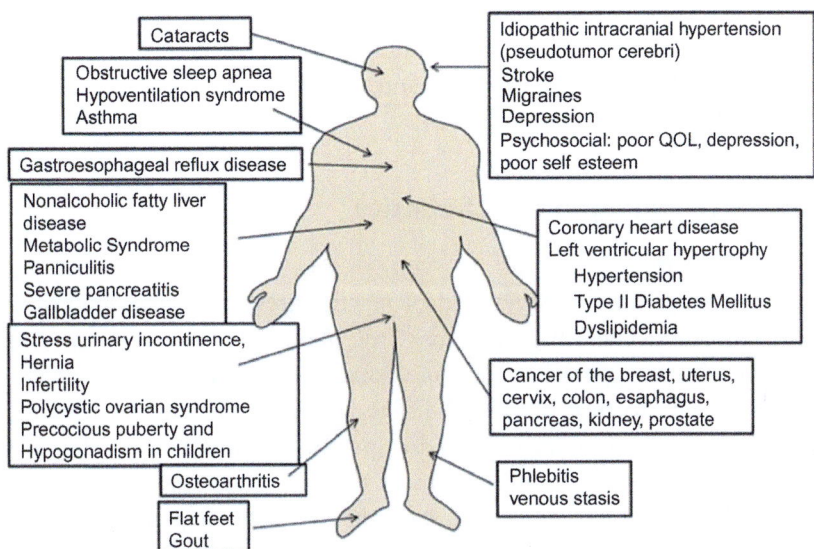

Comorbidities associated with obesity. QOL, quality of life.

Fig. 8 The many comorbidities of obesity [20].

States, the combined prevalence of diabetes and prediabetes is over 50% [22]. Although only a subset of obese people develops T2D, obesity is a major risk factor for T2D, and rates of T2D prevalence have paralleled those of obesity [23].

Obesity and cancer

Pan et al. [24] found that:
- Obese and overweight people had respective risks of 34% and 9% higher for all 19 cancers combined compared with subjects with a body mass index of less than $25 \, kg/m^2$ [24].
- Obese people had an increased risk of non-Hodgkin's lymphoma, leukemia, multiple myeloma, and cancers of the kidney, colon, rectum, breast (in postmenopausal women), ovary, pancreas, and prostate [24].
- Another study showed that in men, a $5 \, kg/m^2$ increase in BMI was strongly associated with esophageal adenocarcinoma and with thyroid, colon, and renal cancers. In women, strong associations between a $5 \, kg/m^2$ increase in BMI and esophageal adenocarcinoma and with endometrial, gallbladder, and renal cancers were noted [25].
- Among postmenopausal women in the United Kingdom, 5% of all cancers (about 6000 annually) are attributable to being overweight or obese [26].

These observations provide strong evidence for the positive association between obesity and overall cancer and some site-specific cancers. If the association were causal, overweight and obesity would be responsible for 7.7% of overall cancer incidence [24].

Failures in management of obesity

Poor training

Current management strategies and/or practice prevention steps are proving to be ineffective. There has been very little implementation of comprehensive, policy-based approaches [27]. Additionally, health professionals are often poorly prepared to treat obesity [28]. They receive little nutritional training and are not prepared to assess diet and/or provide nutritional counseling [29].

A study that surveyed physicians at the University of Michigan [30] showed that few were confident in their ability to change patient behaviors. Only 10.8% of trainees and 17.3% of attending physicians reported that high self-efficacy for changing patients' diet-related behaviors with a similar pattern was observed related to self-efficacy to change patients' behaviors related to exercise.

Physicians were also asked about training in counseling by asking to agree with the following statement: "I received adequate training in lifestyle counseling patients." Only 12.7% of trainees and 23.5% for attending physicians agreed that they had received adequate training in counseling on diet. Only 13.7% of trainees and 17.3% of attending physicians agreed that they had received adequate training in counseling on exercise.

Practitioner bias

Obesity also affects provider's attitudes toward their patients. Physicians are reported to be one of the most frequent sources of weight bias [31]. In fact, research has shown that negative stereotypes and stigma exist within a diverse group of healthcare providers including physicians, nurses, dieticians, and psychologists [32]. In 2010, the British Public Health Minister advocated for calling patients "fat" because "obese" did not have the necessary emotional impact. Her reasoning was that patients would be less worried about their weight if they were simply referred to as obese.

Weight stigmatization like this can lead to heightened risk of psychological distress, maladaptive eating behaviors, exercise avoidance, reduced healthcare utilization, and poorer outcomes in weight loss treatment [32]. So regardless of the effectiveness of any diet, exercise, or pharmaceutical approach, these biases can negate them.

Primary care providers engage in less patient-centered communication with patients they believe are not likely to be adherent [33]. A common explicitly endorsed provider stereotype about patients with obesity is that they are less likely to be adherent to treatment or self-care recommendations, are lazy, undisciplined, and weak-willed. Primary care providers have reported less respect for patients with obesity compared with those without [34,35], and low respect has been shown to predict less positive affective communication and information giving [36]. They may also allocate time differently, spending less time educating obese patients about their health [37].

Finally, physicians may fail to refer for diagnostic testing or to consider treatment options beyond advising the patient to lose weight [38], jumping to the conclusion that obesity is the root cause of the patient's presenting symptoms.

Primary care nursing also falls victim to preexisting beliefs or prejudice toward obese patients. Brown showed that of 546 UK nurses surveyed in 2006 that only 8.2% believed that obese patients were motivated to change, while agreeing with statements that working with population was rewarding and to feeling empathy toward obese patients [39]. The emotional conflict demonstrated by this survey crystalizes the challenges practitioners face as they attempt to manage these patients despite the harsh societal prejudgments ingrained in our collective psyche.

A moving article, "Voices of Patients with Obesity" articulately states what patients are looking for from their doctors. Thirty years after classifying obesity as a disease, we are still failing to provide even basic care and understanding. As one of the authors of this articles pleads, "I know you are behind, that you are dealing with patients with cancer and heart disease, rare diseases, and sinus infections. I know you need more than my allotted 15 minutes. But I am here today, and if you don't have time to help me with a plan, who does?" [40].

Practitioners have to be the bulwark against the seemingly unstoppable tide of obesity. It starts with us.

References

[1] Fontaine KR, et al. Years of life lost due to obesity. JAMA 2003;289(2):187–93.
[2] Hawkes C, Fanzo J. Nourishing the SDGs: global nutrition report 2017. Bristol: Development Initiatives Poverty Research Ltd; 2017.
[3] United States. Dietary Guidelines Advisory Committee. Dietary guidelines for Americans, 2010. No. 232. US Department of Health and Human Services, US Department of Agriculture; 2010.
[4] Blüher M. Obesity: global epidemiology and pathogenesis. Nat Rev Endocrinol 2019;15(5):288–98.
[5] Couzin J. A heavyweight battle over CDC's obesity forecasts. Science 2005;770–1.
[6] Mann CC. Provocative study says obesity may reduce US life expectancy: the rising incidence of obesity, especially among children and teenagers, is leading to a variety of diseases that could depress average life span. Science 2005;307(5716):1716–8.
[7] Kim DD, Basu A. Estimating the medical care costs of obesity in the United States: systematic review, meta-analysis, and empirical analysis. Value Health 2016;19(5):602–13.
[8] von Lengerke T, Krauth C. Economic costs of adult obesity: a review of recent European studies with a focus on subgroup-specific costs. Maturitas 2011;69(3):220–9.
[9] Agha M, Agha R. The rising prevalence of obesity: part a: impact on public health. Int J Surg Oncol 2017;2(7), e17.
[10] De Lorenzo A, et al. Obesity: a preventable, treatable, but relapsing disease. Nutrition 2020;71, 110615.
[11] Tanner M. Obesity is not a disease. Natl Rev 2013. Online.
[12] Nesse RM. On the difficulty of defining disease: a Darwinian perspective. Med Health Care Philos 2001;4(1):37–46.
[13] Kahan S, Zvenyach T. Obesity as a disease: current policies and implications for the future. Curr Obes Rep 2016;5(2):291–7.
[14] Jaacks LM, et al. The obesity transition: stages of the global epidemic. Lancet Diabetes Endocrinol 2019;7(3):231–40.
[15] Ward ZJ, et al. Projected US state-level prevalence of adult obesity and severe obesity. N Engl J Med 2019;381(25):2440–50.

[16] Hossain P, Kawar B, El Nahas M. Obesity and diabetes in the developing world—a growing challenge. N Engl J Med 2007;356(3):213–5.
[17] Bell JA, et al. Healthy obesity and risk of accelerated functional decline and disability. Int J Obes (Lond) 2017;41(6):866–72.
[18] Endalifer ML, Diress G. Epidemiology, predisposing factors, biomarkers, and prevention mechanism of obesity: a systematic review. J Obes 2020;2020.
[19] Chaput J-P, et al. Findings from the Quebec family study on the etiology of obesity: genetics and environmental highlights. Curr Obes Rep 2014;3(1):54–66.
[20] Upadhyay J, et al. Obesity as a disease. Med Clin 2018;102(1):13–33.
[21] Zimmet P, Alberti KG, Shaw J. Global and societal implications of the diabetes epidemic. Nature 2001;414:782–7.
[22] Menken A, et al. Prevalence of and trends in diabetes among adults in the United States, 1988–2012. JAMA 2015;314(10):1021–9.
[23] Kahn SE, Hull RL, Utzschneider KM. Mechanisms linking obesity to insulin resistance and type 2 diabetes. Nature 2006;444(7121):840–6.
[24] Pan SY, Johnson KC, Ugnat A-M, Wen SW, Mao Y, The Canadian Cancer Registries Epidemiology Research Group. Association of obesity and cancer risk in Canada. Am J Epidemiol 2004;159(3):259–68.
[25] Renehan AG, et al. Body-mass index and incidence of cancer: a systematic review and meta-analysis of prospective observational studies. The lancet 2008;371(9612):569–78.
[26] Reeves GK, et al. Cancer incidence and mortality in relation to body mass index in the Million Women Study: cohort study. BMJ 2007;335(7630):1134.
[27] Roberto CA, et al. Patchy progress on obesity prevention: emerging examples, entrenched barriers, and new thinking. The Lancet 2015;385(9985):2400–9.
[28] Dietz WH, et al. Management of obesity: improvement of health-care training and systems for prevention and care. The Lancet 2015;385(9986):2521–33.
[29] Kris-Etherton PM, et al. Nutrition competencies in health professionals' education and training: a new paradigm. Adv Nutr 2015;6(1):83–7.
[30] Howe M, et al. Patient-related diet and exercise counseling: do providers' own lifestyle habits matter? Prev Cardiol 2010;13(4):180–5.
[31] Puhl RM, Brownell KD. Confronting and coping with weight stigma: an investigation of overweight and obese adults. Obesity 2006;14(10):1802–15.
[32] Puhl R, Peterson JL, Luedicke J. Motivating or stigmatizing? Public perceptions of weight-related language used by health providers. Int J Obes (Lond) 2013;37(4):612–9.
[33] Jr S, Richard L, Gordon H, Haidet P. Physicians' communication and perceptions of patients: is it how they look, how they talk, or is it just the doctor? Soc Sci Med 2007;65(3):586–98.
[34] Hebl MR, Xu J. Weighing the care: physicians' reactions to the size of a patient. Int J Obes (Lond) 2001;25(8):1246–52.
[35] Huizinga MM, et al. Physician respect for patients with obesity. J Gen Intern Med 2009;24(11):1236.
[36] Beach MC, et al. Are physicians' attitudes of respect accurately perceived by patients and associated with more positive communication behaviors? Patient Educ Couns 2006;62(3):347–54.
[37] Bertakis KD, Azari R. The impact of obesity on primary care visits. Obes Res 2005;13(9):1615–23.
[38] Persky S, Eccleston CP. Medical student bias and care recommendations for an obese versus non-obese virtual patient. Int J Obes (Lond) 2011;35(5):728–35.
[39] Brown I, et al. Management of obesity in primary care: nurses' practices, beliefs and attitudes. J Adv Nurs 2007;59(4):329–41.
[40] Johnstone J, et al. What I wish my doctor really knew: the voices of patients with obesity. Ann Fam Med 2020;18(2):169–71.

CHAPTER 3

Inflammation: A multifaceted and omnipresent phenomenon

Ronald Tyszkowski[a] and Raman Mehrzad[b]

[a]Private Practice, Allied Health, Women and Infants Hospital, Providence, RI, United States
[b]Division of Plastic and Reconstructive Surgery, Rhode Island Hospital, The Warren Alpert School of Brown University, Providence, RI, United States

Inflammation

Acute inflammation is a defensive physiological response occurring in vascularized tissues to protect the host against injuries [1]. It is a "multifactorial network of chemical signals" that "initiate and maintain a host response designed to heal the afflicted tissue" [2]. The characteristic "cardinal signs" of inflammation, described by the Roman physician Celsus in the first century, rubor (redness), tumor (swelling), calor (heat), and dolor (pain), are the macroscopic manifestation of changes that occur at molecular and cellular levels in inflamed tissues [3].

Activation and directed migration of leukocytes (neutrophils, monocytes, and eosinophils) occurs from the venous system to the sites of tissue injury [2] Polymorphonuclear neutrophils (PMNs) kill pathogens by engulfing them via phagocytosis and/or destroying them by excreting microbicidal proteins and reactive oxygen species [3]. These cells then undergo programmed death or apoptosis.

Attraction of monocytes, via chemotactic factors, follows. They differentiate into macrophages (MΦs), which perform efferocytosis or clearing of the apoptotic cells. These macrophages are the main source of growth factors and cytokines, which we will see in other chapters, have far reaching effects on surrounding cells and physiologic processes.

There is no discrimination between microbial and host targets, so collateral damage to host tissues is unavoidable [4]. This is among the many reasons for the destructive effects of chronic inflammation where the inflammation exudate may remain and continue to damage healthy tissue.

Initiation of acute inflammation can also occur in response to injury second to physical, chemical, or noxious stimuli ("Sterile agents") following cellular stress or damage [5]. Systemic chronic inflammation (SCI) is typically initiated by damage-associated molecular patterns (DAMPs) similar to traumatically induced acute inflammation. Its presence increases with age, as evidenced by increased circulating levels of inflammation modulators such as cytokines and chemokines [6].

Allostasis and allostatic load

Allostasis ("achieving stability through change") is the process by which the body responds to daily stressors and maintains homeostasis [7]. Normal allostatic response is short term in nature and self-resolving (Figs. 1 and 2). This process is integral to survival, but if the allostatic response is insufficient to counteract the environmental stressors or does not shut off it results in allostatic overload [8]. SCI is an example of allostatic overload.

Inflammation triggers

See Fig. 3.

Obesity

Obesity is a significant inflammatory agent. Trends in obesity, which had leveled off briefly in 2009–12, project to 50% of adults by 2030. In the United States, rates of obesity will surpass 50% by 2030 in 29 states and not below 35% in any

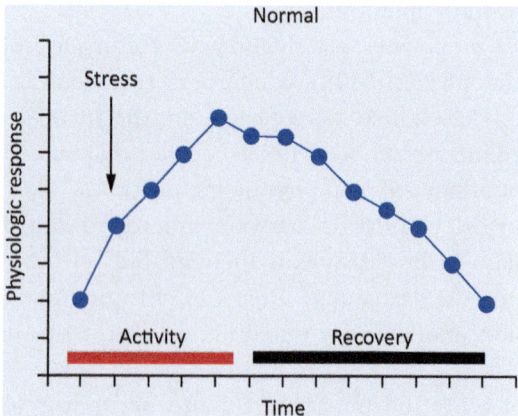

Fig. 1 A normal physiologic response to stress (allostasis) in which the system returns to a normal level of activity following neutralization of the stressor [8].

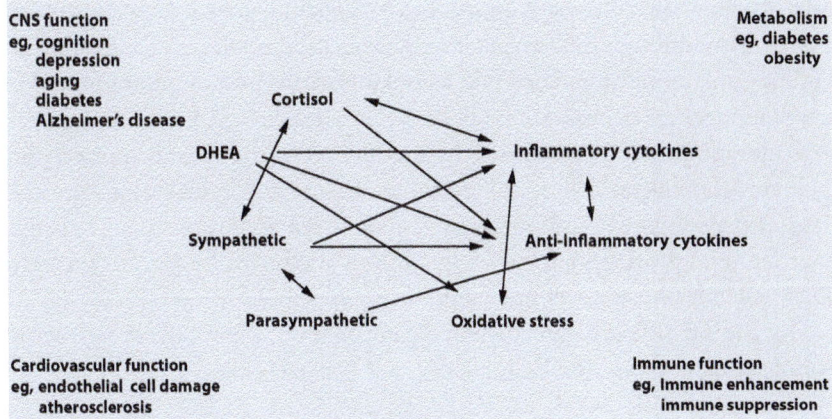

Fig. 2 Mediators of allostasis exist in a nonlinear network, in which different mediators act to affect each other [8]. For example, sympathetic nervous system activity activates inflammatory cytokines, and parasympathetic nervous system activity activates antiinflammatory cytokines. And as shown, parasympathetic and sympathetic activities modulate each other.

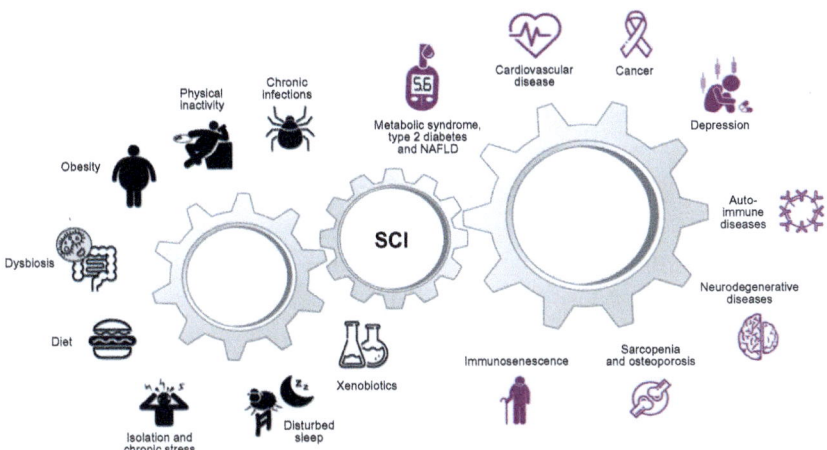

Fig. 3 Several causes of low-grade systemic chronic inflammation (SCI) and their consequences have been identified. As shown on the left of the figure, the most common triggers of SCI (in counterclockwise direction) include chronic infections, physical inactivity, (visceral) obesity, intestinal dysbiosis, diet, social isolation, psychological stress, disturbed sleep and disrupted circadian rhythm, and exposure to xenobiotics such as air pollutants, hazardous waste products, industrial chemicals, and tobacco smoking. As shown on the right, the consequences of SCI (in clockwise direction) include metabolic syndrome, type 2 diabetes, nonalcoholic fatty liver disease (NAFLD), cardiovascular disease, cancer, depression, autoimmune diseases, neurodegenerative diseases, sarcopenia, osteoporosis, and immunosenescence [6].

state [9]. The state of obesity promotes a proinflammatory state via two pathways, which, through different methods, facilitate the release of inflammatory and immune modulators known as adipokines; these include proinflammatory adipokines; tumor necrosis factor alpha and interleukin 6. Additionally and perhaps more importantly, it reduces the production of the antiinflammatory adipokine, Adiponectin. The modification of the normal levels of inflammatory modulators combined with subsequent endothelial and microvascular changes contributes to the development of significantly dysfunctional physiologic states. These include alteration of lipid and glucose metabolism (significantly predisposing the physiologic state to perpetuate obesity), a prolonged and default proinflammatory state, insulin resistance, and hypertension.

Physical activity

Contraction of skeletal muscles, through physical activity, results in the secretion of cytokines and myokines, which can have the effect of decreasing systemic inflammation [10]. Conversely, physical inactivity can lead to increased levels of C-reactive protein (CRP) and proinflammatory cytokines [11]. Physiologic states associated with low physical activity can promote several inflammation-related pathophysiological states, including insulin resistance, dyslipidemia, endothelial dysfunction, high blood pressure, and loss of muscle mass [12]. These in turn increase risk for cardiovascular disease, type 2 diabetes, osteoporosis, various types of cancer, depression, dementia, in individuals who are chronically inactive [12].

The relationship between decreased physical activity and obesity is complex. As mentioned previously, obesity has an intricate relationship with chronic inflammation through many layers of physiologic effect. Decreased activity promotes an increased chance of weight gain, particularly visceral adipose tissue (VAT), which is a major trigger for inflammation [13]. VAT is an active endocrine, immunological, and metabolic organ composed of various cells, which promote obesity-related inflammation and all of its disease state promotion. Additionally, spillover of deposited lipids into other organs significantly promotes organ-specific pathologies (Fig. 4).

Dysbiosis

Dysbiosis is the substitution of the normal gut flora to a dysfunctional array of organisms that can promote disease states. Changes in gut microbiota seem to influence the outcome of multiple inflammatory pathways, in older adults, and may contribute to systemic chronic inflammation [14].

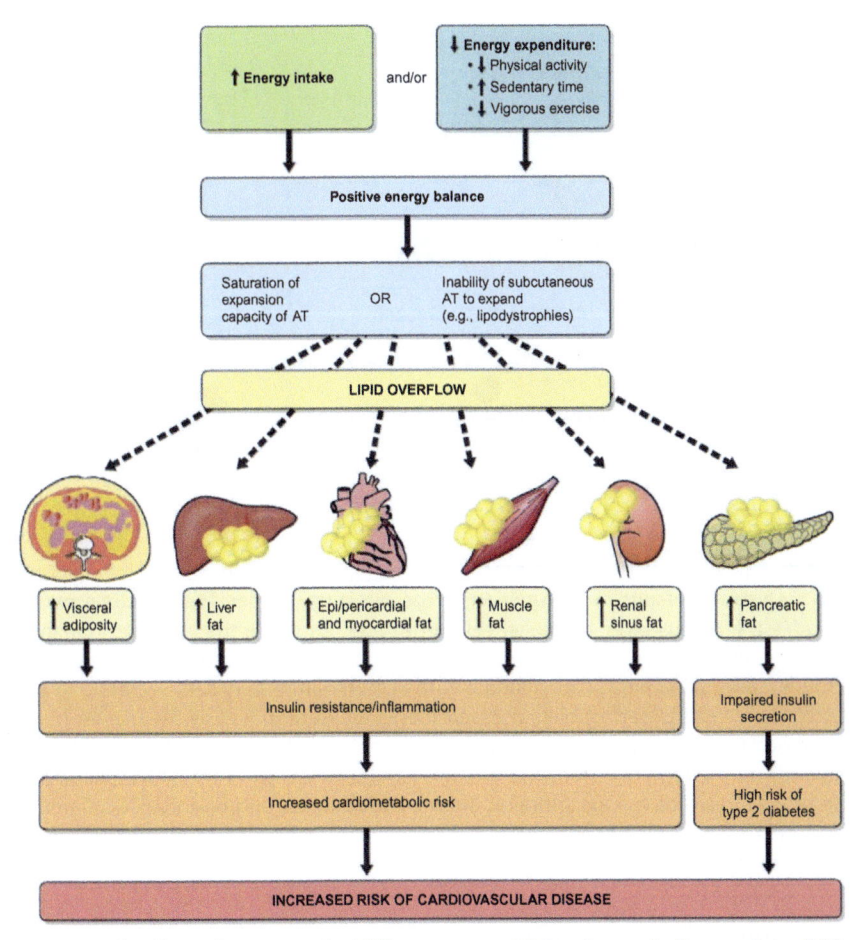

Fig. 4 Lipid spillover from excessive VAT promotes additional organic disease states [13].

Additionally, dysbiosis has been positively correlated with increased fat mass, proinflammatory biomarkers, and insulin resistance [15]. Extrapolating out, obesity has been linked to changes in the gut biome, which is associated with increased intestinal permeability and endotoxemia [16,17]. Zonulin is a protein that regulates intestinal permeability. Elevated levels of zonulin seem to predict inflammation and physical frailty [18] and are found in increased levels in obese children and adults, as well as in patients with type 2 diabetes, fatty liver disease, coronary heart disease, polycystic ovary syndrome, autoimmune diseases, and cancer [17].

Organisms in the gut biome exist in a delicate ecosystem, which has immense influence over proper system-wide physiologic function. We are just beginning to understand the causes of its upset and the dramatic effects of its

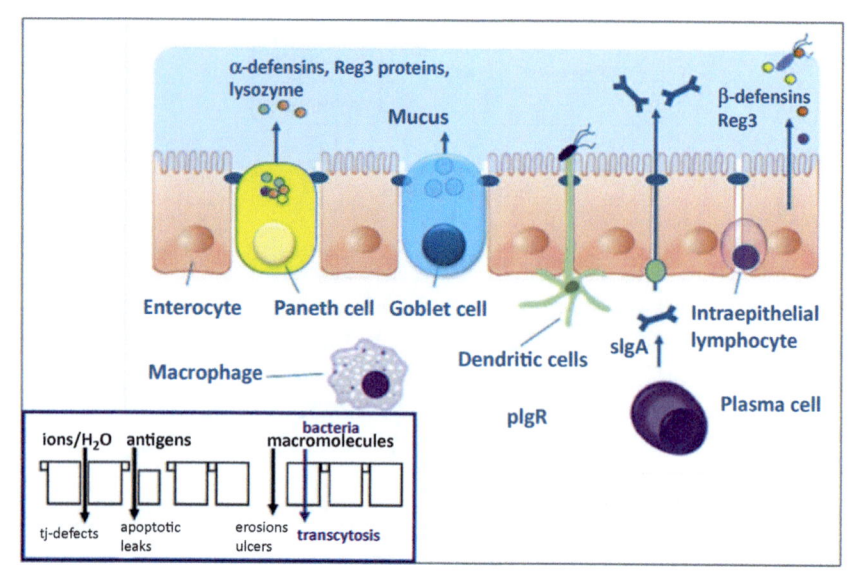

Fig. 5 Dysbiosis results in dysfunction of the intestinal barrier. The intestinal barrier includes the mucus layer, epithelial cells, tight junctions (TJ), the ability to transport luminal content and react to noxious stimuli by secretion of chloride and antimicrobial peptides, and the lamina propria innate with acquired immunity cells secreting Ig and cytokines. Intestinal permeability measurements are determined by the marker molecules used for measurement, since the type of molecules that pass the intestinal barrier depends on the type of lesion, and the deleterious effects can vary [19]. Leakage into the blood stream of various antigenic agents can instigate and/or enhance inflammatory and immunologic activity.

dysfunction. Alterations in intestinal permeability can also result from biome disruption and may have far reaching physiologic consequences (Fig. 5).

Diet

A poor diet can promote SCI in a variety of ways.
- Dietary factors can promote increased intestinal permeability resulting in SCI and low-grade endotoxemia. These factor include decreased consumption of fruit and vegetables, as well as increased consumption of refined grains, alcohol, and ultraprocessed foods [20–24]
- High-glycemic-load foods, such as isolated sugars and refined grains, which are common ingredients in most ultraprocessed foods, can cause increased oxidative stress that activates inflammatory genes [25]
- Salt has been shown to influence macrophages to express a highly inflammatory phenotype and to decrease expression and antiinflammatory activity of T regulatory cells [26]. Additionally, salt intake can contribute

to dysbiosis and its associated inflammation promoting consequences discussed elsewhere in this chapter [26].
- Poor nutrient intake secondary to ingestion of processed or refined foods to the exclusion of fruits and vegetables can result in low levels of micronutrients such as zinc and magnesium [27,28], as well as long-chain omega 3 fatty acids. Omega 3 fatty acids, EHA (eicosapentaenoic acid), and DHA (docosahexaenoic acid) are precursors to agents of inflammation resolution such as resolvins, maresins, and protectins [29].

Chronic stress

Psychological stressors have a real-time effect on physiologic function. Omnipresent job stress can cause physiologic changes [30] that disrupt the ability for glucocorticoids to effectively downregulate inflammatory activity. This is in part due to acquired decreased sensitivity of receptors secondary to the consistent presences of elevated cortisol. Long-term inability to manage acute inflammatory reactions secondary to these chronically high levels of glucocorticoids can lead to systemic chronic inflammation and subsequent poor health [31].

Societal changes have also caused radical shifts in diet and lifestyle. Living circumstances are now very different from the ones that shaped human physiology for most of evolution. "This is believed to have created an evolutionary mismatch in humans—characterized by an increasing separation from their ecological niche—and this mismatch, in turn, has been hypothesized to be a major cause of SCI" [6].

Disturbed sleep

Evidence suggests that there is a connection between proinflammatory cytokine activity and altered sleep patterns and duration [32]. In particular, plasma CRP levels are shown to be elevated in individuals with sleep apnea, which fragments sleep via pauses in breathing [33]. CRP is a plasma protein that participates in the systemic response to inflammation [34] with evidence that it can play a role in the development of atherosclerosis [35]. It is a useful marker for the study of the effects of sleep loss on inflammation, as it shows no circadian (day/night) variation [36].

CRP levels have been shown to increase in a patient group deprived of sleep as compared with control (Fig. 6). As a result, levels can rise above that considered to be a risk factor for cardiovascular disease [37]. Additionally, patients with insomnia have shown increased levels of interleukin-6, an

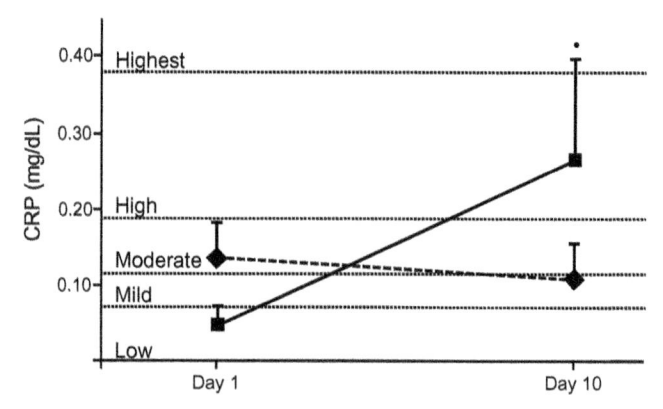

Fig. 6 Mean (± SEM) changes in plasma CRP concentration in four subjects undergoing 10 days of partial sleep deprivation (*black cube*) and five control subjects (*black diamond*). The dotted line represents the boundaries for cardiovascular risk [37].

inflammatory cytokine [38]. This study suggested that levels of interleukin-6 can vary not only in response to quantity of sleep (duration) but quality, in that a low amount of slow wave sleep increased the presence of the cytokine.

Chronic infections

Chronic infections contribute to SCI, but are not primary causative agents. The effect of lifelong infections caused by cytomegalovirus, Epstein–Barr virus, hepatitis C virus and other infectious agents on SCI and immune dysregulation remains controversial [6]. However, emerging evidence appears to support the hypothesis that chronic infection can contribute to the development of Alzheimer's disease, Parkinson's disease, and other age-associated pathologies [39,40].

Xenobiotics

Xenobiotics are substances that we are often unavoidably exposed to in our environment. They include air pollutants, hazardous waste products, and industrial chemicals. The US Centers for Disease Control and Prevention national biomonitoring program issued a report that included data showing that almost all Americans have detectable levels of a wide variety of environmental chemicals in their bodies, including many with known endocrine disrupting, neurotoxic, and carcinogenic activities [41].

Exposure to these substances either early or later in life is linked to multiple systemic chronic inflammation-related pathologies (Fig. 7), including asthma, COPD, cancer, obesity, and type 2 diabetes.

Table 1. Environmental Exposures Associated with Chronic Noncommunicable Diseases

Disease	Exposure During Fetal Development or Early Life	Exposure in Later Life
Asthma	Tobacco smoke Ambient air pollution Household chemicals Bisphenol A	Tobacco smoke Ambient air pollution Household air pollution Ecological exposure to PCBs
COPD	Tobacco smoke Ambient air pollution	Tobacco smoke Ambient air pollution Household air pollution
Obesity	Tobacco smoke Bisphenol A POPs	Bisphenol A POPs Gastrointestinal dysbiosis
Type 2 diabetes	No data	POPs Bisphenol A/phthalates Ambient air pollution
Metabolic syndrome	Endocrine-disrupting chemicals	POPs Ambient air pollution
Hypertension	Tobacco smoke Organochlorine pesticides	Tobacco smoke POPs Ambient air pollution Arsenic (drinking water)
Cardiovascular diseases	Tobacco smoke	Tobacco smoke POPs Ambient air pollution Household air pollution Ambient noise
Low IQ	Tobacco smoke POPs Heavy metals PAHs Organophosphate pesticides Brominated flame retardants	Heavy metals POPs
ADHD/ASD	Heavy metals POPs Bisphenol A/phthalates	Tobacco smoke Bisphenol A/phthalates
Neurodegenerative disorders	No data	Heavy metals Air pollution herbicides
Cancers	Tobacco smoke UV radiation Arsenic	Ambient air pollution Arsenic POPs Many carcinogens

For full details of the exposures, their effects, and references, see Supplementary Tables 1-5 in the online supplement.
ADHD, attention-deficit/hyperactivity disorder; ASD, autistic spectrum disorder; COPD, chronic obstructive pulmonary disease; PAHs, polycyclic aromatic hydrocarbons; PCBs, polychlorinated biphenyls; POPs, persistent organic pollutants; UV, ultraviolet.

Fig. 7 Xenobiotic exposure and chronic noncommunicable disease [41].

The presence of these substances produces a proinflammatory effect through various means. They can act as cytotoxins, cause oxidative stress, or act as endocrine disruptors, starting in utero [6,42,43].

In conclusion, inflammation is a very effective tool for the maintenance of homeostasis in the human body. It is a ubiquitous response to a multitude of environmental stimuli. However, it is the challenge of the clinician to aid the patient in modulating the response, in some cases, and stopping the progression to SCI, in all cases. The data consistently links SCI to most chronic disease states. If SCI can be arrested earlier in its progression, a proactive rather than reactive approach to disease management can be attempted to the best interest and outcome for our patients.

References

[1] Majno G, Joris I. Apoptosis, oncosis, and necrosis. An overview of cell death. Am J Pathol 1995;146(1):3.
[2] Coussens LM, Werb Z. Inflammation and cancer. Nature 2002;420(6917):860–7.
[3] Serhan CN, Recchiuti A. Pro-resolving lipid mediators (SPMs) and their actions in regulating miRNA in novel resolution circuits in inflammation. Front Immunol 2012;3:298.
[4] Serhan CN, Savill J. Resolution of inflammation: the beginning programs the end. Nat Immunol 2005;6(12):1191–7.
[5] Netea MG, et al. A guiding map for inflammation. Nat Immunol 2017;18(8):826–31.
[6] Furman D, et al. Chronic inflammation in the etiology of disease across the life span. Nat Med 2019;25(12):1822–32.
[7] Sterling P. Allostasis: a new paradigm to explain arousal pathology. In: Handbook of Life Stress, Cognition and Health. John Wiley & Sons; 1988.
[8] McEwen BS. Protective and damaging effects of stress mediators: central role of the brain. Dialogues Clin Neurosci 2006;8(4):367.
[9] Ward ZJ, et al. Projected US state-level prevalence of adult obesity and severe obesity. N Engl J Med 2019;381(25):2440–50.
[10] Fiuza-Luces C, et al. Exercise benefits in cardiovascular disease: beyond attenuation of traditional risk factors. Nat Rev Cardiol 2018;15(12):731–43.
[11] Fedewa MV, Hathaway ED, Ward-Ritacco CL. Effect of exercise training on C reactive protein: a systematic review and meta-analysis of randomised and non-randomised controlled trials. Br J Sports Med 2017;51(8):670–6.
[12] Booth FW, Roberts CK, Laye MJ. Lack of exercise is a major cause of chronic diseases. Compr Physiol 2011;2(2):1143–211.
[13] Tchernof A, Després J-P. Pathophysiology of human visceral obesity: an update. Physiol Rev 2013.
[14] Franceschi C, et al. Inflammaging: a new immune–metabolic viewpoint for age-related diseases. Nat Rev Endocrinol 2018;14(10):576–90.
[15] Aron-Wisnewsky J, et al. Major microbiota dysbiosis in severe obesity: fate after bariatric surgery. Gut 2019;68:70–82.
[16] Cani PD, Jordan BF. Gut microbiota-mediated inflammation in obesity: a link with gastrointestinal cancer. Nat Rev Gastroenterol Hepatol 2018;15:671–82.

[17] Sturgeon C, Fasano A. Zonulin, a regulator of epithelial and endothelial barrier functions, and its involvement in chronic inflammatory diseases. Tissue Barriers 2016;4, e1251384.
[18] Qi Y, et al. Intestinal permeability biomarker zonulin is elevated in healthy aging. J Am Med Direc Assoc 2017;18:810.e1–4.
[19] Bischoff SC, Barbara G, Buurman W, et al. Intestinal permeability—a new target for disease prevention and therapy. BMC Gastroenterol 2014;14:189.
[20] Bishehsari F, et al. Alcohol and gut-derived inflammation. Alcohol Res 2017;38:163–71.
[21] Richards JL, Yap YA, McLeod KH, Mackay CR, Mariño E. Dietary metabolites and the gut microbiota: an alternative approach to control inflammatory and autoimmune diseases. Clin Trans Immunol 2016;5, e82.
[22] Zmora N, Bashiardes S, Levy M, Elinav E. The role of the immune system in metabolic health and disease. Cell Metab 2017;25:506–21.
[23] Chassaing B, Van de Wiele T, De Bodt J, Marzorati M, Gewirtz AT. Dietary emulsifiers directly alter human microbiota composition and gene expression ex vivo potentiating intestinal inflammation. Gut 2017;66:1414–27.
[24] Lerner A, Matthias T. Changes in intestinal tight junction permeability associated with industrial food additives explain the rising incidence of autoimmune disease. Autoimmun Rev 2015;14:479–89.
[25] Dickinson S, Hancock DP, Petocz P, Ceriello A, Brand-Miller J. High-glycemic index carbohydrate increases nuclear factor-kappaB activation in mononuclear cells of young, lean healthy subjects. Am J Clin Nutr 2008;87:1188–93.
[26] Muller DN, Wilck N, Haase S, Kleinewietfeld M, Linker RA. Sodium in the microenvironment regulates immune responses and tissue homeostasis. Nat Rev Immunol 2019;19:243–54.
[27] Nielsen FH. Effects of magnesium depletion on inflammation in chronic disease. Curr Opin Clin Nutr Metab Care 2014;17:525–30.
[28] Bonaventura P, Benedetti G, Albarède F, Miossec P. Zinc and its role in immunity and inflammation. Autoimmun Rev 2015;14:277–85.
[29] Calder PC. Omega-3 fatty acids and inflammatory processes: from molecules to man. Biochem Soc Trans 2017;45:1105–15.
[30] Chandola T, Brunner E, Marmot M. Chronic stress at work and the metabolic syndrome: prospective study. BMJ 2006;332:521–5.
[31] Cohen S, et al. Chronic stress, glucocorticoid receptor resistance, inflammation, and disease risk. Proc Natl Acad Sci U S A 2012;109:5995–9.
[32] Simpson N, Dinges DF. Sleep and inflammation. Nutr Rev 2007;65(Suppl. 3):S244–52.
[33] Shamsuzzaman ASM, et al. Elevated C-reactive protein in patients with obstructive sleep apnea. Circulation 2002;105(21):2462–4.
[34] Black S, Kushner I, Samols D. C-reactive protein. J Biol Chem 2004;279(47):48487–90.
[35] Jialal S, Devaraj SK, Venugopal SK. C-reactive protein: risk marker or mediator in atherothrombosis? Hypertension 2004;44(1):6–11.
[36] Meier-Ewert HK, et al. Absence of diurnal variation of C-reactive protein concentrations in healthy human subjects. Clin Chem 2001;47(3):426–30.
[37] Meier-Ewert HK, et al. Effect of sleep loss on C-reactive protein, an inflammatory marker of cardiovascular risk. J Am Coll Cardiol 2004;43(4):678–83.
[38] Burgos I, et al. Increased nocturnal interleukin-6 excretion in patients with primary insomnia: a pilot study. Brain Behav Immun 2006;20(3):246–53.
[39] Smeyne RJ, et al. Infection and risk of Parkinson's disease. J Parkinsons Dis 2020;1–13. Preprint.
[40] Bu X-L, et al. A study on the association between infectious burden and Alzheimer's disease. Eur J Neurol 2015;22(12):1519–25.

[41] Fourth National Report on Human Exposure to Environmental Chemicals. Updated Tables, August 2014. Atlanta, GA: US Department of Health and Human Services Centres for Disease Control and Prevention; 2014. p. 11.
[42] Sly PD, et al. Health consequences of environmental exposures: causal thinking in global environmental epidemiology. Ann Glob Health 2016;82:3–9.
[43] Renz H, et al. An exposome perspective: early-life events and immune development in a changing world. J Allergy Clin Immunol 2017;140:24–40.

CHAPTER 4

Pathophysiology of obesity

Jacqueline J. Chu[a] and Raman Mehrzad[b]
[a]College of Medicine, The Ohio State University, Columbus, OH, United States
[b]Division of Plastic and Reconstructive Surgery, Rhode Island Hospital, The Warren Alpert School of Brown University, Providence, RI, United States

Structure of adipose tissue

First and foremost, it is important to recognize that adipose tissue function and morphology vary. One simple way of dividing the types of adipose tissue is subcutaneous versus visceral, as determined by location in the compartments of the human body. As will be discussed later, this distinction reflects differences not only in distribution but also in function, especially when comparing lean and obese body states. Subcutaneous adipose is fat that is found just beneath the skin and is concentrated in the gluteofemoral, back, and anterior abdominal wall [1]. On the other hand, visceral adipose surrounds internal organs and is mainly found intraabdominally, in the omentum and mesentery. Visceral adipose tissue, more so than subcutaneous adipose tissue, is thought to be the major contributor of obesity-related health complications, including diabetes and cardiovascular disease, and this explains why anthropometric measures of abdominal obesity such as waist circumference, which indirectly measures amount of visceral adipose, have been shown to be more accurate measures of health risk than BMI [2–4].

Adipose tissue can also generally be divided into white and brown types, as determined by the histological presence of uncoupling protein 1 (UCP1) and multilocular vacuoles [5]. Throughout the human body, white and brown adipose are distributed in depots. Most fat in the human body is white adipose. Depots of brown adipose have only recently been identified in adult humans through studies using positron emission tomography-computed tomography (PET-CT), defying older literature positing that brown adipose was present in other mammalian species and human infants only [6–8]. In adults, brown adipose is primarily concentrated in cervical, supraclavicular, axillary, and paravertebral regions, with disappearance of interscapular and perirenal brown adipose depots that are commonly found in infants and other mammals, such as mice [9].

Unlike white adipose cells, which are unilocular and primarily function to store lipids in large vacuoles, brown adipose cells consist of many small vacuoles and a dense population of mitochondria and use UCP1 to consume fatty acids to produce heat in response to cold exposure, a process called nonshivering thermogenesis [10]. In addition to thermogenesis, there is evidence demonstrating that brown adipose may also play a role in energy, especially glucose, homeostasis. Multiple studies have demonstrated associations between brown adipose activity and lower BMI and lower rates of diabetes [11–14], and there is evidence that this effect is at least in part due to the role brown adipose has in insulin-induced glucose uptake and regulation of glucose metabolism [15–17]. This newly discovered role of brown adipose has brought additional complexity to our understanding of the impact of adipose tissue on energy homeostasis, which was originally centered on white adipose tissue only [18].

Complicating the picture, researchers have also identified a potentially distinct set of adipose cells called beige or brite (brown-in-white) adipose, which function similarly to brown adipose but reside among white adipose tissue [19]. In comparison to classic brown adipose cells found in human infants and mice, these beige adipose cells do not express UCP1 or have thermogenic properties unless they are exposed to certain stimuli in a process called "browning." These stimuli are numerous and include cold exposure, exercise, and a large number of hormones and other signaling molecules [9].

In addition, while classic brown adipose cells differentiate from the dermomyotome precursors expressing *En1*, *Myf5*, and *Pax7*, the same cell lineage as skeletal muscle, mouse studies have demonstrated that beige adipose cells are derived from a heterogeneous group of precursors distinct from those of classic brown adipose and white adipose cells [20]. Using these transcriptional markers from mouse studies, researchers have also demonstrated that supraclavicular brown adipose depots of adult humans consist of cells that most resemble beige adipose, rather than classic brown adipose, implying that brown adipose depots in adults were created through activation and recruitment of beige adipose [21,22]. This ability of beige adipose to be recruited via various stimuli has important medical applications, as it can potentially be harnessed as a treatment for obesity and diabetes.

Phenotype of obesity

The WHO defines *obesity* as "abnormal or excessive fat accumulation that may impair health" that is caused by an energy imbalance, such that more calories are consumed than used [23]. The major health risks associated with obesity include cardiovascular disease and diabetes, and individuals who have biomarkers that indicate progression toward these diseases are defined to have *metabolic syndrome* [24]. The precise definitions of these two terms are still under debate, and there is much current research on the measures and thresholds that offer the most validity and reliability for screening and diagnosing individuals with these conditions.

In terms of metabolic syndrome, most experts agree that a combination of obesity, hyperinsulinemia, hyperglycemia or poor glucose tolerance, dyslipidemia, and/or hypertension is indicative of metabolic syndrome and should be included in its diagnostic criteria [24]. In 2009, a joint task force created harmonized criteria of metabolic syndrome; however, the task force was unable to decide how to incorporate obesity into the criteria given the variability of data on the thresholds that should be used to indicate increased cardiometabolic risk [24].

While BMI, a function of height and weight, is a simple and commonly used tool to determine the presence of obesity, with BMI of 30 the common cutoff used [23], a large number of studies have shown that BMI may not offer a complete picture of cardiometabolic health risk and should be supplemented or even replaced by other anthropometric measures [25,26]. This has been partially demonstrated by the presence of obese individuals who are "metabolically healthy," such that, despite a BMI in the obese range, these individuals experience fewer metabolic sequelae and fewer abnormalities in markers of metabolic function [27]. Conversely, there are individuals with normal-range BMI who nonetheless have poor cardiometabolic health, such as South Asians, leading organizations such as the American Diabetic Association to revise BMI threshold for this group when screening for diabetes [28,29].

Essentially, the relationship between obesity and metabolic health is extremely complex and cannot be strictly determined by weight or adipose tissue mass. In this section, we will discuss the characteristics of the obesity phenotype and how they can contribute to the development of metabolic syndrome.

Ectopic fat deposition

As mentioned previously, the role of visceral adipose tissue in metabolic consequences of obesity is the likely the reason why BMI can be an inaccurate indicator of health risk, and the accumulation of visceral vs. subcutaneous adipose tissue likely explains the existence of metabolically healthy and metabolically unhealthy obesity [30]. Virtue and Vidal-Puig proposed that the development of metabolic consequences of obesity can essentially be understood as a limit of adipose expandability [31]. Adipose expansion occurs generally through hyperplasia, the increase in the number of adipocytes, or hypertrophy, the increase in the size of adipocytes [32]. In childhood, adipocytes can undergo both hyperplasia and hypertrophy; however, in adulthood, hypertrophy becomes the predominant method of expanding in response to increases in fat storage needs [33]. In obesity, in the face of chronic energy excess, adipocytes eventually reach the limit of their ability to undergo hypertrophy, leading to cell stress that causes adipocyte dysfunction, including resistance to insulin signaling, and stimulate adipocyte stem cells to differentiate and generate new adipocytes (hyperplasia) [34]. The exact cause of cell stress in adipocyte hypertrophy is unclear, but is likely a combination of hypoxia, accumulation of toxic metabolites from lipid breakdown, adipocyte cell death, and mechanical stress [35].

Researchers theorize that subcutaneous adipose tissue easily expands through hypertrophy but is limited in its ability to undergo hyperplasia [36,37]. In metabolic unhealthy obesity, subcutaneous adipose reaches its limit to store fat, resulting in excess fats being stored in ectopic locations, including the liver, skeletal muscle, and the visceral adipose tissue [38]. Ectopic fat deposition in tissues such as the liver and skeletal muscle leads to lipotoxicity as the deposited fats are broken down into toxic metabolites such as ceramides, which has insulin suppressing effects [39]. The increased deposition of fat in visceral adipose also contributes to lipotoxicity in these tissues because visceral adipose has low capacity for fat storage and tends to break down and release more fatty acids [40]. Because visceral adipose is intra-abdominal, released fatty acids can directly enter the portal circulation to the liver, building on existing lipotoxicity [41].

The validity of this adipose expandability theory can be most clearly seen in patients with lipodystrophies, a set of genetic or acquired conditions in which individuals are unable to develop or maintain subcutaneous adipose tissue [42]. Many different mutations have been identified in genetic causes of lipodystrophies, but common to all causes is either a defect in adipocyte hyperplasia or a defect in adipocyte lipid intake and storage. As a result, these individuals have profound accumulation of fat in ectopic depots such as the liver, skeletal muscle, and pancreas. Lipodystrophies, therefore, almost always result in metabolic conditions, including severe insulin resistance or diabetes, hyperlipidemia, and fatty liver disease [43]. Conversely, treatments such as PPAR-gamma agonists, which stimulate adipocyte hyperplasia, have shown promise in reversing the metabolic stigmata of lipodystrophies [44].

Chronic inflammation

While the above "limited expandability" theory explains some of the contribution of visceral adipose tissue to metabolic syndrome development in obese individuals, the main contribution of visceral adipose is likely its contribution to chronic, low-grade inflammation that disrupts the normal metabolic functions of tissues throughout the body. This has been demonstrated by the ability of antiinflammatory drugs such as salicylates to improve insulin sensitivity and the elevated levels of inflammatory markers, such as TNF-alpha and IL-1 beta, in individuals with type 2 diabetes [45,46]. Additionally, Herrero et al. showed that treatment of insulin resistance with antiinflammatory agents was effective in obese mice but not effective in these lipodystrophic mice [47]. This further implicates the role of inflammation in obesity's metabolic sequelae and demonstrates the differential pathways leading to metabolic dysfunction in lipodystrophy and obesity.

As mentioned previously, continued adipocyte hypertrophy eventually leads to cell stress signals, which indicate cell damage or dysfunction and trigger inflammatory responses [48]. Inflammatory responses in acute situations such as infection are usually self-resolving once the infection clears and are important for tissue healing; however, inflammation induced in situations such as adipocyte hypertrophy is chronic as the signals for cell stress are unresolving with continued energy excess. Therefore, in obesity, a vicious cycle of inflammatory signaling and adipocyte stress and dysfunction propagates and persists [49]. This inflammatory signaling is able to influence metabolism at a local and systemic level, leading to insulin resistance and metabolic syndrome. Current research indicates that visceral adipose inflammation appears to be much more related to the development of metabolically unhealthy obesity than subcutaneous adipose inflammation [49–52].

In healthy adipose tissue, immune cells are a vital component to adipocyte function and interact with adipocytes to maintain energy homeostasis. In lean conditions, immune cells take on a type 2 immune response, which is generally antiinflammatory and insulin-sensitizing [49]. However, as obesity develops and cell stress increases, immune cells begin taking on a type 1 immune response, which is proinflammatory and promotes insulin resistance [53]. For reasons that are not fully understood, visceral adipose more easily shifts to the proinflammatory immune response, potentially explaining the greater importance of visceral adipose in terms of metabolic health risks [54].

Insulin resistance

As demonstrated in the previous sections, obesity causes insulin resistance at an adipocyte and systemic level. Insulin is a major anabolic regulator of energy balance and plays important roles in glucose and lipid metabolism [55]. In terms of glucose metabolism, insulin is secreted by the pancreas in response to high glucose concentrations in the bloodstream, as would occur after food intake, and stimulates glucose intake in tissues, especially in the skeletal muscle and adipose tissue. In addition, it acts on the liver to increase glucose storage as glycogen. In this manner, insulin reduces glucose levels in circulation and insulin resistance thus results in hyperglycemia. In terms of lipid metabolism, insulin is crucial for increasing lipid uptake by adipose tissue and skeletal muscle and decreasing lipid release by adipose tissue. Consequently, when insulin effects are lost, the opposite occurs, resulting in increased lipid release by the adipose tissue and hyperlipidemia.

In the context of obesity, Reilly et al. theorize that insulin resistance develops as a protective response to chronic energy intake that overwhelms the ability of adipocytes to accommodate the excess lipids [35]. By resisting insulin signaling, adipocytes reduce the uptake of new lipids while offloading lipids into the bloodstream, thus relieving cell stress from adipocyte hypertrophy. Insulin resistance systemically may also be helpful as it similarly prevents lipid uptake and subsequent increases in toxic lipid metabolites.

Loss of Brown adipose tissue

The previous sections primary discussed white adipose tissue dysfunction in obesity; however, increasing evidence indicates that brown adipose tissue function and quantity are also affected in the obese individual. As previously discussed, adipose tissue can undergo "beiging" and take on the characteristics of brown adipose tissue. During obesity, the opposite can occur, resulting in brown adipose tissue that becomes "whitened" and loses its metabolic functions [56]. Brown adipose lipid metabolism for thermogenesis is primarily stimulated by catecholamine signaling, but, in obesity, adipose tissue develops catecholamine resistance, potentially as a homeostatic response to uncontrolled lipid metabolism resulting from insulin resistance [35]. This becomes harmful for brown adipose since catecholamines are also responsible for production of VEGF, a growth factor that stimulates the development of new blood vessels [57]. Brown adipose mitochondrial function and thermogenesis rely heavily on adequate tissue oxygenation, which is jeopardized with the loss of VEGF-induced vasculature development. As a result of this hypoxic stress, mitochondria become dysfunctional and are eventually lost, leading to loss of brown adipose thermogenesis and decreases in total body energy expenditure, despite chronic energy excess [56].

Endocrine action of adipocytes in lean and obese states

Thus far, adipose tissue has taken a rather passive role in the regulation of metabolism and energy balance in the body, with its actions mostly responses to cell stress, inflammation, and insulin. However, adipose tissue is actually an extremely active endocrine organ with a physiologic role in systemic modulation of energy balance. This section will describe the functions of the two main hormones secreted by adipose tissue—leptin and adiponectin—and describe how these functions are affected by obesity development. In addition, this section will discuss the endocrine role of adipocyte-generated microRNAs (miRNAs), which is a relatively new finding in the field of adipocyte biology.

Leptin

In normal physiology, leptin is secreted by white adipose tissue in response to food intake, with higher levels secreted during meals [58]. In addition, its levels are proportional to fat mass; more fat mass correlates with greater leptin secretion [58]. Leptin acts primarily through central nervous system regulation at the hypothalamus and brainstem. At the hypothalamus, leptin acts on the appetite center located in the arcuate nucleus and suppresses appetite and food intake [59]. The importance of the role of leptin for appetite is clear in individuals with congenital leptin deficiency. These individuals are hyperphagic and obese, and treatment with leptin replacement leads to resolution of hyperphagia and weight loss [60]. At the brainstem, leptin is responsible for regulating sympathetic and parasympathetic nervous system signals, impacting glucose and lipid metabolism in target tissues. In skeletal muscle and the liver, these signals were shown to improve insulin sensitivity, resulting in increased glucose uptake [61,62]. However, in adipose tissue, leptin inhibits insulin signaling, suppressing glucose uptake [63]. Additionally, leptin actions on the sympathetic nervous system and catecholamine signaling result in increased lipid breakdown in adipose tissue [64].

Leptin can also act directly on target tissues to regulate metabolism. Leptin binding at the liver leads to increased fatty acid oxidation and decreased lipid generation in the liver [65]. Direct action on the adipose tissue also leads to increased fatty acid oxidation and inhibits adipocyte expansion through hyperplasia [66]. Based on these collective functions of leptin, researchers theorize that leptin serves as adipocytes' negative homeostatic signal, indicating to the body that fat stores are in abundance and pushing the balance toward energy expenditure rather than energy intake [67].

In obese individuals, leptin levels are high since leptin secretion is proportional to fat mass, but target tissues become resistant to leptin effects on metabolism [68]. In the brain, leptin signaling is inhibited by defective transport of leptin across the blood-brain barrier and blockade of downstream signaling pathways in neurons of the hypothalamus. Similarly, in tissues such as adipose, skeletal muscle, and liver, leptin downstream signaling pathways are also inhibited. Currently, the cause of leptin resistance is not clear, but researchers theorize that it may be a combination of intracellular feedback inhibition of leptin signaling, ER stress, and inflammation [69].

While leptin resistance develops in terms metabolism, high leptin levels in obesity still contribute to chronic inflammation through stimulation of proinflammatory cytokine secretion, activation of type 1 immune responses, and inhibition of antiinflammatory or immunosuppressive responses [70]. This proinflammatory milieu then stimulates even more leptin secretion from adipose tissues. As a result, leptin and, thus, obesity have been shown to be associated with development of autoimmune diseases, such as lupus, rheumatoid arthritis, and inflammatory bowel disease [71,72]. The effect of leptin on inflammation may also explain the higher incidence of autoimmune diseases in women; estrogen promotes leptin secretion while testosterone inhibits it, and indeed, women can have 2–3 times the amount of circulating leptin as men do [71,73,74].

Adiponectin

Adiponectin is also secreted by white adipose tissue, but, unlike leptin, adiponectin levels decrease with increasing fat mass [75,76]. Based on this phenomenon, researchers theorize that adiponectin, unlike leptin, signals starvation and thus promotes reduction in energy utilization and mobilization and drives increases in energy storage [77]. In the body, the effects of adiponectin on metabolism are driven by adiponectin binding to AdipoR1 and AdipoR2 receptors, which can be found almost ubiquitously [65]. In the skeletal muscle and adipose tissue, adiponectin binding improves insulin signaling, resulting in increased glucose intake and storage and decreased glucose availability in circulation [78]. Additionally, it inhibits breakdown of glycogen in the liver, further promoting glucose storage [78]. In the adipose, adiponectin promotes energy storage through decreasing lipid breakdown and release into circulation, and most importantly, it promotes adipose tissue expansion through hyperplasia, which increases energy storage capacity and prevents ectopic fat accumulation in other tissues [65].

The actions of adiponectin are at least partially mediated by its effects on ceramide levels in target tissues [79,80]. Ceramides are metabolites that are generated through lipid breakdown, and they stimulate proinflammatory cytokine production and interfere with insulin signaling. Adiponectin counteracts these effects by increasing production of ceramidase, which converts ceramides into molecules called sphingosines that promote cell survival.

In obesity, adiponectin levels are decreased, leading to loss of its antiinflammatory, insulin-sensitizing effects, and this has been shown to contribute to metabolic diseases such as type 2 diabetes and atherosclerosis [81].

MicroRNAs (miRNAs)

MicroRNAs are short segments of noncoding RNAs that can modify gene expression posttranscription [82]. They can be characterized as endogenous or exogenous, depending on their site of action; while endogenous miRNAs act within the cell, exogenous miRNAs are packaged into exosomes and released from cells into circulation to regulate gene expression systemically [82]. Adipocytes have been shown to secrete a large number of miRNAs to modulate tissues critical to metabolism, and obesity has been shown to alter miRNA secretion, leading to metabolic consequences [83]. For example, adipose-derived miRNAs miR-155, miR27a, and miR-34a have all been implicated in activating proinflammatory cytokine secretion and type 1 immune responses in macrophages in adipose tissue, and these have all been shown to be upregulated in obese patients [83]. Other miRNAs, such as miR-103 and miR-143, were shown to promote adipocyte hyperplasia and were downregulated in obesity [84]. Systemically, a number of potential adipose-derived miRNAs may modulate insulin sensitivity in the liver and muscle through noninflammatory mechanisms [85].

Putting it together: Treatment for obesity and metabolic syndrome

The previous sections have provided an overview of the phenotypic changes that occur with obesity and the active role that adipose tissue plays in the development of metabolic diseases. Empowered with this understanding of adipocyte dysfunction in obesity, investigators have tested a variety of different strategies to tackle obesity, with varying levels of success. In the following section, we will discuss the challenges of obesity treatment and new treatment modalities for obesity and metabolic syndrome.

Restoring energy balance

Obesity is ultimately an issue of chronic positive energy balance, such that energy intake and energy expenditure are imbalanced. Hill et al. propose that obesity is challenging to treat because the body is evolutionarily designed to defend and preserve body weight [86]. In the context of modern society's sedentary lifestyles, this results in mismatching of energy expenditure and energy intake. In lean individuals with high levels of physical activity, this high energy expenditure drives increased intake to meet energy demand. However, low physical activity and low energy expenditure do not have the same effect on decreasing energy intake and, in fact, the extreme food restriction required to maintain that balance would be unsustainable, resulting in positive energy balance and eventual obesity. These individuals are in an "unregulated zone" of energy balance, in which energy expenditure is unable to drive energy intake. Additionally, the body's basal metabolic energy expenditure decreases with decreasing body mass, meaning that sustained weight loss would require constant food restriction if not coupled with consistent physical activity. Obesity treatment can, therefore, be extremely difficult since it requires lifelong behavioral modifications.

Harnessing Brown adipose tissue

Investigators have attempted to increase brown adipose tissue activity as a means of promoting weight loss in obesity through increasing energy expenditure. However, beta-adrenergic agonists have not been successful in activating brown adipose tissue in humans, thus far, and can have severe cardiac effects [87,88]. Additionally, researchers theorize that increasing nonshivering thermogenesis through brown adipose stimulation may lead to compensatory, weight-preserving mechanisms that drop basal metabolic rate, resulting in no overall changes in energy balance [89].

Resolving inflammation

Given the important role of chronic inflammation in the development of insulin resistance and metabolic syndrome, researchers have sought out methods to counteract or resolve adipose inflammation. Thus far, antiinflammatory drugs have shown mixed results [35]. Tested medications include ant-TNF drugs, IL-1beta antagonists, and salicylates. Generally, these medications have shown expected effects on its inflammatory target but no impact on insulin resistance. On the other hand, diabetic drugs metformin and thiazolidinediones may have antiinflammatory actions, but there is still insufficient evidence that their antidiabetic effects are mediated through antiinflammatory pathways.

Since some component of adipose inflammation, especially in visceral adipose, is related to gut microbiota-induced inflammation, researchers have also focused on antiinflammatory nutrition and diets [90]. These diets primarily focus on high-fiber, low-carbohydrate foods, which promote the growth of commensal gut bacteria with antiinflammatory effects. Similarly, other researchers have focused on the use of probiotic supplements to reduce obesity-mediated inflammation. This research is still in early stages, with most studies conducted on animal models.

Resolving endocrine dysfunction

Similarly, the use of drugs to improve adipocyte endocrine dysfunction is in early development. Leptin has been successfully used to treat obesity due to lipodystrophy or congenital leptin deficiency; however, these patients lack leptin production, while obese patients have high leptin levels and leptin resistance [91]. The attention has therefore been focused on improving leptin sensitivity, and mouse studies have demonstrated some promise in terms of reducing insulin resistance [92,93]. Adiponectin treatment has also been investigated, and multiple therapies have potential, including statins, thiazolidinediones, recombinant adiponectin, and adiponectin receptor agonists [94]. However, most have only been studied in animal models, and thiazolidinediones, the most well-studied drug for this context, can have severe side effects, such as heart failure, and can actually lead to weight gain [78].

Conclusion

In this chapter, we reviewed the biology of adipose tissue, with a focus on the dysfunction that occurs in obesity. New strategies tackling obesity and obesity-associated metabolic sequelae have attempted to modify and correct dysfunctional components of adipose tissue, but there have been no clear successes. Restoring energy balance and ameliorating the systemic consequences of obesity continue to be challenges and warrant further research.

References

[1] Ibrahim MM. Subcutaneous and visceral adipose tissue: structural and functional differences. Obes Rev 2010;11(1):11–8. https://doi.org/10.1111/j.1467-789X.2009.00623.x.

[2] Shah RV, Murthy VL, Abbasi SA, et al. Visceral adiposity and the risk of metabolic syndrome across body mass index: the MESA study. JACC Cardiovasc Imaging 2014;7(12):1221–35. https://doi.org/10.1016/j.jcmg.2014.07.017.

[3] Alberti KG, Zimmet P, Shaw J. Metabolic syndrome—a new world-wide definition. A Consensus Statement from the International Diabetes Federation. Diabet Med 2006;23(5):469–80. https://doi.org/10.1111/j.1464-5491.2006.01858.x.

[4] National Cholesterol Education Program Expert Panel on Detection E. Treatment of high blood cholesterol in a. third report of the National Cholesterol Education Program (NCEP) expert panel on detection, evaluation, and treatment of high blood cholesterol in adults (adult treatment panel III) final report. Circulation 2002;106(25):3143–421. https://www.ncbi.nlm.nih.gov/pubmed/12485966.

[5] Wang W, Seale P. Control of brown and beige fat development. Nat Rev Mol Cell Biol 2016;17(11):691–702. https://doi.org/10.1038/nrm.2016.96.

[6] Ravussin E, Galgani JE. The implication of brown adipose tissue for humans. Annu Rev Nutr 2011;31:33–47. https://doi.org/10.1146/annurev-nutr-072610-145209.

[7] Yeung HW, Grewal RK, Gonen M, Schoder H, Larson SM. Patterns of (18) F-FDG uptake in adipose tissue and muscle: a potential source of false-positives for PET. J Nucl Med 2003;44(11):1789–96. https://www.ncbi.nlm.nih.gov/pubmed/14602861.

[8] Hany TF, Gharehpapagh E, Kamel EM, Buck A, Himms-Hagen J, von Schulthess GK. Brown adipose tissue: a factor to consider in symmetrical tracer uptake in the neck and upper chest region. Eur J Nucl Med Mol Imaging 2002;29(10):1393–8. https://doi.org/10.1007/s00259-002-0902-6.

[9] Sidossis L, Kajimura S. Brown and beige fat in humans: thermogenic adipocytes that control energy and glucose homeostasis. J Clin Invest 2015;125(2):478–86. https://doi.org/10.1172/JCI78362.

[10] Cinti S. White, brown, beige and pink: a rainbow in the adipose organ. Curr Opinion Endocr Metab Res 2019;4:29–36. https://doi.org/10.1016/j.coemr.2018.07.003.

[11] Matsushita M, Yoneshiro T, Aita S, Kameya T, Sugie H, Saito M. Impact of brown adipose tissue on body fatness and glucose metabolism in healthy humans. Int J Obes (Lond) 2014;38(6):812–7. https://doi.org/10.1038/ijo.2013.206.

[12] Ouellet V, Routhier-Labadie A, Bellemare W, et al. Outdoor temperature, age, sex, body mass index, and diabetic status determine the prevalence, mass, and glucose-uptake activity of 18F-FDG-detected BAT in humans. J Clin Endocrinol Metab 2011;96(1):192–9. https://doi.org/10.1210/jc.2010-0989.

[13] Brendle C, Werner MK, Schmadl M, et al. Correlation of Brown adipose tissue with other body fat compartments and patient characteristics: a retrospective analysis in a large patient cohort using PET/CT. Acad Radiol 2018;25(1):102–10. https://doi.org/10.1016/j.acra.2017.09.007.

[14] Pfannenberg C, Werner MK, Ripkens S, et al. Impact of age on the relationships of brown adipose tissue with sex and adiposity in humans. Diabetes 2010;59(7):1789–93. https://doi.org/10.2337/db10-0004.

[15] Orava J, Nuutila P, Lidell ME, et al. Different metabolic responses of human brown adipose tissue to activation by cold and insulin. Cell Metab 2011;14(2):272–9. https://doi.org/10.1016/j.cmet.2011.06.012.

[16] Stanford KI, Middelbeek RJ, Townsend KL, et al. Brown adipose tissue regulates glucose homeostasis and insulin sensitivity. J Clin Invest 2013;123(1):215–23. https://doi.org/10.1172/JCI62308.

[17] Hao Q, Yadav R, Basse AL, et al. Transcriptome profiling of brown adipose tissue during cold exposure reveals extensive regulation of glucose metabolism. Am J Physiol Endocrinol Metab 2015;308(5):E380–92. https://doi.org/10.1152/ajpendo.00277.2014.
[18] Luo L, Liu M. Adipose tissue in control of metabolism. J Endocrinol 2016;231(3):R77–99. https://doi.org/10.1530/JOE-16-0211.
[19] Shabalina IG, Petrovic N, de Jong JM, Kalinovich AV, Cannon B, Nedergaard J. UCP1 in brite/beige adipose tissue mitochondria is functionally thermogenic. Cell Rep 2013;5(5):1196–203. https://doi.org/10.1016/j.celrep.2013.10.044.
[20] Ikeda K, Maretich P, Kajimura S. The common and distinct features of Brown and Beige adipocytes. Trends Endocrinol Metab 2018;29(3):191–200. https://doi.org/10.1016/j.tem.2018.01.001.
[21] Wu J, Bostrom P, Sparks LM, et al. Beige adipocytes are a distinct type of thermogenic fat cell in mouse and human. Cell 2012;150(2):366–76. https://doi.org/10.1016/j.cell.2012.05.016.
[22] Lidell ME, Betz MJ, Dahlqvist Leinhard O, et al. Evidence for two types of brown adipose tissue in humans. Nat Med 2013;19(5):631–4. https://doi.org/10.1038/nm.3017.
[23] WHO. Obesity and Overweight., April 1, 2020, https://www.who.int/news-room/fact-sheets/detail/obesity-and-overweight.
[24] Alberti KG, Eckel RH, Grundy SM, et al. Harmonizing the metabolic syndrome: a joint interim statement of the international diabetes federation task force on epidemiology and prevention; National Heart, Lung, and Blood Institute; American Heart Association; world heart federation; international atherosclerosis society; and International Association for the Study of obesity. Circulation 2009;120(16):1640–5. https://doi.org/10.1161/CIRCULATIONAHA.109.192644.
[25] Bener A, Yousafzai MT, Darwish S, Al-Hamaq AO, Nasralla EA, Abdul-Ghani M. Obesity index that better predict metabolic syndrome: body mass index, waist circumference, waist hip ratio, or waist height ratio. J Obes 2013;2013. https://doi.org/10.1155/2013/269038, 269038.
[26] Janssen I, Katzmarzyk PT, Ross R. Waist circumference and not body mass index explains obesity-related health risk. Am J Clin Nutr 2004;79(3):379–84. https://doi.org/10.1093/ajcn/79.3.379.
[27] Smith GI, Mittendorfer B, Klein S. Metabolically healthy obesity: facts and fantasies. J Clin Invest 2019;129(10):3978–89. https://doi.org/10.1172/JCI129186.
[28] Gujral UP, Pradeepa R, Weber MB, Narayan KM, Mohan V. Type 2 diabetes in South Asians: similarities and differences with white Caucasian and other populations. Ann NY Acad Sci 2013;1281:51–63. https://doi.org/10.1111/j.1749-6632.2012.06838.x.
[29] Misra A. Ethnic-specific criteria for classification of body mass index: a perspective for Asian Indians and American Diabetes Association position statement. Diabetes Technol Ther 2015;17(9):667–71. https://doi.org/10.1089/dia.2015.0007.
[30] Dobson R, Burgess MI, Sprung VS, et al. Metabolically healthy and unhealthy obesity: differential effects on myocardial function according to metabolic syndrome, rather than obesity. Int J Obes (Lond) 2016;40(1):153–61. https://doi.org/10.1038/ijo.2015.151.
[31] Virtue S, Vidal-Puig A. Adipose tissue expandability, lipotoxicity and the Metabolic Syndrome—an allostatic perspective. Biochim Biophys Acta 2010;1801(3):338–49. https://doi.org/10.1016/j.bbalip.2009.12.006.
[32] Vishvanath L, Gupta RK. Contribution of adipogenesis to healthy adipose tissue expansion in obesity. J Clin Invest 2019;129(10):4022–31. https://doi.org/10.1172/JCI129191.
[33] Spalding KL, Arner E, Westermark PO, et al. Dynamics of fat cell turnover in humans. Nature 2008;453(7196):783–7. https://doi.org/10.1038/nature06902.

[34] Wang QA, Tao C, Gupta RK, Scherer PE. Tracking adipogenesis during white adipose tissue development, expansion and regeneration. Nat Med 2013;19(10):1338–44. https://doi.org/10.1038/nm.3324.
[35] Reilly SM, Saltiel AR. Adapting to obesity with adipose tissue inflammation. Nat Rev Endocrinol 2017;13(11):633–43. https://doi.org/10.1038/nrendo.2017.90.
[36] Kim SM, Lun M, Wang M, et al. Loss of white adipose hyperplastic potential is associated with enhanced susceptibility to insulin resistance. Cell Metab 2014;20(6):1049–58. https://doi.org/10.1016/j.cmet.2014.10.010.
[37] Guillermier C, Fazeli PK, Kim S, et al. Imaging mass spectrometry demonstrates age-related decline in human adipose plasticity. JCI Insight 2017;2(5). https://doi.org/10.1172/jci.insight.90349, e90349.
[38] Gyllenhammer LE, Alderete TL, Toledo-Corral CM, Weigensberg M, Goran MI. Saturation of subcutaneous adipose tissue expansion and accumulation of ectopic fat associated with metabolic dysfunction during late and post-pubertal growth. Int J Obes (Lond) 2016;40(4):601–6. https://doi.org/10.1038/ijo.2015.207.
[39] Bays H, Mandarino L, DeFronzo RA. Role of the adipocyte, free fatty acids, and ectopic fat in pathogenesis of type 2 diabetes mellitus: peroxisomal proliferator-activated receptor agonists provide a rational therapeutic approach. J Clin Endocrinol Metab 2004;89(2):463–78. https://doi.org/10.1210/jc.2003-030723.
[40] Ali AH, Koutsari C, Mundi M, et al. Free fatty acid storage in human visceral and subcutaneous adipose tissue: role of adipocyte proteins. Diabetes 2011;60(9):2300–7. https://doi.org/10.2337/db11-0219.
[41] Item F, Konrad D. Visceral fat and metabolic inflammation: the portal theory revisited. Obes Rev 2012;13(Suppl 2):30–9. https://doi.org/10.1111/j.1467-789X.2012.01035.x.
[42] Mann JP, Savage DB. What lipodystrophies teach us about the metabolic syndrome. J Clin Invest 2019;129(10):4009–21. https://doi.org/10.1172/JCI129190.
[43] Huang-Doran I, Sleigh A, Rochford JJ, O'Rahilly S, Savage DB. Lipodystrophy: metabolic insights from a rare disorder. J Endocrinol 2010;207(3):245–55. https://doi.org/10.1677/JOE-10-0272.
[44] Fiorenza CG, Chou SH, Mantzoros CS. Lipodystrophy: pathophysiology and advances in treatment. Nat Rev Endocrinol 2011;7(3):137–50. https://doi.org/10.1038/nrendo.2010.199.
[45] Kim JK, Kim YJ, Fillmore JJ, et al. Prevention of fat-induced insulin resistance by salicylate. J Clin Invest 2001;108(3):437–46. https://doi.org/10.1172/JCI11559.
[46] Donath MY, Shoelson SE. Type 2 diabetes as an inflammatory disease. Nat Rev Immunol 2011;11(2):98–107. https://doi.org/10.1038/nri2925.
[47] Herrero L, Shapiro H, Nayer A, Lee J, Shoelson SE. Inflammation and adipose tissue macrophages in lipodystrophic mice. Proc Natl Acad Sci U S A 2010;107(1):240–5. https://doi.org/10.1073/pnas.0905310107.
[48] Haczeyni F, Bell-Anderson KS, Farrell GC. Causes and mechanisms of adipocyte enlargement and adipose expansion. Obes Rev 2018;19(3):406–20. https://doi.org/10.1111/obr.12646.
[49] Wu H, Ballantyne CM. Metabolic inflammation and insulin resistance in obesity. Circ Res 2020;126(11):1549–64. https://doi.org/10.1161/CIRCRESAHA.119.315896.
[50] Verboven K, Wouters K, Gaens K, et al. Abdominal subcutaneous and visceral adipocyte size, lipolysis and inflammation relate to insulin resistance in male obese humans. Sci Rep 2018;8(1):4677. https://doi.org/10.1038/s41598-018-22962-x.
[51] Wouters K, Gaens K, Bijnen M, et al. Circulating classical monocytes are associated with CD11c(+) macrophages in human visceral adipose tissue. Sci Rep 2017;7:42665. https://doi.org/10.1038/srep42665.

[52] Alexopoulos N, Katritsis D, Raggi P. Visceral adipose tissue as a source of inflammation and promoter of atherosclerosis. Atherosclerosis 2014;233(1):104–12. https://doi.org/10.1016/j.atherosclerosis.2013.12.023.
[53] McLaughlin T, Ackerman SE, Shen L, Engleman E. Role of innate and adaptive immunity in obesity-associated metabolic disease. J Clin Invest 2017;127(1):5–13. https://doi.org/10.1172/JCI88876.
[54] Wernstedt Asterholm I, Tao C, Morley TS, et al. Adipocyte inflammation is essential for healthy adipose tissue expansion and remodeling. Cell Metab 2014;20(1):103–18. https://doi.org/10.1016/j.cmet.2014.05.005.
[55] Wilcox G. Insulin and insulin resistance. Clin Biochem Rev 2005;26(2):19–39. https://www.ncbi.nlm.nih.gov/pubmed/16278749.
[56] Shimizu I, Walsh K. The whitening of Brown fat and its implications for weight Management in Obesity. Curr Obes Rep 2015;4(2):224–9. https://doi.org/10.1007/s13679-015-0157-8.
[57] Shimizu I, Aprahamian T, Kikuchi R, et al. Vascular rarefaction mediates whitening of brown fat in obesity. J Clin Invest 2014;124(5):2099–112. https://doi.org/10.1172/JCI71643.
[58] Park HK, Ahima RS. Physiology of leptin: energy homeostasis, neuroendocrine function and metabolism. Metabolism 2015;64(1):24–34. https://doi.org/10.1016/j.metabol.2014.08.004.
[59] Vong L, Ye C, Yang Z, Choi B, Chua Jr S, Lowell BB. Leptin action on GABAergic neurons prevents obesity and reduces inhibitory tone to POMC neurons. Neuron 2011;71(1):142–54. https://doi.org/10.1016/j.neuron.2011.05.028.
[60] Farooqi IS, Jebb SA, Langmack G, et al. Effects of recombinant leptin therapy in a child with congenital leptin deficiency. N Engl J Med 1999;341(12):879–84. https://doi.org/10.1056/NEJM199909163411204.
[61] Roman EA, Reis D, Romanatto T, et al. Central leptin action improves skeletal muscle AKT, AMPK, and PGC1 alpha activation by hypothalamic PI3K-dependent mechanism. Mol Cell Endocrinol 2010;314(1):62–9. https://doi.org/10.1016/j.mce.2009.08.007.
[62] German J, Kim F, Schwartz GJ, et al. Hypothalamic leptin signaling regulates hepatic insulin sensitivity via a neurocircuit involving the vagus nerve. Endocrinology 2009;150(10):4502–11. https://doi.org/10.1210/en.2009-0445.
[63] D'Souza AM, Neumann UH, Glavas MM, Kieffer TJ. The glucoregulatory actions of leptin. Mol Metab 2017;6(9):1052–65. https://doi.org/10.1016/j.molmet.2017.04.011.
[64] Zeng W, Pirzgalska RM, Pereira MM, et al. Sympathetic neuro-adipose connections mediate leptin-driven lipolysis. Cell 2015;163(1):84–94. https://doi.org/10.1016/j.cell.2015.08.055.
[65] Stern JH, Rutkowski JM, Scherer PE. Adiponectin, leptin, and fatty acids in the maintenance of metabolic homeostasis through adipose tissue crosstalk. Cell Metab 2016;23(5):770–84. https://doi.org/10.1016/j.cmet.2016.04.011.
[66] Wagoner B, Hausman DB, Harris RB. Direct and indirect effects of leptin on preadipocyte proliferation and differentiation. Am J Physiol Regul Integr Comp Physiol 2006;290(6):R1557–64. https://doi.org/10.1152/ajpregu.00860.2005.
[67] Harris RB. Direct and indirect effects of leptin on adipocyte metabolism. Biochim Biophys Acta 2014;1842(3):414–23. https://doi.org/10.1016/j.bbadis.2013.05.009.
[68] Sainz N, Barrenetxe J, Moreno-Aliaga MJ, Martinez JA. Leptin resistance and diet-induced obesity: central and peripheral actions of leptin. Metabolism 2015;64(1):35–46. https://doi.org/10.1016/j.metabol.2014.10.015.
[69] Myers Jr MG, Leibel RL, Seeley RJ, Schwartz MW. Obesity and leptin resistance: distinguishing cause from effect. Trends Endocrinol Metab 2010;21(11):643–51. https://doi.org/10.1016/j.tem.2010.08.002.

[70] Iikuni N, Lam QL, Lu L, Matarese G, La Cava A. Leptin and inflammation. Curr Immunol Rev 2008;4(2):70–9. https://doi.org/10.2174/157339508784325046.
[71] Vadacca M, Margiotta DP, Navarini L, Afeltra A. Leptin in immuno-rheumatological diseases. Cell Mol Immunol 2011;8(3):203–12. https://doi.org/10.1038/cmi.2010.75.
[72] Versini M, Jeandel PY, Rosenthal E, Shoenfeld Y. Obesity in autoimmune diseases: not a passive bystander. Autoimmun Rev 2014;13(9):981–1000. https://doi.org/10.1016/j.autrev.2014.07.001.
[73] Jenks MZ, Fairfield HE, Johnson EC, Morrison RF, Muday GK. Sex steroid hormones regulate leptin transcript accumulation and protein secretion in 3T3-L1 cells. Sci Rep 2017;7(1):8232. https://doi.org/10.1038/s41598-017-07473-5.
[74] Hellstrom L, Wahrenberg H, Hruska K, Reynisdottir S, Arner P. Mechanisms behind gender differences in circulating leptin levels. J Intern Med 2000;247(4):457–62. https://doi.org/10.1046/j.1365-2796.2000.00678.x.
[75] Straub LG, Scherer PE. Metabolic messengers: adiponectin. Nat Metab 2019;1(3):334–9. https://doi.org/10.1038/s42255-019-0041-z.
[76] Arita Y, Kihara S, Ouchi N, et al. Paradoxical decrease of an adipose-specific protein, adiponectin, in obesity. Biochem Biophys Res Commun 1999;257(1):79–83. https://doi.org/10.1006/bbrc.1999.0255.
[77] Lee B, Shao J. Adiponectin and energy homeostasis. Rev Endocr Metab Disord 2014;15(2):149–56. https://doi.org/10.1007/s11154-013-9283-3.
[78] Achari AE, Jain SK. Adiponectin, a therapeutic target for obesity, diabetes, and endothelial dysfunction. Int J Mol Sci 2017;18(6). https://doi.org/10.3390/ijms18061321.
[79] Turer AT, Scherer PE. Adiponectin: mechanistic insights and clinical implications. Diabetologia 2012;55(9):2319–26. https://doi.org/10.1007/s00125-012-2598-x.
[80] Chavez JA, Summers SA. A ceramide-centric view of insulin resistance. Cell Metab 2012;15(5):585–94. https://doi.org/10.1016/j.cmet.2012.04.002.
[81] Freitas Lima LC, Braga VA, do Socorro de Franca Silva M, et al. Adipokines, diabetes and atherosclerosis: an inflammatory association. Front Physiol 2015;6:304. https://doi.org/10.3389/fphys.2015.00304.
[82] O'Brien J, Hayder H, Zayed Y, Peng C. Overview of micro RNA biogenesis, mechanisms of actions, and circulation. Front Endocrinol (Lausanne) 2018;9:402. https://doi.org/10.3389/fendo.2018.00402.
[83] Ji C, Guo X. The clinical potential of circulating micro RNAs in obesity. Nat Rev Endocrinol 2019;15(12):731–43. https://doi.org/10.1038/s41574-019-0260-0.
[84] Xie H, Lim B, Lodish HF. Micro RNAs induced during adipogenesis that accelerate fat cell development are downregulated in obesity. Diabetes 2009;58(5):1050–7. https://doi.org/10.2337/db08-1299.
[85] Kim Y, Kim OK. Potential roles of adipocyte extracellular vesicle-derived miRNAs in obesity-mediated insulin resistance. Adv Nutr 2020. https://doi.org/10.1093/advances/nmaa105.
[86] Hill JO, Wyatt HR, Peters JC. Energy balance and obesity. Circulation 2012;126(1):126–32. https://doi.org/10.1161/CIRCULATIONAHA.111.087213.
[87] Trayhurn P. Brown adipose tissue-a therapeutic target in obesity? Front Physiol 2018;9:1672. https://doi.org/10.3389/fphys.2018.01672.
[88] Vosselman MJ, van der Lans AA, Brans B, et al. Systemic beta-adrenergic stimulation of thermogenesis is not accompanied by brown adipose tissue activity in humans. Diabetes 2012;61(12):3106–13. https://doi.org/10.2337/db12-0288.
[89] Chechi K, Nedergaard J, Richard D. Brown adipose tissue as an anti-obesity tissue in humans. Obes Rev 2014;15(2):92–106. https://doi.org/10.1111/obr.12116.
[90] Muscogiuri G, Cantone E, Cassarano S, et al. Gut microbiota: a new path to treat obesity. Int J Obes Suppl 2019;9(1):10–9. https://doi.org/10.1038/s41367-019-0011-7.

[91] Myers Jr MG, Heymsfield SB, Haft C, et al. Challenges and opportunities of defining clinical leptin resistance. Cell Metab 2012;15(2):150–6. https://doi.org/10.1016/j.cmet.2012.01.002.

[92] Lee J, Liu J, Feng X, et al. Withaferin a is a leptin sensitizer with strong antidiabetic properties in mice. Nat Med 2016;22(9):1023–32. https://doi.org/10.1038/nm.4145.

[93] Zhao S, Zhu Y, Schultz RD, et al. Partial leptin reduction as an insulin sensitization and weight loss strategy. Cell Metab 2019;30(4):706–719 e6. https://doi.org/10.1016/j.cmet.2019.08.005.

[94] Nigro E, Scudiero O, Monaco ML, et al. New insight into adiponectin role in obesity and obesity-related diseases. Biomed Res Int 2014;2014. https://doi.org/10.1155/2014/658913, 658913.

CHAPTER 5

Consequences of inflammation in obesity

Mercy Adewale[a], Danielle Ruediger[a,#], and Jessica A. Zaman[b]
[a]Albany Medical College, Albany, NY, United States
[b]Department of Surgery, Albany Medical Center, Albany, NY, United States

Introduction

Obesity, defined as a body mass index greater than or equal to $30\,kg/m^2$, is a consistently growing public-health crisis globally. In the United States, it is estimated that more than 40% of the adult population falls into the obese category, making it one of the most prevalent and costly diseases in the country [1]. As the prevalence of obesity has increased over the past few decades (Fig. 1), significant research has been done to better categorize the disease and understand what it means for the health of the body.

Today, it is commonly accepted that obesity represents a state of chronic inflammation. Adipose tissue, once believed to only be a site of passive energy storage and a mechanism for organ protection, is a complex, dynamic, heterogeneous endocrine organ. Adipose tissue comprises adipocytes, connective tissue, fibroblasts, endothelial cells, stem cells, and many immune cells, including T cells, macrophages, and dendritic cells [3,4]. Via these various cell types, adipose tissue can communicate and influence other organs through its release of adipokines, cytokines, and free fatty acids (FFAs). Adipokines are bioactive peptides that have many effects including glucose and energy homeostasis and balancing pro- and antiinflammatory states. Cytokines are immune modulating peptides. Adipose tissue has been shown to secrete monocyte-chemotactic protein 1 (MCP-1), IL-8, IL-6, IL-1, angiotensin II, TNF-alpha, and IL-10, among others, which all play an important role in immune function [5].

Obesity involves adipocyte hypertrophy, which results in an imbalance of adipokines and cytokine secretion, which tends to favor the proinflammatory state [6] (Fig. 2). Obesity affects the balance of

[#]Current address: Department of Surgery, Kaweah Delta Health Care District, Visalia, CA, United States

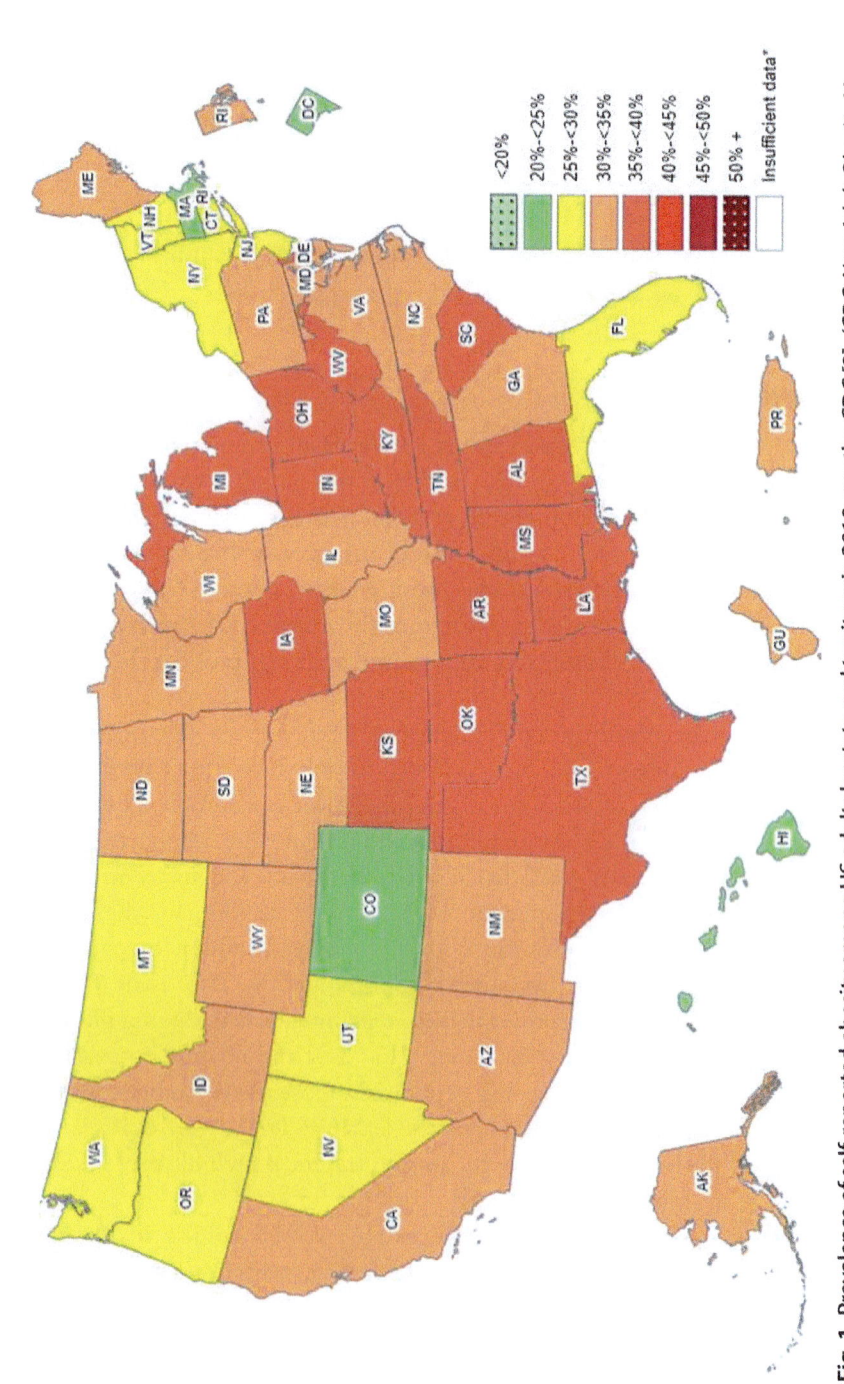

Fig. 1 Prevalence of self-reported obesity among US adults by state and territory in 2019, per the CDC [2]. (CDC. New Adult Obesity Maps. Centers for Disease Control and Prevention https://www.cdc.gov/obesity/data/prevalence-maps.html (2020).)

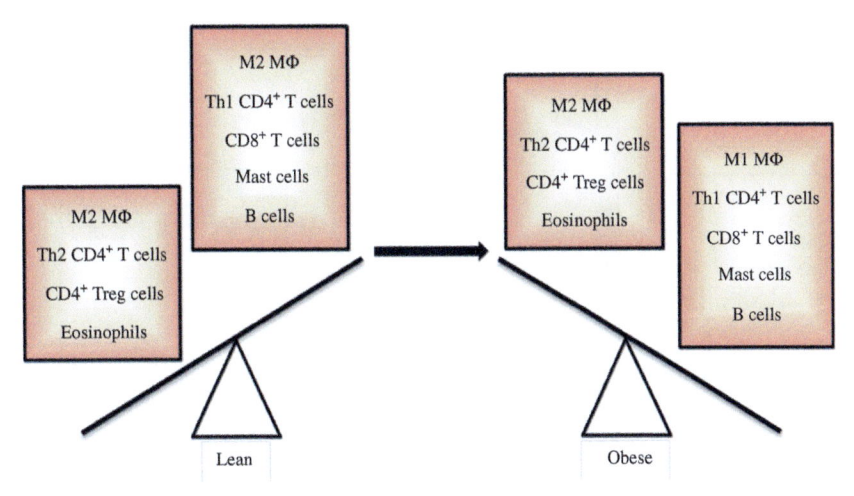

```
                    ┌─────────────────┐
                    │     M2 MΦ       │
                    │  Th1 CD4⁺ T cells│
                    │   CD8⁺ T cells  │        ┌─────────────────┐
                    │    Mast cells   │        │     M2 MΦ       │
   ┌──────────────┐ │     B cells     │        │  Th2 CD4⁺ T cells│    ┌─────────────────┐
   │    M2 MΦ     │ └─────────────────┘        │  CD4⁺ Treg cells│    │     M1 MΦ       │
   │ Th2 CD4⁺ T cells│                         │   Eosinophils   │    │ Th1 CD4⁺ T cells│
   │ CD4⁺ Treg cells │                         └─────────────────┘    │   CD8⁺ T cells  │
   │  Eosinophils │                                                   │    Mast cells   │
   └──────────────┘                                                   │     B cells     │
                                                                      └─────────────────┘
                          Lean                         Obese
```

Fig. 2 Immune cell populations in lean and obese states. Note that obesity is characterized by more M1 macrophages, which are proinflammatory [6]. *(Khodabandehloo H, Gorgani-Firuzjaee S, Panahi G, Meshkani R. Molecular and cellular mechanisms linking inflammation to insulin resistance and β-cell dysfunction. Transl Res 2016;167:228–56.)*

important adipokines, such as leptin and adiponectin, which have opposing effects on the immune system. Leptin is proinflammatory as it upregulates phagocytic function, stimulates proliferation and differentiation of monocytes, modulates activation of NK lymphocytes, and induces secretion of proinflammatory cytokines [7]. Adiponectin is an antiinflammatory adipokine that opposes the actions of leptin [8]. In states of obesity, enlarging adipocytes also secrete important cytokines including MCP-1, which attracts monocytes to adipose tissue [9]. Monocytes then differentiate into adipose tissue macrophages or ATMs. ATMs play a major role in producing the proinflammatory state seen in obesity. Macrophages in obesity tend to be M1 macrophages, or proinflammatory macrophages, which secrete TNF-alpha, IL-6, and IL-1, as opposed to M2 macrophages, which secrete antiinflammatory cytokines such as IL-10 [10] (Fig. 3).

There are many mechanisms by which obesity initiates a state of chronic inflammation, and understanding how this inflammatory state impacts the different organ systems of the body is crucial to understanding how obesity affects overall health.

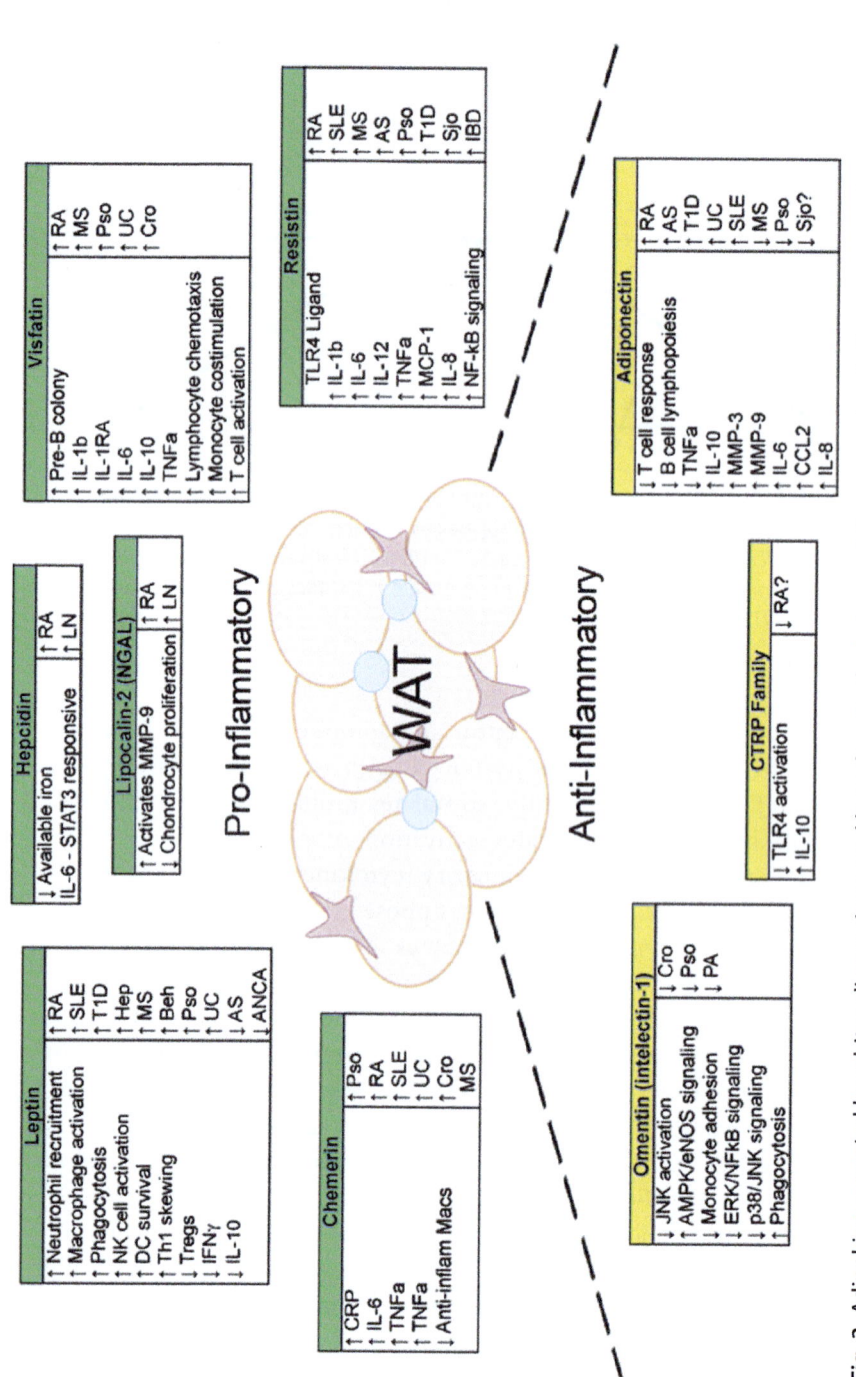

Fig. 3 Adipokines secreted by white adipose tissue and how they tip the balance of the pro- and antiinflammatory environment [11]. (Hutcheson J. Adipokines influence the inflammatory balance in autoimmunity. Cytokine 2015;75:272–9.)

Mechanism of inflammation

Tissue inflammatory process can be subdivided into acute inflammation and chronic inflammation. Both processes are defined by the type of response to internal or external stimuli such as toxins, necrotic cells, and tissue injury. Inducers of inflammation such as pathogen-associated molecular patterns (PAMPS) bind to toll-like receptors (TLRs) or nucleotide-binding oligomerization-domain protein (NLRs), which are then activated to stimulate cytokine release [12]. Major inflammatory cytokines, tissue necrotic factor alpha (TNF-a), IL-6, and IL-1 induce endothelial changes, which facilitate the entry of immune cells to the site of injury [13]. Likewise, inflammasomes, which are innate immune complexes that recognize dead cell bodies, extracellular ATP, and uric acid crystals stimulate the activation of caspase-1, which is responsible for cleaving cytokine precursors such as IL-1B. Caspase 1-induced inflammation is associated with cyto-protection, cell survival, and regenerative processes [14].

In acute inflammation, cellular response to tissue injury is short term and localized to the site of injury. Tissue injury can be triggered by trauma, infection, necrosis, immune reaction, and foreign bodies such as silica or asbestos. Vascular endothelial cells become vasodilated, which allow for increased blood flow to injury site and localized leukocyte concentration. Leukocytes and plasma proteins travel to the injury site and are selectively extravasated into the lumen by endothelial-cell selectins and integrins. Once leukocytes are activated by microbial products, they phagocytose and eliminate necrotic tissues by releasing reactive oxygen species, proteinase 3, cathepsin G, and elastase [12]. The expected outcome of acute inflammation is the resolution of tissue injury, repair and regeneration of cells, or progression to chronic inflammation.

Chronic inflammation occurs if initial tissue injury is not resolved by acute inflammation, thereby requiring a more robust and extended inflammatory response from lymphocytic cells. Hence, chronic inflammation is characterized by an extended period (months to years) of cytokine stimulation, healing of necrotic tissue, fibrosis, and scar formation. The hallmark of chronic inflammation involves the infiltration of lymphocytic T and B cells. B cells are further activated to secrete plasma proteins [15]. Lymphocytes respond to cellular injury by activating cytokines including IL-1 and TNF-a, which populate tissue injury sites. As mentioned, triggers of chronic inflammation are persistent infections, immune reactions, foreign bodies, and toxins. Persistent infections are often due to microbes that are resistant to clearance, such as *Mycobacterium tuberculosis*, *Treponema pallidum*, and certain viruses and fungi, all of which stimulate T lymphocyte-mediated response. Immune-mediated inflammatory response occurs when inappropriate immune mediators are activated against self-antigens, which could lead to autoimmune conditions such as myasthenia gravis, rheumatoid arthritis, ulcerative colitis, or allergic reaction, which is described as an exaggerated immune response to environmental stimuli such as for asthma. Immune-mediated processes can exhibit mixed acute and chronic inflammatory pattern since it requires repeated bouts of inflammation with no complete resolution. In prolonged inflammation, IL-1B and TNF-a reduce erythropoietin release from the kidney [15]. TNF-a also triggers macrophage-induced phagocytosis of circulating erythrocytes. Furthermore, acute-phase reactant, hepcidin inhibits ferroportin-mediated release of iron stores from macrophages and absorption of iron into circulation form the intestine. In this scenario, serum iron and total iron-binding capacity (TIBC) are low, while serum ferritin is high. This is called anemia of chronic disease [15].

The cellular mediators and cytokines in chronic inflammation ultimately function to activate macrophages. Macrophages are matured monocytes that circulate in the blood, connective tissues, or organs, e.g., the liver has Kupffer cells, spleen and lymph nodes have histiocytes, central nervous system (CNS) has microglial cells, lungs have alveolar macrophages [16]. They are also known to be part of the reticuloendothelial system. Tissue macrophages are activated by diverse stimuli either via classical pathway or alternative pathway. Classical pathway is induced by microbial products such as endotoxin T-cell-derived signals and foreign crystals to produce IFN-y, lysosomal enzymes, reactive oxygen species, nitrogen oxide to kill their target. Classically activated macrophages are important to host defense against ingested microbes and many chronic inflammatory reactions [16]. On the other hand, the alternative pathway is initiated by cytokines other than IFN-y, IL-4, and IL-13 produced by T-reg cells. The goal is to promote repair by secreting growth factors for angiogenesis, fibroblast, and stimulate collagen synthesis.

As mentioned earlier, lymphocytic cells play a major role in chronic inflammation. B and T lymphocytes are mobilized in the setting of infection or nonimmune-mediated inflammation. The activation of T and B cells is part of the adaptive immune response in infections and immunologic disease. B lymphocytes can mature into plasma cells, which secrete antibodies; T lymphocytes are activated to secrete cytokines. Th1 cells secrete IFN-y, which activates the classical pathway of macrophage activation. Th2 cells secrete

IL-4, IL-5, and IL-13, which activate eosinophils and alternative pathway and TH17 secretes IL-17, TNF, which regulates inflammation and recruits neutrophils and monocytes [16]. Lymphocytes and macrophages interact bidirectionally to propagate inflammation. Macrophages present antigens to CD4T lymphocytes, which are then activated to secrete cytokines that promote inflammation. Other cells involved in chronic inflammation are eosinophils and mast cells [16]. Eosinophils use the IgE-mediated process to battle parasites. Eosinophilic granules contain major basic protein, a charged cationic protein that is toxic to parasites causing epithelial cell necrosis. Mast cells exacerbate IgE-mediated antibody response in people prone to allergic reaction. Mast cells are sentinel cells widely distributed in connective tissues throughout the body.

Chronic inflammation can occur in granulomatous diseases. Granulomatous inflammation consists of macrophages, fibroblasts, and lymphocytes. They form under three conditions, namely: persistent T-cell activation, immune-mediated process such as Chron's disease, sarcoidosis, and berylliosis.

In conclusion, acute and chronic inflammatory processes are initiated to resolve tissue injury and restore cellular function. Exacerbation of chronic inflammation exists in certain disease conditions ultimately destroying cellular integrity.

Inflammatory processes in cardiovascular diseases and its relation to obesity

Cardiac inflammatory response occurs in atherosclerotic disease of the coronary arteries, which can result in ischemia and myocardial injury. Less frequently, ischemic heart disease (IHD) can result from increased demand such as in hypertension, decreased preload as seen in shock, and reduced oxygenation (pneumonia, CHF, anemia). Inflammation plays a critical role in the pathogenesis of coronary atherosclerosis disease. Atherosclerosis is characterized as intimal blockage by plaques, which can be stable or prone to rupture causing thrombosis. Risk factors of atherosclerosis include genetics, age (> 40), gender (men and postmenopausal women), hyperlipidemia, hypertension, smoking, diabetes mellitus. Once endothelial injury occurs, inflammatory response, primarily driven by C-reactive protein (CRP), stimulates plaque formation and progression. First, there is increased endothelial permeability and leukocytic infiltration, oxidized LDL, and cholesterol crystals migrate into the site of injury forming plaques, platelets adhere, and monocytes accumulate to form foam cells, which release inflammatory cytokines (IL-1). Recruited T-cells are activated in the growing intimal lesions, propagate IFN-y release and activation of smooth muscle cell proliferation forming stable atheroma [16].

Obesity is a modifiable risk factor of coronary atherosclerosis disease. White adipose tissue releases adipokines, which promote insulin resistance, endothelial dysfunction, hypercoagulability, and chronic inflammation. Obesity increases inflammatory adipocytokines (TNF-a, IL-6, MCP-1, Leptin, and Resitin), thereby propagating atherosclerotic disease [17] (Fig. 4).

Deposition of adipose in different anatomical regions has differing consequences. That is, subcutaneous adipose tissue is more metabolically protective, while pericardial and other visceral deposits associate strongly with incidence of coronary artery disease [18]. There is also genetic evidence supporting obesity-associated coronary artery disease as obese monozygotic twins had increased deposits of epicardium adipose tissue and inflammatory marker, CRP [18].

In summary, inflammation is an essential process in the formation of atherosclerotic plaque in coronary arteries evidenced by marked release of CRP, IL-1, and IFN-Y proinflammatory cytokines. Moreover, obesity and other metabolic syndromes such as hyperlipidemia and type 2 DM result in endothelial injury and subsequently, plaque formation.

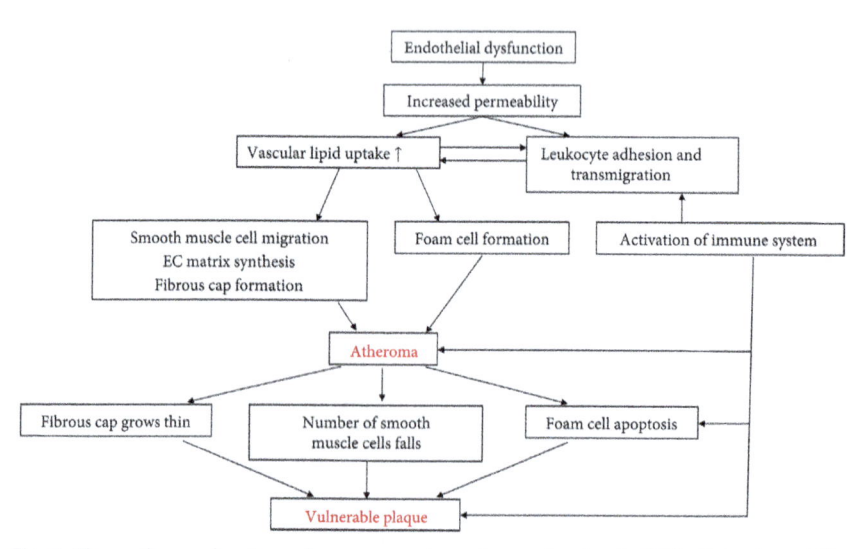

Fig. 4 The pathomechanism of coronary artery disease in obesity [17]. *(Csige I, et al. The impact of obesity on the cardiovascular system. J Diabetes Res 2018;3407306.)*

Inflammatory processes in endocrine diseases and its relation to obesity

Obesity is a significant risk factor for type II diabetes that causes a state of chronic low-grade inflammation, which is in part due to the accumulation of macrophages in adipose tissue in the obese state. Specifically, it is M1 macrophages that accumulate in adipose tissue of obese individuals. These macrophages are known to secrete proinflammatory cytokines including TNF-alpha, IL-6, and IL-1 [6]. TNF-alpha is a potent immunoregulatory cytokine that activates the MAPK and NF-kappaB signaling pathways resulting in release of other inflammatory cytokines. It has been demonstrated that obese individuals have 2.5-fold more TNF-alpha in their adipose tissue than lean individuals [19]. Along with initiating release of inflammatory cytokines, TNF-alpha also inhibits insulin receptor tyrosine kinase activity in both skeletal muscle and adipose tissue, which results in insulin resistance, one of the hallmarks of type II diabetes [20,21]. Aside from obesity's role in exacerbating insulin resistance, obesity also affects beta-cell function, another important factor that contributes to type II diabetes. Recall that beta cells are endocrine cells in the pancreatic islets of Langerhans that secrete insulin. The chronic inflammatory state that exists in obesity has been shown to affect pancreatic islets, specifically by macrophage expansion of resident intra-islet macrophages. The effects of increased macrophages in the islet include elevated proinflammatory cytokines and depressed antiinflammatory cytokines [22,23]. Additionally, islet inflammation has negative consequences on beta-cells, specifically inflammation leads to decreased beta-cell mass and impaired glucose-stimulated insulin secretion, both of which contribute to the progression of type II diabetes [24]. The link between obesity, insulin resistance, and beta-cell dysfunction is well defined by the chronic inflammatory state of obesity (Fig. 5).

While obesity's role in type II diabetes is one of the most significant effects of obesity on the endocrine system, it is important to recognize that obesity also plays a role in the progression of endocrine cancers, such as breast, thyroid, pancreatic, and prostate cancers. There are many factors linking obesity and cancer progression. A link with growing interest demonstrates adiponectin or APN as having a role in carcinogenesis. Although controversial, APN has been demonstrated to have a protective effect on cancer progression [26]. APN has antiinflammatory, antiatherogenic, proapoptotic, and antiproliferative properties [27]. Obese individuals have decreased levels of APN as compared with nonobese individuals, and thus, obese individuals may have less activation of these anticancer pathways. For

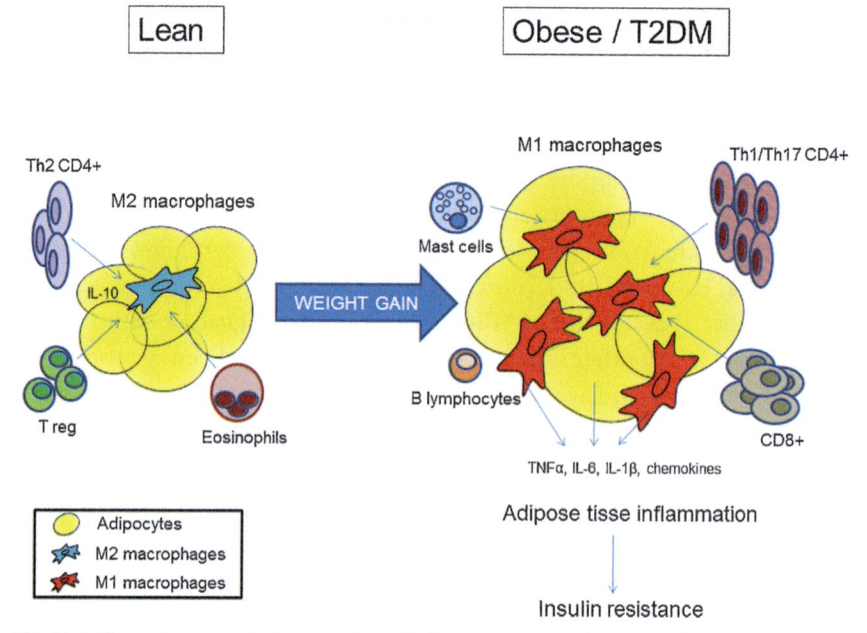

Fig. 5 Adipocytes secrete increased proinflammatory cytokines in the setting of obesity, which leads to adipose tissue inflammation and subsequent insulin resistance [25]. (Esser N, Legrand-Poels S, Piette J, Scheen AJ, Paquot N. Inflammation as a link between obesity, metabolic syndrome and type 2 diabetes. Diabet Res Clin Pract 2014;105:141–50.)

example, in premenopausal women with breast cancer, baseline APN levels helped to predict recurrence of breast cancer with a 12% reduction in the risk of breast neoplastic events per unit increase of APN [28]. Aside from APN, obesity can promote cancer through hyperinsulinemia, increased oxidative stress, and chronic low-grade inflammation [29,30].

Uterine cancer has been implicated as the cancer with the greatest relative risk of death in obese individuals compared with nonobese individuals—some studies report the RR as high as 6.3 with a P value of <0.001 [31]. Insulin resistance, a consequence of obesity and chronic inflammation, is a risk factor for endometrial cancer, a type of uterine cancer [32]. The high insulin levels seen in insulin resistance promote cell proliferation and survival via the PI3K and MAPK pathways, which play a role in cell proliferation and apoptosis [32]. Additionally, decreased levels of adiponectin, as seen in obesity, are associated with endometrial cancer [33,34]. Again, adiponectin is an antiinflammatory adipokine. Leptin, a proinflammatory adipokine, also plays a role in endometrial cancer. Studies demonstrate leptin's role in stimulating endometrial proliferation, which contributes to endometrial cancer progression [35,36].

Obesity and the chronic inflammatory state that it induces have important health consequences on the endocrine system including contributing to the progression of type II diabetes as well as several endocrine and reproductive organ cancers.

Inflammatory processes in gastrointestinal diseases and its relation to obesity

The gastrointestinal system comprises several organs that are intimately connected to visceral adipose tissue or VAT. This adipose tissue has been implicated in the proinflammatory state seen in obesity, which may contribute to several gastrointestinal diseases including gastroesophageal reflux disease, Barrett's esophagus, fatty liver disease, viral hepatitis, acute pancreatitis, gallbladder diseases, inflammatory bowel disease, and several GI cancers [37,38] (Fig. 6). The mechanism by which obesity and its associated chronic low-grade inflammatory state play a role in these GI diseases is often via adipokines, which are molecules secreted directly by adipocytes. Obesity is associated with an imbalance in these adipokines, which ultimately favors a proinflammatory state.

Inflammatory bowel disease represents a group of diseases marked by chronic relapsing and remitting inflammation in the GI tract. Crohn's disease involves transmural inflammation, or inflammation in all layers of the

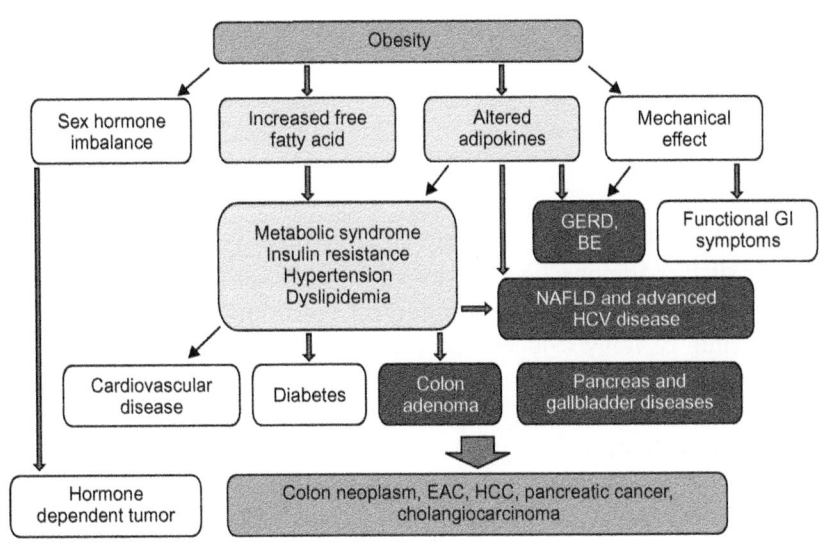

Fig. 6 The effects of obesity on the gastrointestinal system [37]. *(Nam SY. Obesity-related digestive diseases and their pathophysiology. Gut Liver 2017;11:323–34.)*

gut wall, while ulcerative colitis is only inflammation of the mucosa and superficial submucosa. There is no association between obesity and ulcerative colitis, but there is growing evidence that obesity may be associated with increased risk of Crohn's disease; however, this remains controversial [39,40]. As with other obesity-associated diseases, the onset of obesity in childhood demonstrates greater risk for Crohn's disease [41]. There are many possible explanations for the link between obesity and Crohn's disease, and many of them are related to the proinflammatory state obesity induces [42]. Both visceral adipose tissue and creeping fat, a pathognomonic feature seen in Crohn's disease, have upregulation of genes related to inflammation compared with fats seen in patients without Crohn's disease, even those who are obese [43]. These proinflammatory genes code for NFKB, IL1, IL6, and IL8, among several others. Many of these cytokines are known to be elevated in obese individuals indicating that in Crohn's disease there is even greater elevation in these proinflammatory cytokines commonly associated with the chronic inflammation seen in obesity.

Obesity and its associated chronic inflammatory state also play a role in the development and progression of nonalcoholic fatty liver disease, or NAFLD, which is the most prevalent cause of chronic liver disease worldwide. This disease has increased in prevalence throughout the obesity epidemic with between 75 and 100 million individuals in the United States being affected [44]. It is estimated that 66% of patients greater than 50 years old and affected with diabetes or obesity, also have NAFLD. Nonalcoholic fatty liver disease can progress to nonalcoholic steatohepatitis (NASH) and cirrhosis and is implicated in hepatocellular carcinoma [44]. The association between obesity and NAFLD is well described. In fact, weight loss has been shown to result in improvement in NAFLD and NASH [45]. Obesity, but specifically central adiposity, results in increased free fatty acids from VAT and a chronic low-grade inflammatory state, which are considered two of the most important factors contributing to NAFLD [46]. VAT secretes adipokines such as adiponectin and leptin. In the obese state, there is a relative increase in the amount of circulating leptin, but overall there is leptin resistance. Leptin typically reduces lipid accumulation in nonadipose tissue, but with the leptin resistance seen in obesity, there is increased lipid accumulation in the liver, which is a key feature of NAFLD [46]. VAT also plays a role in the progression from NAFLD to NASH via activation of the intrinsic apoptosis pathway. VAT secretes free fatty acids and adipokines. FFAs can be toxic and activate the intrinsic apoptosis pathway in hepatocytes via JNK, an MAP kinase, which leads to downstream effects resulting in lipoapoptosis.

This process, in combination with the proinflammatory state of obesity, promotes progression from NAFLD to NASH and eventually cirrhosis [47].

Another important group of GI diseases include cancers of the gastrointestinal system. Obesity is associated with increased risk of several GI cancers including esophageal, gastric, pancreatic, gallbladder, and colon cancer [44]. Esophageal cancer, the most strongly associated GI cancer with obesity, has a relative risk of 1.52 and a P value of <0.0001 in men [45,46]. There are several proposed mechanisms that link obesity and these GI cancers—below are just a few of the hypotheses. Gastric and colon cancers grow anatomically close to adipose tissue. Adipocytes near cancer cells can become dedifferentiated into cancer-associated adipocytes, which then secrete adipokines that can stimulate adhesion, migration, and invasion of tumor cells [47] (Fig. 7). In colon cancer, adipocytes release FFAs through lipolysis,

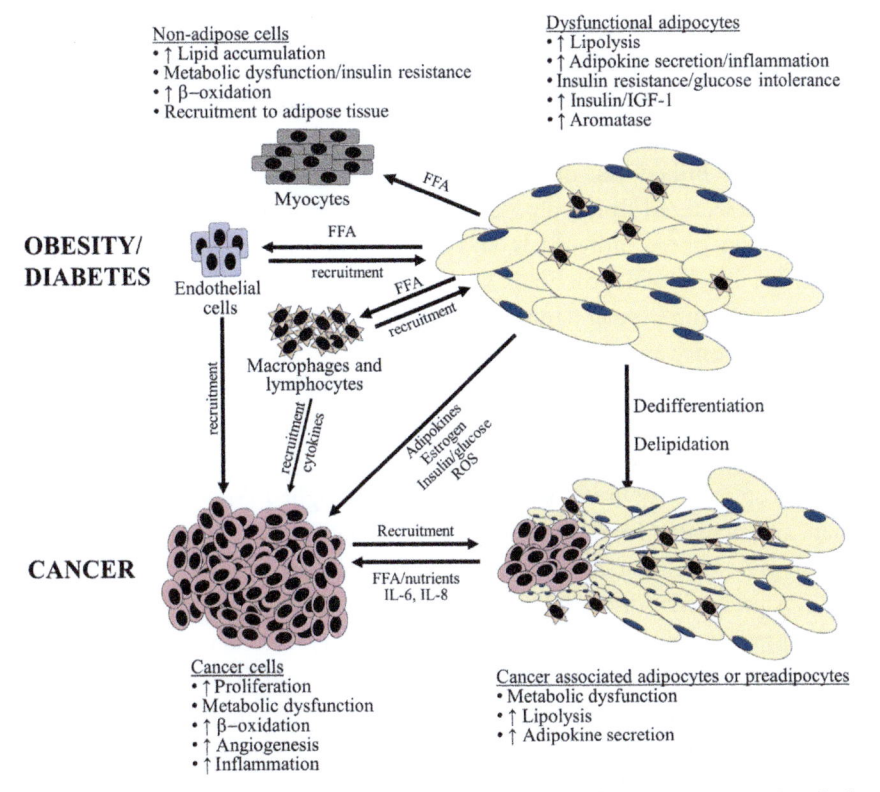

Fig. 7 The interplay between obesity, inflammation, and cancer progression [47]. *(Nieman KM, Romero IL, Van Houten B, Lengyel E. Adipose tissue and adipocytes support tumorigenesis and metastasis. Biochim Biophys Acta 2013;1831:1533–41.)*

which are then used by cancer cells for energy production allowing them to survive in nutrient-deprived conditions [48]. Obesity is associated with increased oxidative stress, which may also contribute to cancer pathogenesis via damaging cell membranes, cytoplasmic proteins, and nuclear DNA [49,50]. More research is needed to fully elucidate the interplay of obesity, the chronic low-grade inflammatory state it induces, and progression of gastrointestinal cancers.

Inflammatory processes in musculoskeletal diseases and its relation to obesity

Rheumatoid arthritis, or RA, is known to be an autoimmune disease. With the establishment that obesity causes a chronic low-grade inflammatory state, the question of whether obesity and obesity-related inflammation played a role in autoimmune diseases, such as RA, became relevant. There are several studies that demonstrate that obesity does increase the risk for developing RA [51,52]. This risk becomes greater in women who were obese at age 18, which demonstrates the relationship between chronic obesity and RA [51]. There are many potential explanations for how obesity and RA are linked, but one potential link is by leptin, a proinflammatory adipokine secreted from adipose tissue [11]. Leptin levels are known to be increased in obese individuals, and several studies have also demonstrated increased levels of leptin in RA patients [53,54]. Leptin and the role it plays in creating a proinflammatory state may help explain the association between obesity and RA.

While RA is known to be a condition highly connected with the immune state, its counterpart osteoarthritis, or OA, is less known for this. However, growing evidence demonstrates that inflammation may contribute to osteoarthritis more than previously thought [55]. Studies show that there are increased levels of circulating TNF-alpha and IL-6 in osteoarthritis, which presents a clear connection between an inflammatory process and OA [56]. As previously discussed, obesity represents a state of chronic low-grade inflammation. Associated with this state are increased levels of proinflammatory cytokines, such as TNF-alpha, IL-1beta, and IL-6, which provides a connection between obesity and OA through the chronic low-grade inflammatory state seen in obesity. In OA, TNF-alpha induces the production of matrix metalloproteinases or MMPs and inhibits the synthesis of proteoglycan and type II collagen [57,58] (Fig. 8). Together this allows TNF-alpha to play a role in cartilage degradation and bone resorption, which are both hallmarks of osteoarthritis. IL-6 and IL-1beta have similar effects on cartilage

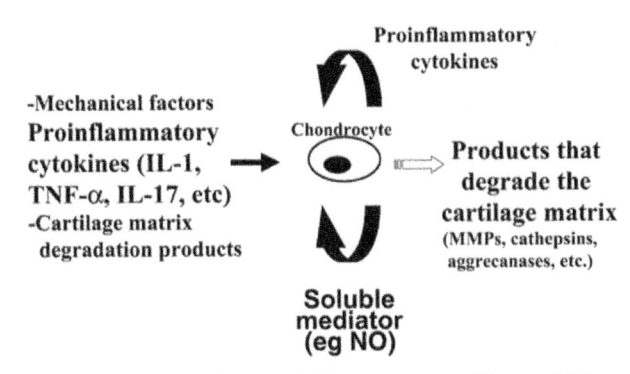

```
                        Proinflammatory
                           cytokines
-Mechanical factors          ⌒
Proinflammatory     Chondrocyte
cytokines (IL-1,       →   ◯   ⇨   Products that
TNF-α, IL-17, etc)                  degrade the
-Cartilage matrix           ⌣       cartilage matrix
degradation products               (MMPs, cathepsins,
                                    aggrecanases, etc.)
                         Soluble
                         mediator
                         (eg NO)
```

Fig. 8 Proposed mechanism by how proinflammatory cytokines, which are elevated in states of obesity, contribute to cartilage breakdown seen in osteoarthritis [57]. *(Goldring SR, Goldring MB. The role of cytokines in cartilage matrix degeneration in osteoarthritis. Clin Orthopaed Relat Res 2004;427:S27.)*

and bone structure, which demonstrates one mechanism by which an obese patient with subsequent chronic inflammation develops OA.

Obesity and its associated chronic low-grade inflammatory state also play a role in intervertebral disc degeneration or IDD, which is a widely prevalent disorder that contributes to the leading cause of pain in US adults [59]. Obesity is a well-described mechanical risk factor of IDD, but growing evidence shows obesity also contributes to the inflammatory state that plays a role in the progression of IDD. Leptin, an important proinflammatory adipokine found to be increased in obesity, and its receptor were found to be present in intervertebral disc tissues [60]. Leptin directly stimulates proliferation of nucleus pulposus and annulus fibrosis cells of the intervertebral disc, and these proliferating cells form clusters, which promote disc degeneration [61,62]. Additionally, leptin increases nitrous oxide production and expression of proinflammatory cytokines and MMPs, which together can initiate degradative and inflammatory pathways in disc cells [63].

Obesity has a negative impact on musculoskeletal diseases such as RA, OA, and IDD. Proinflammatory cytokines and adipokines provide the link between the obesity-induced chronic low-grade inflammatory state and progression of these widely prevalent musculoskeletal diseases.

Inflammatory processes in the central nervous system and their relation to obesity

The pathogenesis of neuroinflammation is hinged on the function of neuronal cells involved and the accumulation of abnormal proteins. As such, clinical presentation depends on the pattern of neuronal dysfunction: those affecting cortical neurons result in memory loss, language deficit, executive dysfunction; those affecting basal ganglia result in movement disorders; those affecting the cerebellum result in ataxia and imbalance; those affecting motor neurons result in weakness [64]. Neuronal insult triggers microglia-induced activation of inflammation, which may result in neurodegeneration or neurogenesis. Microglia are resident macrophages in the CNS that stimulate innate immune response. Acute CNS inflammation can occur due to stroke, hypoxia, or trauma. Upon activation of microglia, release of proinflammatory cytokines increases blood-brain permeability and leukocyte infiltration including T cells and macrophages [65]. Once recruited, leukocytes clear dead cells and increase synaptic connection that promotes neurogenesis via the action of IFN-y, IL-4, IL-6, TNF-α. There are two subtypes of macrophages that regulate inflammation: M1-macrophages stimulate inflammation and apoptosis of injured axons followed by M2-induced antiinflammatory process, which enhance axonal regeneration [66]. Severe neurodegeneration occurs in the setting of unregulated chronic inflammation as seen in Alzheimer's disease, Parkinson's disease, multiple sclerosis, etc. In Alzheimer's disease, accumulation of large deposits of Aβ amyloid alters neurotransmission and increases neuronal toxicity, which eventually leads to irreversible neuronal death and memory loss [64].

Obesity, Type-2 diabetes mellitus, and high-fat diet have been linked to increased neurodegeneration. Adipokines stimulate cytokine release some of which are proinflammatory (IL-6, IL-1b, IL-8, TNF-α Ap2, Adipsin, Leptin, resistin, visfatin) while some are antiinflammatory (IL-10, IL-ra, Omentin-1 Apelin, Adiponectin, CTRPs) [67]. Furthermore, insulin resistance in obese and diabetic patients has been shown to play a significant role in symptomatic neurodegeneration and cognitive decline. For instance, insulin resistance leads to decreased activation of Akt, a protein that regulates signaling cascade in glucose metabolism, and inhibition of GSK3 B, a tau-kinase. Therefore, during insulin resistance, increased GS3-B activation leads to tau-protein hyperphosphorylation, a hallmark of Alzheimer's disease. Hyperinsulinemia also leads to sequestration of insulin-degrading enzyme and decreased Aβ clearance resulting in prolonged neurodegeneration in Alzheimer's disease [68] (Fig. 9).

PPAR α, δ, and γ (most-abundant) are expressed in adult human brains and have been shown to regulate insulin-dependent glucose metabolism localized in the nucleus. Therefore, certain drugs such as PPAR agonists act to prevent neurodegeneration and brain atrophy. They also preserve IR-IGF receptor bearing CNS neurons, cholinergic homeostasis, and myelin gene expression [69].

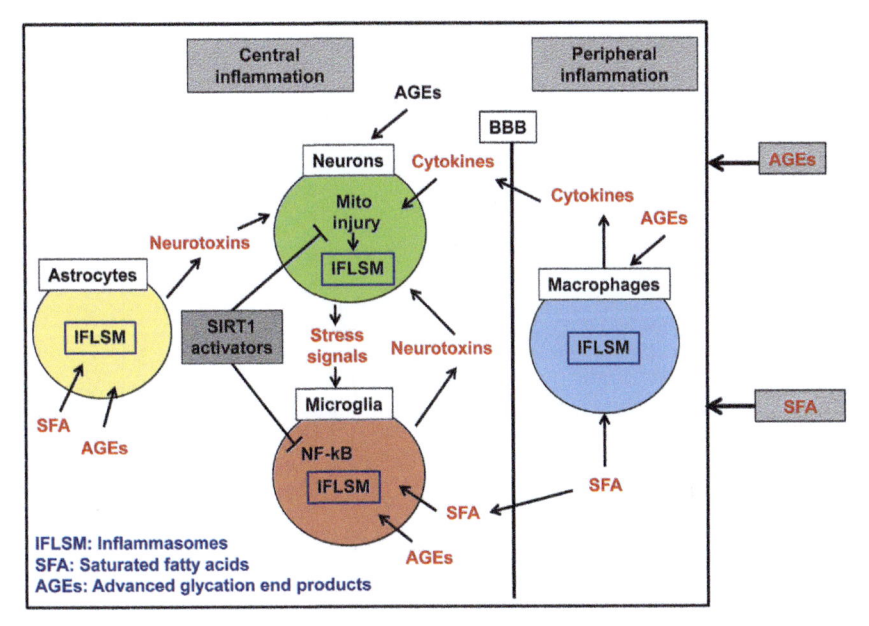

Fig. 9 Neuroinflammation in obesity and diabetes. Cytokines and stress signals released by neurons can further activate injuries to neurons [68]. *(Pugazhenthi S, Qin L, Reddy PH. Common neurodegenerative pathways in obesity, diabetes, and Alzheimer's disease. Biochim Biophys Acta 2017;1863:1037–45.)*

In summary, regulation of neuroinflammation is dependent on microglia-induced cytokine release, M1 and M2 macrophages, and T cells. Chronic inflammation is seen in neurodegenerative diseases such as Alzheimer's disease and can be exacerbated in insulin-resistance metabolic syndromes such as obesity.

Conclusion

Obesity induces a chronic-low grade inflammatory state through a multitude of mechanisms. Important factors include an imbalance of the pro- and antiinflammatory adipokines leptin and adiponectin, increased proinflammatory cytokines such as TNF-alpha, IL-1, and IL-6, and decreased antiinflammatory factors such as IL-10. Together these changes alter the inflammatory state seen in obese individuals. This chronic low-grade inflammatory state impacts many different organ systems including, but not limited to, the cardiovascular system, endocrine organs including reproductive organs, gastrointestinal system, musculoskeletal system, and neurological system (Fig. 10). Each system sees varying effects of obesity. For instance, in the gastrointestinal system obesity plays a role in the development and

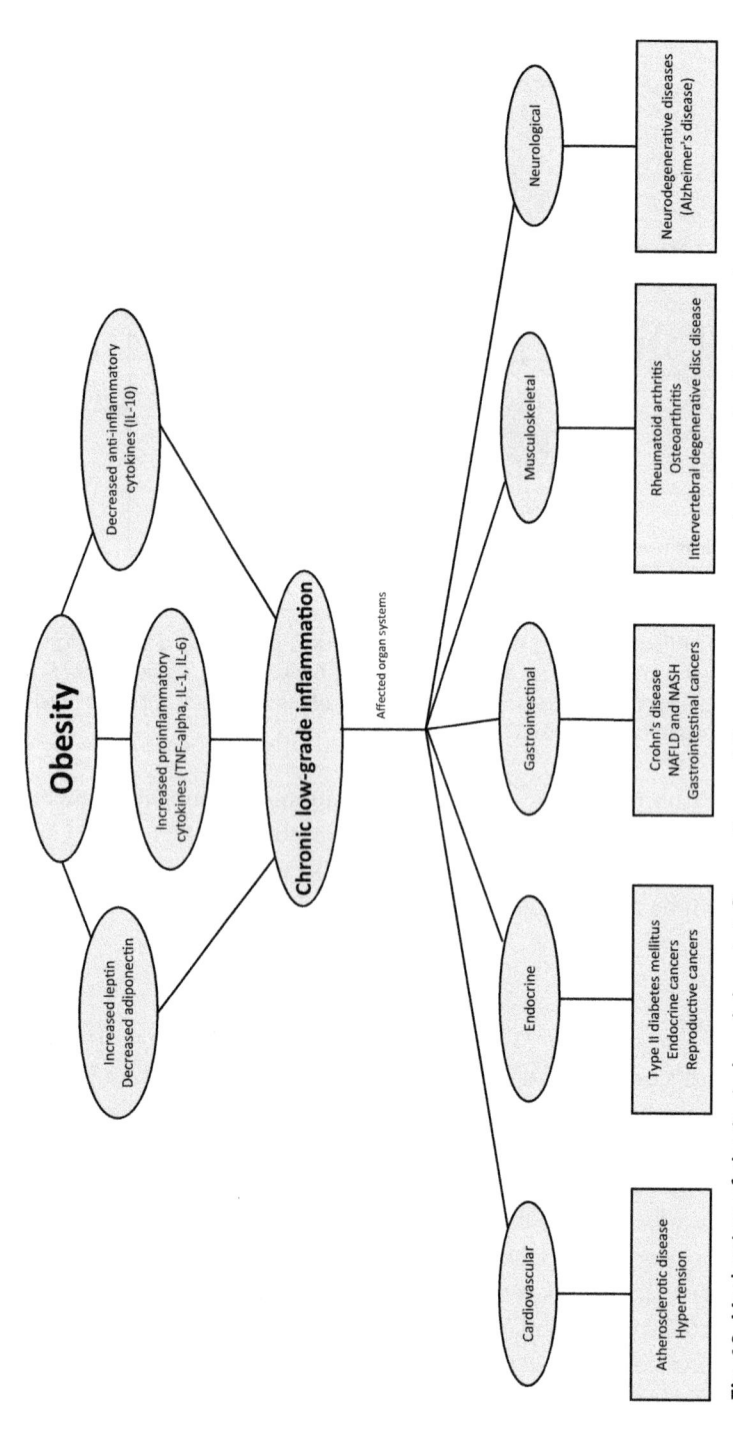

Fig. 10 Mechanism of obesity-induced chronic inflammation and the consequences on the human body. (original image).

progression of Crohn's disease as well as several GI cancers. Within the endocrine system, obesity and its chronic inflammatory state wreak havoc on the pancreas leading to development and progression of type II diabetes mellitus, which lends itself to further complications in the human body not discussed here. Overall, obesity and the chronic low-grade inflammatory state it induces have negative consequences on several body systems, which contribute to the development and progression of many different disease states.

References

[1] Hales CM, Fryar CD, Carroll MD, Freedman DS, Ogden CL. Trends in obesity and severe obesity prevalence in US youth and adults by sex and age, 2007-2008 to 2015-2016. JAMA 2018;319:1723–5.
[2] CDC. New adult obesity maps. Centers for Disease Control and Prevention; 2020. https://www.cdc.gov/obesity/data/prevalence-maps.html.
[3] Rezaee F. Role of adipose tissue in metabolic system disorders. J Diab Metab 2013;01.
[4] Caspar-Bauguil S, et al. Adipose tissues as an ancestral immune organ: site-specific change in obesity. FEBS Lett 2005;579:3487–92.
[5] Wang P, Mariman E, Renes J, Keijer J. The secretory function of adipocytes in the physiology of white adipose tissue. J Cell Physiol 2008;216:3–13.
[6] Khodabandehloo H, Gorgani-Firuzjaee S, Panahi G, Meshkani R. Molecular and cellular mechanisms linking inflammation to insulin resistance and β-cell dysfunction. Transl Res 2016;167:228–56.
[7] Martí A, Marcos A, Martínez JA. Obesity and immune function relationships. Obes Rev 2001;2:131–40.
[8] Koerner A, Kratzsch J, Kiess W. Adipocytokines: leptin—the classical, resistin—the controversial, adiponectin—the promising, and more to come. Best Pract Res Clin Endocrinol Metab 2005;19:525–46.
[9] Christiansen T, Richelsen B, Bruun JM. Monocyte chemoattractant protein-1 is produced in isolated adipocytes, associated with adiposity and reduced after weight loss in morbid obese subjects. Int J Obes (Lond) 2005;29:146–50.
[10] Mantovani A, et al. The chemokine system in diverse forms of macrophage activation and polarization. Trends Immunol 2004;25:677–86.
[11] Hutcheson J. Adipokines influence the inflammatory balance in autoimmunity. Cytokine 2015;75:272–9.
[12] Medzhitov R. Origin and physiological roles of inflammation. Nature 2008;454:428–35.
[13] Varela ML, Mogildea M, Moreno I, Lopes A. Acute inflammation and metabolism. Inflammation 2018;41:1115–27.
[14] Keller M, Rüegg A, Werner S, Beer H-D. Active caspase-1 is a regulator of unconventional protein secretion. Cell 2008;132:818–31.
[15] Germolec DR, Shipkowski KA, Frawley RP, Evans E. Markers of inflammation. Methods Mol Biol 2018;1803:57–79.
[16] Kumar V, Abbas AK, Aster JC, Perkins JA. Robbins basic pathology. Elsevier; 1944. 2018.
[17] Csige I, et al. The impact of obesity on the cardiovascular system. J Diabetes Res 2018;2018:3407306.
[18] Strissel K, Denis G, Nikolajczyk B. Immune regulators of inflammation in obesity-associated type 2 diabetes and coronary artery disease. Curr Opin Endocrinol Diabetes Obes 2014;21.

[19] Kern PA, et al. The expression of tumor necrosis factor in human adipose tissue. Regulation by obesity, weight loss, and relationship to lipoprotein lipase. J Clin Invest 1995;95:2111–9.
[20] Peraldi P, Hotamisligil GS, Buurman WA, White MF, Spiegelman BM. Tumor necrosis factor (TNF)-α inhibits insulin signaling through stimulation of the p55 TNF receptor and activation of sphingomyelinase*. J Biol Chem 1996;271:13018–22.
[21] Hotamisligil GS, Budavari A, Murray D, Spiegelman BM. Reduced tyrosine kinase activity of the insulin receptor in obesity-diabetes. Central role of tumor necrosis factor-alpha. J Clin Invest 1994;94:1543–9.
[22] Ying W, Fu W, Lee YS, Olefsky JM. The role of macrophages in obesity-associated islet inflammation and β-cell abnormalities. Nat Rev Endocrinol 2020;16:81–90.
[23] He W, Yuan T, Maedler K. Macrophage-associated pro-inflammatory state in human islets from obese individuals. Nutr Diabetes 2019;9:36.
[24] Ying W, et al. Expansion of islet-resident macrophages leads to inflammation affecting β cell proliferation and function in obesity. Cell Metab 2019;29:457–474.e5.
[25] Esser N, Legrand-Poels S, Piette J, Scheen AJ, Paquot N. Inflammation as a link between obesity, metabolic syndrome and type 2 diabetes. Diabetes Res Clin Pract 2014;105:141–50.
[26] Tumminia A, et al. Adipose tissue, obesity and adiponectin: role in endocrine Cancer risk. Int J Mol Sci 2019;20.
[27] Dalamaga M, Diakopoulos KN, Mantzoros CS. The role of adiponectin in cancer: a review of current evidence. Endocr Rev 2012;33:547–94.
[28] Macis D, et al. Prognostic effect of circulating adiponectin in a randomized 2 x 2 trial of low-dose tamoxifen and fenretinide in premenopausal women at risk for breast cancer. J Clin Oncol 2012;30:151–7.
[29] Vigneri R, Goldfine ID, Frittitta L. Insulin, insulin receptors, and cancer. J Endocrinol Invest 2016;39:1365–76.
[30] Kompella P, Vasquez KM. Obesity and Cancer: a mechanistic overview of metabolic changes in obesity that impact genetic instability. Mol Carcinog 2019;58:1531–50.
[31] Calle EE, Rodriguez C, Walker-Thurmond K, Thun MJ. Overweight, obesity, and mortality from cancer in a prospectively studied cohort of U.S. adults. N Engl J Med 2003;348:1625–38.
[32] Mu N, Zhu Y, Wang Y, Zhang H, Xue F. Insulin resistance: a significant risk factor of endometrial cancer. Gynecol Oncol 2012;125:751–7.
[33] Dal Maso L, et al. Circulating adiponectin and endometrial cancer risk. J Clin Endocrinol Metab 2004;89:1160–3.
[34] Lin T, Zhao X, Kong W. Association between adiponectin levels and endometrial carcinoma risk: evidence from a dose-response meta-analysis. BMJ Open 2015;5, e008541.
[35] Cymbaluk A, Chudecka-Głaz A, Rzepka-Górska I. Leptin levels in serum depending on body mass index in patients with endometrial hyperplasia and cancer. Eur J Obstet Gynecol Reprod Biol 2008;136:74–7.
[36] Ahn J-H, Choi YS, Choi J-H. Leptin promotes human endometriotic cell migration and invasion by up-regulating MMP-2 through the JAK2/STAT3 signaling pathway. Mol Hum Reprod 2015;21:792–802.
[37] Nam SY. Obesity-related digestive diseases and their pathophysiology. Gut Liver 2017;11:323–34.
[38] Chang M-L, Yang Z, Yang S-S. Roles of adipokines in digestive diseases: markers of inflammation, metabolic alteration and disease progression. Int J Mol Sci 2020;21.
[39] Mendall MA, Gunasekera AV, John BJ, Kumar D. Is obesity a risk factor for Crohn's disease? Dig Dis Sci 2011;56:837–44.
[40] Rahmani J, et al. Body mass index and risk of inflammatory bowel disease: a systematic review and dose-response meta-analysis of cohort studies of over a million participants. Obes Rev 2019;20:1312–20.

[41] Jensen CB, et al. Childhood body mass index and risk of inflammatory bowel disease in adulthood: a population-based cohort study. Am J Gastroenterol 2018;113:694–701.
[42] Kredel LI, Siegmund B. Adipose-tissue and intestinal inflammation—visceral obesity and creeping fat. Front Immunol 2014;5:462.
[43] Zulian A, et al. Visceral adipocytes: old actors in obesity and new protagonists in Crohn's disease? Gut 2012;61:86–94.
[44] Lauby-Secretan B, et al. Body fatness and Cancer—viewpoint of the IARC working group. N Engl J Med 2016;375:794–8.
[45] Friedenreich CM, Ryder-Burbidge C, McNeil J. Physical activity, obesity and sedentary behavior in cancer etiology: epidemiologic evidence and biologic mechanisms. Mol Oncol 2021;15:790–800.
[46] Renehan AG, Tyson M, Egger M, Heller RF, Zwahlen M. Body-mass index and incidence of cancer: a systematic review and meta-analysis of prospective observational studies. Lancet 2008;371:569–78.
[47] Nieman KM, Romero IL, Van Houten B, Lengyel E. Adipose tissue and adipocytes support tumorigenesis and metastasis. Biochim Biophys Acta 2013;1831:1533–41.
[48] Wen Y-A, et al. Adipocytes activate mitochondrial fatty acid oxidation and autophagy to promote tumor growth in colon cancer. Cell Death Dis 2017;8, e2593.
[49] Ulrich CM, Himbert C, Holowatyj AN, Hursting SD. Energy balance and gastrointestinal cancer: risk, interventions, outcomes and mechanisms. Nat Rev Gastroenterol Hepatol 2018;15:683–98.
[50] Kim YJ, Kim E-H, Hahm KB. Oxidative stress in inflammation-based gastrointestinal tract diseases: challenges and opportunities. J Gastroenterol Hepatol 2012;27:1004–10.
[51] Lu B, et al. Being overweight or obese and risk of developing rheumatoid arthritis among women: a prospective cohort study. Ann Rheum Dis 2014;73:1914–22.
[52] Dar L, et al. Are obesity and rheumatoid arthritis interrelated? Int J Clin Pract 2018;72.
[53] Otero M, et al. Changes in plasma levels of fat-derived hormones adiponectin, leptin, resistin and visfatin in patients with rheumatoid arthritis. Ann Rheum Dis 2006;65:1198–201.
[54] Del Prete A, Salvi V, Sozzani S. Adipokines as potential biomarkers in rheumatoid arthritis. Mediators Inflamm 2014;2014, e425068. https://www.hindawi.com/journals/mi/2014/425068/.
[55] Robinson WH, et al. Low-grade inflammation as a key mediator of the pathogenesis of osteoarthritis. Nat Rev Rheumatol 2016;12:580–92.
[56] Stannus O, et al. Circulating levels of IL-6 and TNF-α are associated with knee radiographic osteoarthritis and knee cartilage loss in older adults. Osteoarthr Cartil 2010;18:1441–7.
[57] Goldring SR, Goldring MB. The role of cytokines in cartilage matrix degeneration in osteoarthritis. Clin Orthop Relat Res 2004;427:S27.
[58] Wang T, He C. Pro-inflammatory cytokines: the link between obesity and osteoarthritis. Cytokine Growth Factor Rev 2018;44:38–50.
[59] Deyo RA, Mirza SK, Martin BI. Back pain prevalence and visit rates: estimates from U.S. national surveys, 2002. Spine (Phila Pa 1976) 2006;31:2724–7.
[60] Gruber HE, Ingram JA, Hoelscher GL, Hanley EN. Leptin expression by annulus cells in the human intervertebral disc. Spine J 2007;7:437–43.
[61] Zhao C-Q, Liu D, Li H, Jiang L-S, Dai L-Y. Expression of leptin and its functional receptor on disc cells: contribution to cell proliferation. Spine (Phila Pa 1976) 2008;33:E858–64.
[62] Li Z, et al. Leptin induces cyclin D1 expression and proliferation of human nucleus pulposus cells via JAK/STAT, PI3K/Akt and MEK/ERK pathways. PLoS One 2012;7, e53176.
[63] Segar AH, Fairbank JCT, Urban J. Leptin and the intervertebral disc: a biochemical link exists between obesity, intervertebral disc degeneration and low back pain-an in vitro study in a bovine model. Eur Spine J 2019;28:214–23.

[64] Robbins Basic Pathology, https://www.us.elsevierhealth.com/robbins-basic-pathology-9780323353175.html.
[65] de Araújo Boleti AP, et al. Neuroinflammation: an overview of neurodegenerative and metabolic diseases and of biotechnological studies. Neurochem Int 2020;136, 104714.
[66] Yong HYF, Rawji KS, Ghorbani S, Xue M, Yong VW. The benefits of neuroinflammation for the repair of the injured central nervous system. Cell Mol Immunol 2019;16:540–6.
[67] Aguilar-Valles A, Inoue W, Rummel C, Luheshi GN. Obesity, adipokines and neuroinflammation. Neuropharmacology 2015;96:124–34.
[68] Pugazhenthi S, Qin L, Reddy PH. Common neurodegenerative pathways in obesity, diabetes, and Alzheimer's disease. Biochim Biophys Acta 2017;1863:1037–45.
[69] de la Monte SM, Longato L, Tong M, Wands JR. Insulin resistance and neurodegeneration: roles of obesity, type 2 diabetes mellitus and non-alcoholic steatohepatitis. Curr Opin Investig Drugs 2009;10:1049–60.

CHAPTER 6

Inflammation and obesity

Ronald Tyszkowski[a] and Raman Mehrzad[b]
[a]Private Practice, Allied Health, Women and Infants Hospital, Providence, RI, United States
[b]Division of Plastic and Reconstructive Surgery, Rhode Island Hospital, The Warren Alpert School of Brown University, Providence, RI, United States

Obesity and inflammation

As we observe the multitude of negative physiologic effects of obesity on the human body, we see that promotion of a proinflammatory state may be the most insidious. Obesity, as a chronic condition, promotes an equally chronic state of inflammation. As a general risk factor for disease, obesity amplifies the effects of multiple inflammatory stimulators, rapidly accelerating their deleterious effects. The inflammatory process in turn results in physiologic effects that can perpetuate the obese state and make its reversal more difficult. In this chapter, we will track the pathway from obesity to Inflammation and examine the end results.

Preexisting physiologic states related to obesity promote pathways to inflammation. The state of obesity promotes a proinflammatory state via two pathways which, through different methods, facilitate the release of inflammatory and immune modulators known as adipokines; these include proinflammatory adipokines; tumor necrosis factor alpha, and interleukin 6. Additionally and perhaps more importantly, it reduces the production of the antiinflammatory adipokine, Adiponectin. The modification of the normal levels of inflammatory modulators combined with subsequent endothelial and microvascular changes contributes to the development of significantly dysfunctional physiologic states. These include alteration of lipid and glucose metabolism (significantly predisposing the physiologic state to perpetuate obesity), a prolonged and default proinflammatory state, insulin resistance, and hypertension. The sum total of these states results in Metabolic Syndrome. Metabolic syndrome being defined as a condition of increased risk for cardiovascular disease and type 2 diabetes mellitus [1].

As a means to understand obesity-regulated inflammation, we will review the unique anatomy and physiology of adipose tissue, the effects of obesity on adipose tissue, the major cytokines and their mechanisms of action in the inflammatory pathway, the tissue changes that occur in response to sustained inflammation, and finally, the links to pathologic changes.

Changes in adipose tissue

The origin of the obesity-mediated inflammatory response is within the adipose tissue itself. Adipose tissue is a complex and highly active metabolic and endocrine organ and not simply a storage unit. It is composed of adipocytes (fat cells), connective tissue, nerve tissue, stromovascular cells, and immune cells [2]. As much as 50% of nuclei and protein synthetic components found in adipose tissue are located in nonadipocytic cells [3], which are responsible for a significant percentage of proteins secreted into the body [2].

Adipose tissue can be divided into two major types: brown and white [4]. Brown adipose tissue plays a role in thermogenesis, and its function as a metabolic modulator is still being defined [5]. White adipose tissue, on the other hand, plays a greater role in the regulation of physiological and pathological processes including immunity and inflammation [6]. It is this role as an endocrine organ that positions white adipose tissue as a major agent of physiologic dysfunction particularly as the morphologic changes secondary to obesity occur.

Overnutrition leads to adipocyte hypertrophy and is positively correlated with an increased adipocyte death [7] through constriction and secondary tissue hypoxia. Monocyte infiltration of the adipose tissue in response to cellular death correlates with a global increase in body mass and local adipocyte hypertrophy. This infiltration seems to be a significant trigger for the related inflammatory state, as monocytes are transformed by the "endocrine and metabolic milieu" present in the adipose tissue [8]. They change from a noninflammatory macrophage to a lipid engorged foam cell. These cells then in turn produce adipokines (e.g., IL-6 and TNF-α) that promote pathological changes associated with obesity, insulin resistance, and endothelial dysfunction [8].

Changes in the structure and distribution of adipose tissue in response to obesity significantly affect the nature and quantity of adipokine secretion and subsequently, systemic physiology. It is safe to assume that the obese state is consistent with an altered and most probably amplified inflammatory state.

Adipokines: Origins and effects

Adipokines are cytokines, defined as polypeptides that can act as autocrine and/or paracrine cell regulators. These cellular modulators of inflammation and immunity are secreted by adipose tissue and can act in either a pro- or an antiinflammatory manner. Receptors for adipokines are present in the cell membranes of adipocytes, which allow for autocrine and paracrine function, i.e., these cells can alter structure and function of themselves and the cells around them. Adipocytes, or fat cells, secrete these adipokines in proportion to their volume. Increased volume also shifts the balance toward a predominately proinflammatory function. Inasmuch as high volume adipocytes are pathognomonic of obesity, the connection between the two becomes clearer [9].

Tumor necrosis factor alpha

Tumor Necrosis Factor alpha presents as a cytokine having multiple roles throughout many systems of the body. Most germane to this discussion is its role as a primary "mediator of cellular and molecular events essential to the full development of an inflammatory /immune response" [10].

It is expressed by adipocytes and stromovascular cells [11], is found in increased amounts in obese humans, and is positively correlated with insulin resistance [12]. Additionally, there appears to be a hierarchy of cytokines, such that TNF-α can orchestrate the synthesis, secretion, and activity of other cytokines, thereby amplifying its effects [13]. In vitro and In vivo studies have shown that although TNF-α does have direct endocrine effect on metabolic processes such as glucose uptake, glucose metabolism, and fatty acid oxidation (among others) [14], its indirect effects on other actors and adipose-tissue hormones are where its greatest effects can be seen, particularly in regard to its promotion of insulin resistance [2]. In adipose tissue, it suppresses gene expression related to uptake and storage of glucose and nonesterfied fatty acids [14].

The promotion of increased or sustained TNF-α expression from adipocytes in the obese state as it relates to amplified or sustained proinflammatory states can also challenge the management of inflammatory disorders. Select immune-related inflammatory diseases (IMIDs) can be treated with anti-TNF-α agents. However, the efficacy of these agents is significantly reduced in the obese patient. Overall, management of IMIDs is a greater challenge in the obese patient and has been associated "with more severe disease activity, inferior quality of life, and higher burden of hospitalization" [15].

Interleukin 6

Interleukin 6 is also recognized as a cytokine. In this case, Interleukin 6 acts to regulate information transfer throughout the body during the inflammatory process [16]. Interestingly, it can act either in a proinflammatory or antiinflammatory manner. Regardless, it is positively correlated with obesity, impaired glucose tolerance and insulin resistance [2]. Both expression of IL-6 and circulating levels decrease with weight loss, and higher concentrations predict the development of type 2 diabetes and cardiovascular disease.

One-third of total circulating IL-6 originates from adipose tissue [17], and it is produced by adipocytes as well as macrophages present in the obese tissue matrix [18].

Adiponectin

Adiponectin is a protein that has regulatory effects on homeostasis, glucose and lipid metabolism, and antiinflammatory action. It is produced exclusively in the adipose tissue [19]. Decreased levels are present in obesity as well as cardiovascular disease, hypertension, and metabolic syndrome [19]. High levels are actually related to weight loss (lastra), and it improves insulin insensitivity [20]. Low levels can be correlated to weight gain and obesity.

As studies into adiponectin continue, its roles in the development of multiple disease states including atherosclerosis, cancer, type 2 diabetes, and fatty liver disease are becoming more apparent. Its decreased presence in the obese state has far-ranging implications in the pathogenesis of multiple chronic and significant illnesses.

Promotion of inflammation in obesity

Overconsumption of calories has been shown to initiate an acute inflammatory response in mice and humans [21]. In lean individuals, a low-level response occurs, which resolves after nutrients are metabolized. However, the response is amplified and resolution less complete in obese individuals. Additionally, food quality may affect intensity and duration of response with high fiber better than high fat [22].

Adipocytes respond to overfeeding by increasing production of kinases (enzymes that catalyze the transfer of phosphate groups from high-energy, phosphate-donating molecules to specific substrates): c-jun N-terminal kinase (JNK), the inhibitor of k kinase (IKK), and the protein kinase R (PKR). In obese men and women, compared with lean, the activation of these kinases can be amplified [23,24]. They in turn can induce the expression of the proinflammatory cytokines.

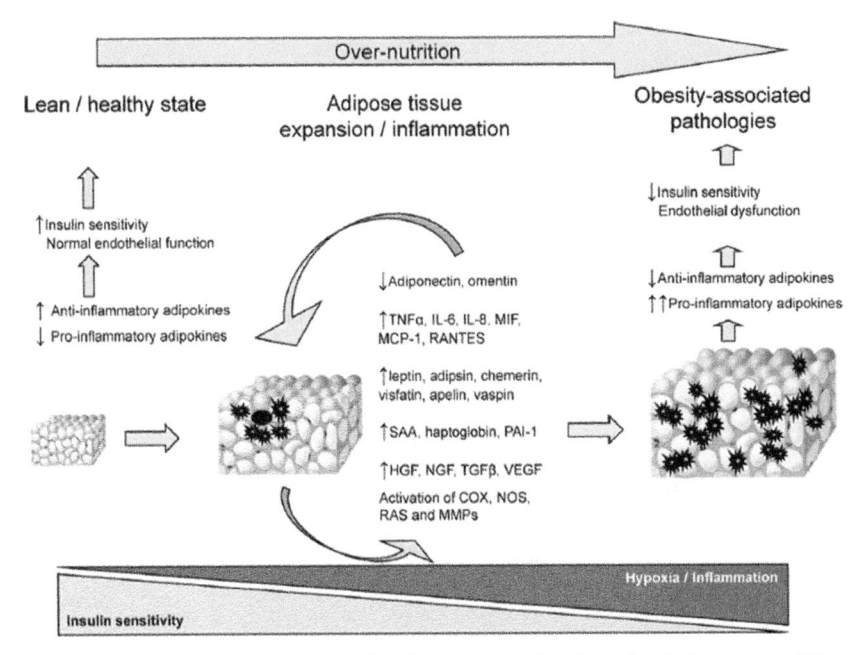

Fig. 1 The continuum from the lean/healthy state to the obese/pathologic state [6].

This reaction further demonstrates the insidiousness of the obese state as it perpetuates itself and its own destructive physiologic changes. When overeating at the same intensity as a lean individual, the obese patients pay a greater price in the amount and duration of inflammatory physiologic changes, along with the damage they may cause.

Fig. 1 demonstrates the continuum from the lean/healthy state to the obese/pathologic state and the subsequent alteration in cytokine concentration breakdown. As adipose tissue expands, the relative concentrations of proinflammatory to antiinflammatory cytokines shift to a proinflammatory dominated state. This increases hypoxia and inflammation and decreases insulin sensitivity, providing fertile ground for the development of obesity-related pathologies.

Insulin resistance

Insulin resistance is one of the most important and dangerous effects of obesity-mediated inflammation. It not only positively correlates with increased incidence of chronic disease, but also promotes and perpetuates obesity through various channels including minimizing the effectiveness of dietary modulation.

Insulin resistance is characterized by lack of response to circulating insulin levels resulting in fasting hyperglycemia. Several pathologic states including lipodystrophy, polycystic ovarian syndrome, nonalcoholic fatty liver disease, and most importantly, type 2 diabetes are accompanied by increased fasting plasma insulin concentrations [25].

The downstream effects of obese-related inflammation set the stage for the multiple pathological states that make up Metabolic Syndrome.

One of the effects of the increased concentration of the three kinases JNK-IKK-PKR is the interference in the normal functioning of insulin. A probable mechanism of action is the phosphorylation, or addition of a phosphate group, to the COOH-terminal end of insulin receptor substrate (IRS) proteins [26]. This phosphorylation inhibits the function of these proteins and interferes with insulin signaling at the cell membrane. It is important to note that this disruption in function occurs via multiple different kinases and different sites of phosphorylation generating a complicated network of effect [26].

microRNA

microRNAs (miRNA) are small noncoding ribonucleic acids (RNAs) that play critical roles in the regulation of host genome expression at the post-transcription level [27].

Obesity, independent of other cardiometabolic risk factors, negatively influences circulating inflammation-related miRNA. Dysregulation of circulating miRNA may contribute mechanistically to the heightened inflammatory state associated with obesity [28].

Endothelial and microvascular dysfunction

"The endothelium is a highly dynamic cell layer that is involved in a multitude of physiologic functions, including the control of vasomotor tone, the trafficking of cells and nutrients, the maintenance of blood fluidity, and the growth of new blood vessels" [29]. Microcirculation, or the blood supply to the endothelium, mimics regular circulation in that its functions include transport of nutrients and removal of toxins. Interaction between local tissue and arterioles determines arteriole diameter, so that tissues can modulate blood flow as needed [30]. An appropriate balance of vasodilators (increasing blood flow) with vasoconstrictors (decreasing blood flow) based on need is essential to proper endothelial function. Nitric oxide (NO), an important vasodilator, plays a key role as it is antiatherogenic and antithrombotic secondary to its ability to relax the surrounding smooth muscle, inhibit platelet aggregation and smooth muscle cell proliferation, and prevent leukocyte adhesion [31]. The reduction of the bioavailability of NO is a significant factor in the development of endothelial dysfunction. Since insulin has a direct effect on the availability of NO in the endothelium, the interference in normal insulin signaling in tissue can initiate a cascade of events leading to endothelial dysfunction, as well as its pathologic sequela.

Endothelial dysfunction is present in obese patients before hypertension or hyperglycemia. It can be shown through an impaired endothelium-dependent vasodilation, reduced arterial compliance, and accelerated atherosclerosis [30]. Decreased levels of adiponectin have been shown to correlate with impaired endothelial vasodilation possibly indicating a link between obesity-related inflammation and endothelial dysfunction [32].

It is important to note here that, in advance of abnormal lab testing or demonstrated elevated blood pressure, the potentially destructive effects of obesity mediated inflammation are taking root. A different classification system for risk evaluation is indicated along with a heightened sense of urgency in this patient population.

Quantifying the ratio of pro to anti inflammatory cytokines may provide insight into where on the progression an obese patient may fall. Subsequently, it may then be possible to stage their inflammatory status in order to quantify the risk for pathology, as well as direct treatment.

Obesity, inflammation, and cancer

The routes from chronic inflammation to cancer have been recognized for over 100 years. Inflammatory cells, such as neutrophils, monocytes, and eosinophils, along with the cytokines they produce can have cancer promoting effects. These effects can include releasing tumor growth and survival factors, promoting angiogenesis and lymphangiogenesis, stimulating DNA changes, remodeling the extracellular matrix, coating tumor cells to make available receptors for disseminating cells via lymphatics and capillaries, and evading host defense mechanisms. Additionally, a chronic state of inflammation and the consistent high concentrations of cytokines may create a desensitization that mutes the natural response to precancerous and cancerous cells [33].

The significant pathological states of increased insulin resistance and resultant hyperinsulinemia, which are positively correlated with obesity and increased BMI, initiate some of the pathways leading to increased cancer risk. Fig. 2 demonstrates three pathways that lead from hyperinsulinemia to increased cancer risk.

```
                    ┌─────────────────────────┐
                    │  Increase Insulin Resistance │
                    │     or Hyperinsulinemia      │
                    └─────────────────────────┘
```

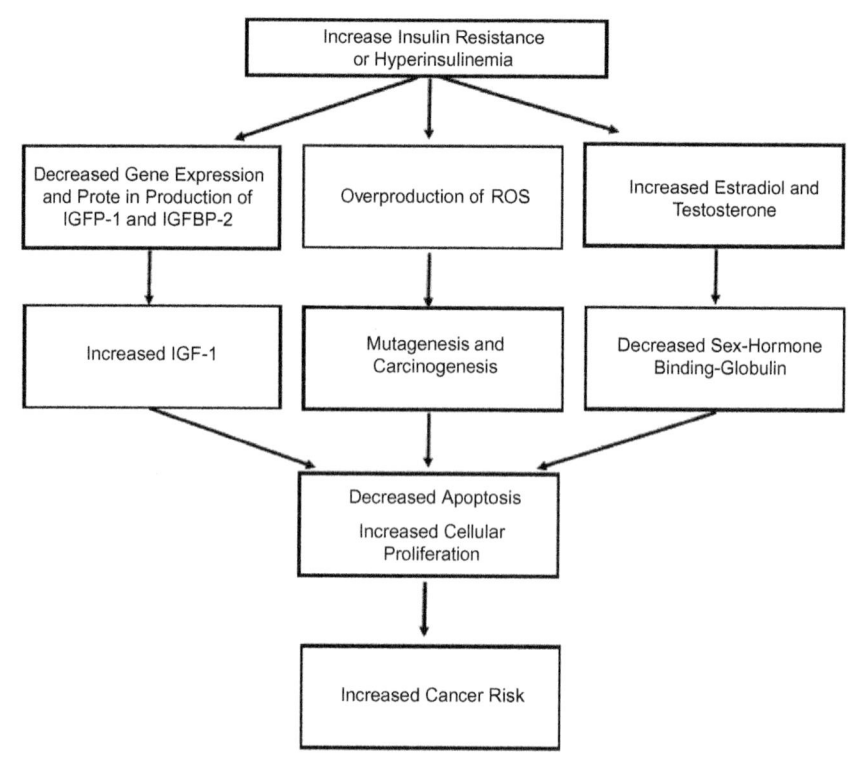

Fig. 2 Potential routes from insulin resistance to cancer. *(Adapted from Amin MN, et al. How the association between obesity and inflammation may lead to insulin resistance and cancer. Diabetes Metab Syndr Clin Res Rev 2019;13 (2);1213–1224.)*

Pathway one: Increased production of insulin-like growth factor binding protein-1 and 2 leads to an increase in Insulin Growth Factor. High serum concentrations of IGF1 are associated with an increased risk of breast, prostate, colorectal, and lung cancers. Physiologically, IGF1 is the major mediator of the effects of the growth hormone; it thus has a strong influence on cell proliferation and differentiation and is a potent inhibitor of apoptosis [34].

Pathway two: Oxidative stress has an accepted role in the etiology of both obesity and cancer [35]. Obesity and type 2 diabetes are associated with increased amounts of reactive oxygen species (ROS), resulting in increased oxidative stress. The increased amounts of ROS may be attributed to the presence of surplus amounts of energy-rich compounds such as glucose and the subsequent metabolic activity they stimulate. Additionally, ROS have been shown to be increased in the adipose tissue of obese mice [36].

Tissues devoid of efficient machinery for ROS removal are particularly vulnerable to develop mutagenesis and carcinogenesis [37].

Pathway three: Multiple studies and meta-analyses have corroborated an inverse relationship between Sex Hormone Binding Globulin (SHGB) and cancer, most specifically breast cancer. Increased levels of IGF-1 downregulate the amounts of circulating SHGB. Less circulating levels of SHBG result in increased levels of estradiol, leading to cellular proliferation and decreased apoptosis specifically in breast endothelium and epithelium. Higher levels of insulin are related to decreased synthesis of SHGB by the liver [38]. Associated physiologic conditions such as hyperinsulinemia, insulin resistance, and dyslipidemia may be major risk factors for colon and breast cancer [39].

The altered secretion of adipokines that is associated with enlargement of the adipocyte (which is also positively correlated with increased BMI) is related to cancer as well. These secreted factors can directly promote mammary tumorigenesis through induction of antiapoptotic transcriptional programs and protooncogene stabilization [40]. Additionally, the endocrine effects of the adipokines secreted by the adipocyte participate in a highly complex cross talk with surrounding tumor cells, promoting tumor progression [41].

The presence of increased and/or decreased levels of adipokines including the ones discussed in this chapter (TNF-α, IL-6, Adiponectin) has been shown in multiple studies to be associated with increased cancer incidence though various tissues, including prostate, breast, and GI tract.

In the patients already diagnosed with cancer, higher amounts of circulating IL-6 also increase mortality. IL-6 promotes tumorigenesis, angiogenesis, invasiveness, metastasis and inhibits apoptosis [42,43]. It also protects cancer cells from therapy-induced DNA damage and oxidative stress by facilitating the repair and induction of counter signaling pathways [43].

Conversely, decreased amounts of Adiponectin (adiponectinemia) are related to increased cancer rates. Adiponectin exhibits antiatherogenic, proapoptotic, and antiproliferative properties and is inversely correlated with the development of several types of malignancies later in life [41]. Actual adiponectin, adiponectin analogues, and precursor molecules to adiponectin are being evaluated as potential treatments.

Additionally, other studies have postulated that adipose tissue may act as a reservoir of potentially carcinogenic substances. The substances, including organopesticides and polychlorinated biphenyls (PCBs), have been linked to increased risk of breast cancer, prostate cancer, and lymphoma [44].

References

[1] Emanuela F, et al. Inflammation as a link between obesity and metabolic syndrome. J Nutr Metab 2012;2012.
[2] Kershaw EE, Flier JS. Adipose tissue as an endocrine organ. J Clin Endocrinol Metab 2004;89(6):2548–56.
[3] Kern PA, et al. Adipose tissue tumor necrosis factor and interleukin-6 expression in human obesity and insulin resistance. Am J Physiol Endocrinol Metab 2001;280(5):E745–51.
[4] Curat CA, et al. From blood monocytes to adipose tissue-resident macrophages: induction of diapedesis by human mature adipocytes. Diabetes 2004;53(5):1285–92.
[5] Cannon B, Nedergaard JAN. Brown adipose tissue: function and physiological significance. Physiol Rev 2004;84:277–359.
[6] Karastergiou K, Mohamed-Ali V. The autocrine and paracrine roles of adipokines. Mol Cell Endocrinol 2010;318(1–2):69–78.
[7] Weisberg SP, McCann D, Desai M, Rosenbaum M, Leibel RL, Ferrante Jr AW. Obesity is associated with macrophage accumulation in adipose tissue. J Clin Invest 2003;112(12):1796–808.
[8] Lumeng CN, Bodzin JL, Saltiel AR. Obesity induces a phenotypic switch in adipose tissue macrophage polarization. J Clin Invest 2007;117(1):175–84.
[9] Skurk T, Alberti-Huber C, Herder C, Hauner H. Relationship between adipocyte size and adipokine expression and secretion. J Clin Endocrinol Metab 2007;92(3):1023–33.
[10] Strieter RM, Kunkel SL, Bone RC. Role of tumor necrosis factor-alpha in disease states and inflammation. Crit Care Med 1993;21(10 Suppl):S447–63.
[11] Fain JN, Madan AK, Hiler ML, Cheema P, Bahouth SW. Comparison of the release of Adipokines by adipose tissue, adipose tissue matrix, and adipocytes from visceral and subcutaneous abdominal adipose tissues of obese humans. Endocrinology 2004;145(5):2273–82.
[12] Hotamisligil GS, Shargill NS, Spiegelman BM. Adipose expression of tumor necrosis factor-alpha: direct role in obesity-linked insulin resistance. Science 1993;259(5091):87–91.
[13] Coppack S. Pro-inflammatory cytokines and adipose tissue. Proc Nutr Soc 2001;60(3):349–56.
[14] Ruan H, Miles PD, Ladd CM, Ross K, Golub TR, Olefsky JM, Lodish HF. Profiling gene transcription in vivo reveals adipose tissue as an immediate target of tumor necrosis factor-alpha: implications for insulin resistance. Diabetes 2002;51(11):3176–88.
[15] Singh S, et al. Obesity and response to anti-tumor necrosis factor-α agents in patients with select immune-mediated inflammatory diseases: a systematic review and meta-analysis. PLoS ONE 2018;13(5), e0195123.
[16] Devlin TM, editor. Textbook of Biochemistry with Clinical Correlations. John Wiley & Sons; 2010.
[17] Fontana L, Eagon JC, Trujillo ME, Scherer PE, Klein S. Visceral fat adipokine secretion is associated with systemic inflammation in obese humans. Diabetes 2007;56(4):1010–3.
[18] Fernández-Sánchez A, Madrigal-Santillán E, Bautista M, Esquivel-Soto J, Morales-González Á, Esquivel-Chirino C, Durante-Montiel I, Sánchez-Rivera G, Valadez-Vega C, Morales-González JA. Inflammation, oxidative stress, and obesity. Int J Mol Sci 2011;12:3117–32.
[19] Kadowaki T, Yamauchi T. Adiponectin and adiponectin receptors. Endocr Rev 2005;26(3):439–51.
[20] Lastra G, Manrique CM, Hayden MR. The role of beta-cell dysfunction in the cardiometabolic syndrome. J Cardiometab Syndr 2006 Winter;1(1):41–6.
[21] Aljada A, Mohanty P, Ghanim H, Abdo T, Tripathy D, Chaudhuri A, Dandona P. Increase in intranuclear nuclear factor kappaB and decrease in inhibitor kappaB in mononuclear cells after a mixed meal: evidence for a proinflammatory effect. Am J Clin Nutr 2004;79(4):682–90. https://doi.org/10.1093/ajcn/79.4.682. 15051615.

[22] Dandona P, et al. Metabolic syndrome: a comprehensive perspective based on interactions between obesity, diabetes, and inflammation. Circulation 2005;111(11):1448–1454.6.
[23] Solinas G, Karin M. JNK1 and IKKβ: molecular links between obesity and metabolic dysfunction. FASEB J 2010;24(8):2596–611.
[24] Nakamura T, et al. Double-stranded RNA-dependent protein kinase links pathogen sensing with stress and metabolic homeostasis. Cell 2010;140(3):338–348.4.
[25] Petersen MC, Shulman GI. Mechanisms of insulin action and insulin resistance. Physiol Rev 2018;98(4):2133–223.
[26] Boura-Halfon S, Zick Y. Phosphorylation of IRS proteins, insulin action, and insulin resistance. Am J Physiol Endocrinol Metab 2009;296(4):E581–91.
[27] Dai R, Ansar Ahmed S. MicroRNA, a new paradigm for understanding immunoregulation, inflammation, and autoimmune diseases. Transl Res 2011;157(4):163–79.
[28] Hijmans JG, et al. Influence of overweight and obesity on circulating inflammation-related microRNA. Microrna 2018;7(2):148–54.
[29] Aird WC. Endothelium as an organ system. Crit Care Med 2004;32(5):S271–9.
[30] Kraemer-Aguiar LG, Laflor CM, Bouskela E. Skin microcirculatory dysfunction is already present in normoglycemic subjects with metabolic syndrome. Metabolism 2008;57(12):1740–6.
[31] Ritchie SA, et al. The role of insulin and the adipocytokines in regulation of vascular endothelial function. Clin Sci 2004;107(6):519–32.
[32] Tan KCB, et al. Hypoadiponectinemia is associated with impaired endothelium-dependent vasodilation. J Clin Endocrinol Metabol 2004;89(2):765–9.
[33] Coussens LM, Werb Z. Inflammation and cancer. Nature 2002;420(6917):860–7.
[34] Fürstenberger G, Senn H-J. Insulin-like growth factors and cancer. Lancet Oncol 2002;3(5):298–302.
[35] Prieto-Hontoria PL, et al. Role of obesity-associated dysfunctional adipose tissue in cancer: a molecular nutrition approach. Biochim Biophys Acta 2011;1807(6):664–78.
[36] Furukawa S, et al. Increased oxidative stress in obesity and its impact on metabolic syndrome. J Clin Invest 2017;114(12):1752–61.
[37] Ziech D, Franco R, Pappa A, Panayiotidis MI. Reactive oxygen species (ROS)-induced genetic and epigenetic alterations in human carcinogenesis. Mutat Res 2011;711(1–2):167–73.
[38] Amin MN, et al. How the association between obesity and inflammation may lead to insulin resistance and cancer. Diabetes Metab Syndr Clin Res Rev 2019;13(2):1213–24.
[39] Arcidiacono B, et al. insulin resistance and cancer risk: an overview of the pathogenetic mechanisms. Exp Diabetes Res 2012;2012.
[40] Iyengar P, et al. Adipocyte-secreted factors synergistically promote mammary tumorigenesis through induction of anti-apoptotic transcriptional programs and proto-oncogene stabilization. Oncogene 2003;22(41):6408–23.
[41] Macciò A, Madeddu C. Obesity, inflammation, and postmenopausal breast cancer: therapeutic implications. TheScientificWorldJournal 2011;11.
[42] Salgado R, et al. Circulating interleukin-6 predicts survival in patients with metastatic breast cancer. Int J Cancer 2003;103(5):642–6.
[43] Kumari N, et al. Role of interleukin-6 in cancer progression and therapeutic resistance. Tumour Biol 2016;37(9):11553–72.
[44] Irigaray P, et al. Overweight/obesity and cancer genesis: more than a biological link. Biomed Pharmacother 2007;61(10):665–78.

CHAPTER 7

Obesity, inflammation, and aging

Jacqueline J. Chu[a] and Raman Mehrzad[b]
[a]College of Medicine, The Ohio State University, Columbus, OH, Unites States
[b]Division of Plastic and Reconstructive Surgery, Rhode Island Hospital, The Warren Alpert School of Brown University, Providence, RI, United States

Inflammation and aging

Originally posed by Franceschi et al. in 2000, "inflammaging" is a theory that explains the presence of chronic, low-grade inflammation in aging individuals and the relationship between this inflammation and development of aging-associated diseases [1]. In this theory, inflammation, which is how our bodies respond to stressors and disease, is a necessary function for survival that is selected for through evolution; however, as individuals age, cumulative exposure to these stressors leads to a chronic proinflammatory state that becomes detrimental to health. An additional component of this theory explains that individuals who are able to reach old age without many aging-associated diseases have higher levels of antiinflammatory compounds that counteract the effects of the proinflammatory compounds [2]. This section will provide an overview of the various contributors to chronic inflammation in aging based on the inflammaging theory.

Immunosenescence

Immunosenescence refers to aging-related changes to the immune system [3]. As people age, both adaptive and innate immune systems tend to lose efficacy over time, leading to difficulties mounting immune responses against new pathogens. Adaptive immunity, which is responsible for immunologic memory, is especially affected, and a well-known consequence of this is the decreased efficacy of vaccinations in the elderly [4]. In the elderly, a process known as thymic involution occurs, in which progressively fewer naïve T-cells are produced, impacting the ability of the immune system to recognize and remember new threats [5]. At the same time, innate immunity, which is responsible for nonspecific immune responses to a variety of infectious and noninfectious molecules, is dysfunctional, resulting in ineffective clearing of threats and prolonged production of inflammatory cytokines [6,7].

The development of immunosenescence is potentially attributable to chronic exposure to immunogenic antigens (immune-response-inducing molecules) that worsens with aging. In humans, chronic low-grade infection by human cytomegalovirus (HCMV) is proposed as a major contributor to immunosenescence in the adaptive immune system. HCMV is a common infection that increases in prevalence with increasing age and generally remains latent, but persistent, in nonimmunocompromised hosts [8]. Researchers theorize that chronic suppression of HCMV replication eventually leads to depletion of naïve T cells at old age as the T cell repertoire becomes dominated by HCMV-specific T cells at the cost of T cell diversity; this is supported by studies that have demonstrated that HCMV-specific T cells may comprise of 25% of the T cell population [9].

This theory of immunosenescence, inflammation, and aging-related diseases is supported by the health consequences seen in HIV-positive patients, whose disease course is typified by T cell depletion but high levels of proinflammatory molecules due to chronic infection [10]. Like aging individuals, HIV-positive patients have higher risks of developing aging-related diseases, including cardiovascular disease, cancer, and osteoporosis [10].

Gut dysbiosis

The gut microbiome consists of the microbial organisms that inhabit the gastrointestinal tract. While originally thought as merely contributors to digestion, the gut microbiome has now been shown to have effects on autoimmunity, metabolic diseases, and even cognitive function [11–13]. An abundance of research has demonstrated that aging is associated with gut dysbiosis [14]. Old individuals have different gut microbiota than young individuals, with decreased microbial diversity, increased prevalence of opportunistic bacteria types, and loss of commensal bacteria types [15–17]. In addition, there is a difference in microbial diversity among older individuals; those who are more frail and in poorer health have decreased microbial diversity compared with healthier individuals [18]. Inflammation is associated with gut dysbiosis; however, it is unclear whether gut dysbiosis leads to chronic inflammation or vice versa or some combination of both [14,17].

The importance of the gut microbiota on immune system regulation is well established. Healthy gut microbiota, for example, is responsible for the suppression of inflammation and immune responses against antigens found in ingested foods and the stimulation of tissue healing in response to injury caused by inflammation [19]. Systemically, alterations in gut microbiota have been shown to be linked to autoimmune conditions such as rheumatoid arthritis and multiple sclerosis [12]. In terms of the link between gut microbiota and aging, there is support that gut dysbiosis in the elderly leads to the development of aging-related diseases. In the ELDERMET study of 178 elderly subjects in various residential settings, microbiome composition was correlated with greater frailty in addition to higher levels of inflammatory markers such as TNF-alpha, IL-6, IL-8, and CRP [20]. In addition, those living in long-term care residences (high frailty) had significantly lower microbiome diversity.

In Western societies, gut dysbiosis associated with aging is attributed to greater exposure to antibiotics as well as the "Western" diet that is dense in fat and carbohydrates but low in fiber. Antibiotics are known to deplete the gut microbiome, allowing opportunistic bacteria such as *C. diff*, a major cause of hospital-associated diarrhea, to proliferate [21]. Low-fiber diets upset the balance of gut microbiota as commensal bacteria rely on fiber for nutrition. Dietary fiber plays an important role in immune system regulation by gut microbiota since bacterial digestion of fiber produces short-chain fatty acids (SCFAs). SCFA is responsible for local and systemic immune downregulation primarily through induction of regulatory T cell activity [19]. Additionally, even among normally commensal bacteria, the lack of dietary fiber can lead to these bacteria utilizing other sources of nutrition, including the mucous that serves as a protective barrier for the intestinal lining [22]. The intestinal lining, now exposed to antigens from food as well as bacteria, stimulates proinflammatory cytokine production and immune cell responses. The weakened intestinal barrier can also cause "leaky gut," resulting in chronic translocation of bacteria and bacterial components into the bloodstream, triggering chronic systemic inflammation [23,24].

Alternatively, gut dysbiosis may be a consequence of chronic inflammation caused by immunosenescence, which is a theory that is currently not well studied [14,17]. Ineffective and dysregulated innate immune cells in the gut may lead to inflammation of the gut, and researchers propose that this chronic inflammation selects for bacteria that are able to tolerate the oxidative environments generated, resulting in decreased gut biodiversity. Additionally, it may damage the intestinal barrier, leading to the "leaky gut" phenomenon described previously and perpetuated systemic inflammation.

Cell debris

While the immune system is typically thought of as the human body's defense system against infection, it also plays an important housekeeping role for the body by clearing cellular debris, such as toxic metabolites or dead or dying cells [25]. Cells of the innate immune system are able to recognize cellular debris through receptors, called Pattern Recognition Receptors (PRRs), which bind to particular molecular components that are found in cellular debris, called Damage-Associated Molecular Patterns (DAMPs) [26]. Generally, DAMPs are molecules that are usually found within the cell, such as DNA or mRNA, and are thus exposed when cells die. Other DAMPs include reactive oxygen species (ROS) or advanced-glycation end-products (AGEs) that are cytotoxic. In response to DAMPs, innate immune cells release proinflammatory cytokines that trigger the migration of other immune cells to the location of cell damage. Ultimately, macrophages, innate immune cells, phagocytose and degrade the cell debris, thus ending the inflammatory process [27].

Aging increases production of debris that is inadequately cleared by the innate immune system, leading to chronic inflammation. For example, skin aging studies have demonstrated that AGEs accumulate with chronological age [28]. AGE is produced by the glycation (addition of a sugar moiety) of proteins or lipids, and the amount of glycation is associated with the rate of protein or lipid turnover. As a result, long-lived proteins in the skin such as collagen and fibronectin accumulate glycations as individuals age. Glycation can also be induced by UV radiation, to which older individuals would have more cumulative exposure. In addition to increased production of cellular debris, immunosenescence may also play a role; macrophages in an aging innate immune system are less effective at phagocytosis and antiinflammatory signaling [29].

Cell senescence

Cell senescence is a practically permanent state of growth and cell cycle arrest that cells enter to prevent cancer development [30]. Cell senescence is therefore commonly triggered by DNA damage, telomere shortening or damage, mitochondrial damage, and chromatin changes. These all can lead to harmful mutations to the DNA or changes to cell function that can eventually lead to cancer. As individuals age, cells have undergone more cycles of replication and more DNA insults, leading to increased numbers of senescent cells [31]. While these cells no longer replicate, senescent cells are still active and upregulate a set of proinflammatory genes collectively called the Senescence-Associated Secretory Phenotype (SASP). Like with cellular debris, the proinflammatory milieu generated by senescent cells through SASP attracts immune cells such as macrophages that then clear senescent cells from tissue [32,33]. However, the increased number of senescent cells associated with aging along with decreased functionality of macrophages results in accumulation of proinflammatory senescent cells and proinflammatory signaling from immune cells attempting to clear these senescent cells, leading to chronic inflammation [33].

Inflammation and obesity

In the previous section, we described some of the processes that cause chronic inflammation in aging individuals. Obesity is also a chronic inflammatory process and is known to cause metabolic dysfunction through inflammation. In this section, we will briefly discuss how obesity leads to chronic inflammation and metabolic sequelae.

Metabolic inflammation

Obesity is a state of chronic positive energy balance, resulting in expansion of adipose tissue. Adipose tissue stores excess energy intake in the form of lipids and responds to insulin signaling by increasing glucose uptake, increasing uptake of lipids, and decreasing lipid breakdown into free fatty acids [34–36]. In healthy adipose tissue, adipocytes are surrounded by type 2 immune cells that are generally antiinflammatory and release cytokines that promote insulin sensitivity [37]. On the other hand, obesity is characterized by proinflammatory type I immune cells in the adipose tissue. One trigger for this proinflammatory immune shift is changes in gut microbiota and permeability, which occurs, as mentioned previously, as a result of high-fat and low-fiber diets [38]. In addition, as adipocytes continue to increase in size through hypertrophy, cell stress also increases [39]. This is potentially a result of hypoxia as the large adipocytes outgrow their blood supply or mechanical stress as adipocyte growth becomes restricted by the web of extracellular matrix that surrounds adipocytes [37]. The increased cell stress then triggers the recruitment of type I, proinflammatory immune cells. Cytokine release from proinflammatory cells affects insulin signaling pathways in adipose tissue as well as in organs important for metabolism, such as the liver and skeletal muscle, resulting in insulin resistance [40]. Insulin resistance then eventually leads to metabolic conditions such as type-2 diabetes, hyperlipidemia, and hypertension [41].

Adipocyte senescence

Another potential result of adipocyte cell stress is adipocyte senescence, which, as described previously, is a proinflammatory state that can lead to chronic inflammation [42]. In obese individuals, cell stress and inflammation have been shown to be a trigger for adipose tissue expansion through hyperplasia or the generation of more adipocytes through differentiation of adipocyte stem cells (preadipocytes) [43]. Continuous cycles of replication and differentiation, however, trigger cellular senescence in preadipocytes, and indeed, obese individuals have a much larger proportion of senescent preadipocytes than nonobese individuals [44].

Connecting inflammation, obesity, and aging

The previous sections have illustrated how aging and obesity both lead to chronic inflammation throughout the body and may actually share some common pathways. Because of their similarities, researchers have often proposed that obesity can accelerate the aging process, and indeed, obesity has been linked to increased risk in developing multiple aging-related conditions [45]. In this next section, we will describe how, through induction of chronic inflammation, obesity and aging may work synergistically to cause many of the diseases we associate with aging.

Immunocompromise

As discussed previously, immunosenescence is a characteristic of aging individuals and results in weakened immune responses to infections and vaccines. Obesity appears to accelerate immunosenescence with detrimental effects on adaptive immune cell function; studies have demonstrated that vaccines are less effective in obese individuals, and obese individuals have worse outcomes after infection [46–48]. Chronic inflammation caused by dysfunction adipose tissue in obesity has been shown to result in loss of T cells over time. Similar to the effects of HCMV infection, adipose inflammation and continuous activation of T cells progressively diminish the diversity of naïve T cells [49]. This may be because the milieu of cytokines generated by adipose tissue predisposes the development of short-lived effector T cells, which are important for the active clearance of infection, at the cost of memory T cell development [46]. Short-lived effector T cells are not maintained over long periods of time, while memory T cells are. Adipose inflammation therefore results in loss of naïve T cells without the generation of many long-lasting memory T cells. Lastly, in obese individuals, ectopic fat deposition occurs in lymphoid tissues including the thymus, which suppresses naïve T cell development [50].

Insulin resistance

Aging processes can independently cause adipose tissue dysfunction, which exacerbates existing adipose-induced inflammation and contributes to the development of metabolic sequelae [51]. As mentioned previously, obesity can induce preadipocyte senescence as adipocyte cell stress and inflammation exhaust preadipocyte proliferation and differentiation capacity. Preadipocyte proliferation and differentiation are also a normal part of adipose tissue maintenance; in normal physiology, adipocytes turnover at a rate of 10% per year [52]. Preadipocyte senescence and its associated inflammatory profile are therefore an expected consequence of aging [53].

Senescence in aging is unevenly distributed and seems to occur at higher rates in subcutaneous adipose tissue, the fat that people visibly carry on their bodies and the primary compartment of fat storage, rather than visceral adipose tissue, the fat that surrounds intraabdominal organs [54]. As a result, subcutaneous adipose tissue loses its ability to expand through hyperplasia as people age; fats must then be stored in the visceral adipose as well as in nonadipose tissues such as the liver and skeletal muscle [55,56]. Just like in obesity, ectopic fat storage in areas such as the liver and skeletal muscle results in insulin resistance as free fatty acid breakdown in these cells leads to increased levels of toxic ceramides, which inhibits insulin signaling [57,58]. Visceral adipose accumulation worsens this process since it is able to directly release fatty acids into the portal circulation to the liver, given its location in the intraabdominal cavity. For this same reason, visceral adipose is more prone to inflammation since it is in contact with intestinal circulation and proinflammatory molecules released by the gut microbiota, which tends to be dysbiotic in both aging and obesity [43].

Atherosclerosis

Atherosclerosis describes the development of lipid plaques in arteries, and progression of atherosclerosis can lead to cardiovascular disease (myocardial infarction, strokes, etc.). Extensive research has established that atherosclerosis is a chronic inflammatory condition of the vascular endothelium, the layer of tissue that lines the inside of blood vessels [59]. Both obesity and aging have been shown to exacerbate this inflammatory process [60,61].

Lipid plaques are prone to develop at points in the vasculature where endothelial shear stress is low; these areas are generally at curvatures and bifurcations of blood vessels where laminar flow of blood is disrupted [62]. Endothelial cells change in morphology and function in response to levels of shear stress detected by their mechanoreceptors, and over time, endothelial cells at sites of low shear stress no longer express atheroprotective genes and exhibit a proinflammatory phenotype [63]. In straight sections of blood vessels where endothelial cells experience high shear stress, endothelial cells have an elongated, fusiform shape (low vessel wall permeability) and produce high levels of nitric oxide. Nitric oxide plays a crucial role in vasodilation as well as maintenance of an antiinflammatory state through inhibiting expression NF-kB pathways responsible for production of proinflammatory cytokines and immune cell adhesion molecules [63–66].

On the other hand, detection of low endothelial shear stress leads to decreased nitric oxide generation, which consequently increases NF-kB expression [63]. Endothelial cells take on a polygonal morphology (high vessel wall permeability) and upregulate generation of proinflammatory cytokines and immune cell chemoattractants [67]. In addition, endothelial shear stress triggers increased uptake of low-density lipoproteins (LDLs) through increased expression of LDL receptors and increased oxidative stress through increased generation of reactive oxygen species (ROS) [67]. The increased vessel wall permeability combined with increased LDL receptor expression leads to LDL accumulation in the subendothelial space, while the increased generation of ROS modifies the LDL, which is highly antigenic and becomes phagocytosed by macrophages attracted by proinflammatory molecules [68]. These macrophages then die, releasing more proinflammatory mediators and attracting more immune cells to the site. An additional contributor to, as well as consequence of, this atherogenic process is increased rates of endothelial cell apoptosis and turnover. Nitric oxide maintains endothelial cell survival, and reduction of nitric oxide in areas of low endothelial shear stress results in increased endothelial cell death, which is then exacerbated by high levels of oxidative stress generated by ROS [69].

Obesity is a well-established risk factor for cardiovascular disease and acts both directly and indirectly to promote atherosclerosis [70]. In terms of direct action, as mentioned previously, hypertrophic, stressed adipocytes induce the activation of proinflammatory type-1 immune responses, including the secretion of proinflammatory cytokines such as IL-6 and TNF-alpha by macrophages. These cytokines, for endothelial cells, increase the secretion of cell adhesion molecules and immune cell chemoattractants, resulting in worsening immune cell infiltration and action [70]. In terms of indirect action, these same inflammatory mediators are responsible for the induction of systemic insulin resistance, which increases the rate of LDL generation by the liver [70].

Multiple principles of inflammaging are at work in the connection between aging and atherosclerosis. First, endothelial cell senescence naturally occurs with aging, leading to dysfunctional endothelial cells with a proinflammatory phenotype (SASP) [71]. The development of cell senescence is accelerated in atherosclerotic plaques due to the environment of high oxidative stress and inflammation that predisposes to high cell turnover. In addition, the chronic inflammatory state in aging individuals, induced by a variety of mechanisms described previously, predisposes the development of myeloid cells (macrophages and neutrophils) over lymphoid cells (T and B cells) in the bone marrow, resulting in an increased number of available macrophages in the bloodstream to contribute to atherosclerosis [72]. Finally, through the process of aging, hematopoietic stem cells with mutations can accumulate in the bone marrow, and these cells can clonally proliferate and potentially become malignant. The cells generated in this process, called clonal hematopoiesis of indeterminate potential (CHIP), have been found to secrete high amounts of IL-6, contributing to the proinflammatory state of atherosclerosis [72].

Alzheimer's disease

Alzheimer's disease is the most common neurodegenerative disease in the elderly, and it is characterized by the development of protein plaques in the brain. In Alzheimer's disease, amyloid-beta generated normally by neurons accumulates in the extracellular space [73]. While original studies on these diseases have focused on the direct neurotoxicity of these protein plaques, newer research in the area has demonstrated that neuroinflammation stimulated by the presence of these plaques likely is a large contributor to neurotoxicity and disease progression as well [74].

The brain is considered immune privileged; the blood-brain barrier tightly regulates the entry and exit of molecules and cells into the brain, so normally immune cells from the peripheral circulation have no exposure to brain antigens or access to the brain [75]. Indeed, it would actually be quite harmful for inflammatory responses to occur in the brain as damaged neurons regenerate slowly. However, that does not mean that the brain is devoid of immune cells. Microglial cells, the brain counterpart of macrophages in the periphery, are crucial for phagocytosing cell debris as well as maintaining an antiinflammatory environment [75]. Astrocytes, as well, play a role in sustaining the immune privilege of the brain and have been shown to initiate cell death in T cells that manage to pass through the blood–brain barrier [75].

In Alzheimer's disease, amyloid-beta accumulation in the extracellular space likely triggers a chronic inflammatory response in microglial cells, leading to neurotoxicity [76]. In normal physiology, amyloid-beta is regularly produced and is usually cleared through phagocytosis by microglial cells. In this case, amyloid-beta stimulates short-term, acute inflammation that is quickly resolved when microglial cells clear the amyloid. However, a number of different factors, including aging and obesity, can result in sustained proinflammatory responses that injure neurons [76]. In terms of aging, immunosenescence of microglial cells is a likely contributor; aging microglia have different functionality from young microglia, including less effective phagocytosis and, importantly, upregulation of proinflammatory cytokines [77]. In addition, like other senescent cell types, the increased proinflammatory expression may be due to transition to SASP. In terms of obesity, a clear relationship between obesity and Alzheimer's has been established; however, little is known about how these two conditions are connected. One potential theory is that obesity induces insulin resistance, including in the brain, and this then induces changes in blood flow and glucose metabolism that predispose to amyloid deposition [78]. Systemic inflammation induced by obesity may also directly cause neuroinflammation; proinflammatory cytokines may pass into the brain through areas such as the hypothalamus that have a more permeable blood-brain barrier, or they may increase the permeability of the blood-brain barrier, thus allowing for entry of proinflammatory cytokines into the brain [79].

Antiinflammatory intervention for aging-related illnesses

Many elderly individuals remain healthy in old age and develop very few of the conditions discussed previously. Given this phenomenon, researchers have investigated the characteristics that have allowed for healthy longevity in these individuals and have identified an opposing system of antiinflammatory mediators that may counteract and prevent the damage caused by proinflammatory processes. In this section, we will discuss the role and function of these antiinflammatory mediators. In addition, we will discuss how we may harness antiinflammatory interventions to treat aging-related illnesses.

Antiinflammatory mediators in healthy aging and longevity

Through studies on centenarians, researchers have found that, while they had high levels of proinflammatory cytokines, these long-lived individuals also had high levels of antiinflammatory cytokines, including IL-1Ra,

IL-4, IL-10, and TGF-beta [80]. All of these cytokines have been shown to counteract the actions of proinflammatory cytokines; for example, IL-1Ra is a receptor antagonist of IL-1, and IL-4 suppresses type 1 immune responses [81]. IL-10 has been especially well studied in this context and has been correlated with decreased cardiovascular disease risk in centenarians [82,83]. Additional experimental studies have linked high levels of IL-10 with decreased aging-related insulin resistance, but also immunosuppression [84,85].

Targeting inflammation in aging-related illnesses

Many strategies for decreasing age-related inflammation have been evaluated as a way to treat or prevent aging-related illnesses. Antiinflammatory drugs have been assessed for the treatment of insulin resistance, and in fact, many of our existing drugs for treatment of diabetes may have antiinflammatory effects that were not originally recognized [86]. Metformin and thiazolidinediones, especially, have been well studied; both have been shown to decrease production of proinflammatory cytokines and may therefore improve insulin sensitivity partially by reducing inflammation-induced inhibition of insulin signaling [87,88]. More importantly, these medications are now being investigated to be used for treatment of atherosclerosis, as well as neurodegenerative diseases [89–92]. Similarly, statins, which are commonly used for hyperlipidemia and atherosclerosis, may also have previously unrecognized antiinflammatory properties [93]. Statins have been shown to reduce expression of cell-adhesion molecules in endothelial cells, as well as prevent macrophage growth. Finally, the use of antiinflammatory medications for Alzheimer's disease has so far been less successful; however, this may be due to our insufficient understanding of the disease process and the importance of inflammatory activation of microglia for normal physiologic removal of amyloid-beta [94]. Previous trials have used NSAIDs or minocycline, with little success, but other antiinflammatory options are still being evaluated [95–97].

Conclusions

Chronic inflammation is a feature common to both obesity and aging, and, as demonstrated in this chapter, the inflammatory processes of these two conditions build upon each other, leading to or exacerbating aging-related illnesses. Common mechanisms underlying aging-related illnesses involve local immunosenescence and cell senescence in a background of whole-body inflammation. New strategies to treat or prevent aging-related illnesses should thus focus on antiinflammatory interventions that will ameliorate chronic inflammation.

References

[1] Franceschi C, Bonafe M, Valensin S, et al. Inflamm-aging. An evolutionary perspective on immunosenescence. Ann N Y Acad Sci 2000;908:244–54. https://doi.org/10.1111/j.1749-6632.2000.tb06651.x.

[2] Franceschi C, Capri M, Monti D, et al. Inflammaging and anti-inflammaging: a systemic perspective on aging and longevity emerged from studies in humans. Mech Ageing Dev 2007;128(1):92–105. https://doi.org/10.1016/j.mad.2006.11.016.

[3] Aiello A, Farzaneh F, Candore G, et al. Immunosenescence and its hallmarks: how to oppose aging strategically? A review of potential options for therapeutic intervention. Front Immunol 2019;10:2247. https://doi.org/10.3389/fimmu.2019.02247.

[4] Rondy M, El Omeiri N, Thompson MG, Leveque A, Moren A, Sullivan SG. Effectiveness of influenza vaccines in preventing severe influenza illness among adults: a systematic review and meta-analysis of test-negative design case-control studies. J Infect 2017;75(5):381–94. https://doi.org/10.1016/j.jinf.2017.09.010.

[5] Lazuardi L, Jenewein B, Wolf AM, Pfister G, Tzankov A, Grubeck-Loebenstein B. Age-related loss of naive T cells and dysregulation of T-cell/B-cell interactions in human lymph nodes. Immunology 2005;114(1):37–43. https://doi.org/10.1111/j.1365-2567.2004.02006.x.

[6] Shaw AC, Joshi S, Greenwood H, Panda A, Lord JM. Aging of the innate immune system. Curr Opin Immunol 2010;22(4):507–13. https://doi.org/10.1016/j.coi.2010.05.003.

[7] Fulop T, Larbi A, Dupuis G, et al. Immunosenescence and Inflamm-aging as two sides of the same coin: friends or foes? Front Immunol 2017;8:1960. https://doi.org/10.3389/fimmu.2017.01960.

[8] Britt W. Manifestations of human cytomegalovirus infection: proposed mechanisms of acute and chronic disease. Curr Top Microbiol Immunol 2008;325:417–70. https://doi.org/10.1007/978-3-540-77349-8_23.

[9] Khan N, Shariff N, Cobbold M, et al. Cytomegalovirus seropositivity drives the CD8 T cell repertoire toward greater clonality in healthy elderly individuals. J Immunol 2002;169(4):1984–92. https://doi.org/10.4049/jimmunol.169.4.1984.

[10] Deeks SG. HIV infection, inflammation, immunosenescence, and aging. Annu Rev Med 2011;62:141–55. https://doi.org/10.1146/annurev-med-042909-093756.

[11] Fan Y, Pedersen O. Gut microbiota in human metabolic health and disease. Nat Rev Microbiol 2021;19(1):55–71. https://doi.org/10.1038/s41579-020-0433-9.

[12] De Luca F, Shoenfeld Y. The microbiome in autoimmune diseases. Clin Exp Immunol 2019;195(1):74–85. https://doi.org/10.1111/cei.13158.

[13] Saji N, Murotani K, Hisada T, et al. The relationship between the gut microbiome and mild cognitive impairment in patients without dementia: a cross-sectional study conducted in Japan. Sci Rep 2019;9(1):19227. https://doi.org/10.1038/s41598-019-55851-y.

[14] DeJong EN, Surette MG, Bowdish DME. The gut microbiota and unhealthy aging: disentangling cause from consequence. Cell Host Microbe 2020;28(2):180–9. https://doi.org/10.1016/j.chom.2020.07.013.

[15] O'Toole PW, Jeffery IB. Gut microbiota and aging. Science 2015;350(6265):1214–5. https://doi.org/10.1126/science.aac8469.

[16] Odamaki T, Kato K, Sugahara H, et al. Age-related changes in gut microbiota composition from newborn to centenarian: a cross-sectional study. BMC Microbiol 2016;16:90. https://doi.org/10.1186/s12866-016-0708-5.

[17] Buford TW. (dis) trust your gut: the gut microbiome in age-related inflammation, health, and disease. Microbiome 2017;5(1):80. https://doi.org/10.1186/s40168-017-0296-0.
[18] Jackson MA, Jeffery IB, Beaumont M, et al. Signatures of early frailty in the gut microbiota. Genome Med 2016;8(1):8. https://doi.org/10.1186/s13073-016-0262-7.
[19] Belkaid Y, Hand TW. Role of the microbiota in immunity and inflammation. Cell 2014;157(1):121–41. https://doi.org/10.1016/j.cell.2014.03.011.
[20] Claesson MJ, Jeffery IB, Conde S, et al. Gut microbiota composition correlates with diet and health in the elderly. Nature 2012;488(7410):178–84. https://doi.org/10.1038/nature11319.
[21] Lessa FC, Mu Y, Bamberg WM, et al. Burden of *Clostridium difficile* infection in the United States. N Engl J Med 2015;372(9):825–34. https://doi.org/10.1056/NEJMoa1408913.
[22] Makki K, Deehan EC, Walter J, Backhed F. The impact of dietary fiber on gut microbiota in host health and disease. Cell Host Microbe 2018;23(6):705–15. https://doi.org/10.1016/j.chom.2018.05.012.
[23] Tilg H, Zmora N, Adolph TE, Elinav E. The intestinal microbiota fuelling metabolic inflammation. Nat Rev Immunol 2020;20(1):40–54. https://doi.org/10.1038/s41577-019-0198-4.
[24] Desai MS, Seekatz AM, Koropatkin NM, et al. A dietary fiber-deprived gut microbiota degrades the colonic mucus barrier and enhances pathogen susceptibility. Cell 2016;167(5):1339–1353.e21. https://doi.org/10.1016/j.cell.2016.10.043.
[25] Franceschi C, Garagnani P, Vitale G, Capri M, Salvioli S. Inflammaging and 'Garb-aging'. Trends Endocrinol Metab 2017;28(3):199–212. https://doi.org/10.1016/j.tem.2016.09.005.
[26] Gong T, Liu L, Jiang W, Zhou R. DAMP-sensing receptors in sterile inflammation and inflammatory diseases. Nat Rev Immunol 2020;20(2):95–112. https://doi.org/10.1038/s41577-019-0215-7.
[27] Oishi Y, Manabe I. Macrophages in age-related chronic inflammatory diseases. NPJ Aging Mech Dis 2016;2:16018. https://doi.org/10.1038/npjamd.2016.18.
[28] Gkogkolou P, Bohm M. Advanced glycation end products: key players in skin aging? Dermatoendocrinol 2012;4(3):259–70. https://doi.org/10.4161/derm.22028.
[29] Li W. Phagocyte dysfunction, tissue aging and degeneration. Ageing Res Rev 2013;12(4):1005–12. https://doi.org/10.1016/j.arr.2013.05.006.
[30] Di Micco R, Krizhanovsky V, Baker D, d'Adda di Fagagna F. Cellular senescence in ageing: from mechanisms to therapeutic opportunities. Nat Rev Mol Cell Biol 2020. https://doi.org/10.1038/s41580-020-00314-w.
[31] van Deursen JM. The role of senescent cells in ageing. Nature 2014;509(7501):439–46. https://doi.org/10.1038/nature13193.
[32] Hoenicke L, Zender L. Immune surveillance of senescent cells—biological significance in cancer- and non-cancer pathologies. Carcinogenesis 2012;33(6):1123–6. https://doi.org/10.1093/carcin/bgs124.
[33] Tchkonia T, Zhu Y, van Deursen J, Campisi J, Kirkland JL. Cellular senescence and the senescent secretory phenotype: therapeutic opportunities. J Clin Invest 2013;123(3):966–72. https://doi.org/10.1172/JCI64098.
[34] Leto D, Saltiel AR. Regulation of glucose transport by insulin: traffic control of GLUT4. Nat Rev Mol Cell Biol 2012;13(6):383–96. https://doi.org/10.1038/nrm3351.
[35] Sanders FW, Griffin JL. De novo lipogenesis in the liver in health and disease: more than just a shunting yard for glucose. Biol Rev Camb Philos Soc 2016;91(2):452–68. https://doi.org/10.1111/brv.12178.
[36] Duncan RE, Ahmadian M, Jaworski K, Sarkadi-Nagy E, Sul HS. Regulation of lipolysis in adipocytes. Annu Rev Nutr 2007;27:79–101. https://doi.org/10.1146/annurev.nutr.27.061406.093734.

[37] Wu H, Ballantyne CM. Metabolic inflammation and insulin resistance in obesity. Circ Res 2020;126(11):1549–64. https://doi.org/10.1161/CIRCRESAHA.119.315896.
[38] Muscogiuri G, Cantone E, Cassarano S, et al. Gut microbiota: a new path to treat obesity. Int J Obes Suppl 2019;9(1):10–9. https://doi.org/10.1038/s41367-019-0011-7.
[39] Saltiel AR, Olefsky JM. Inflammatory mechanisms linking obesity and metabolic disease. J Clin Invest 2017;127(1):1–4. https://doi.org/10.1172/JCI92035.
[40] McLaughlin T, Ackerman SE, Shen L, Engleman E. Role of innate and adaptive immunity in obesity-associated metabolic disease. J Clin Invest 2017;127(1):5–13. https://doi.org/10.1172/JCI88876.
[41] Wilcox G. Insulin and insulin resistance. Clin Biochem Rev 2005;26(2):19–39. https://www.ncbi.nlm.nih.gov/pubmed/16278749.
[42] Liu Z, Wu KKL, Jiang X, Xu A, Cheng KKY. The role of adipose tissue senescence in obesity- and ageing-related metabolic disorders. Clin Sci (Lond) 2020;134(2):315–30. https://doi.org/10.1042/CS20190966.
[43] Wernstedt Asterholm I, Tao C, Morley TS, et al. Adipocyte inflammation is essential for healthy adipose tissue expansion and remodeling. Cell Metab 2014;20(1):103–18. https://doi.org/10.1016/j.cmet.2014.05.005.
[44] Tchkonia T, Morbeck DE, Von Zglinicki T, et al. Fat tissue, aging, and cellular senescence. Aging Cell 2010;9(5):667–84. https://doi.org/10.1111/j.1474-9726.2010.00608.x.
[45] Tam BT, Morais JA, Santosa S. Obesity and ageing: two sides of the same coin. Obes Rev 2020;21(4). https://doi.org/10.1111/obr.12991, e12991.
[46] Karlsson EA, Beck MA. The burden of obesity on infectious disease. Exp Biol Med (Maywood) 2010;235(12):1412–24. https://doi.org/10.1258/ebm.2010.010227.
[47] Sheridan PA, Paich HA, Handy J, et al. Obesity is associated with impaired immune response to influenza vaccination in humans. Int J Obes (Lond) 2012;36(8):1072–7. https://doi.org/10.1038/ijo.2011.208.
[48] Green WD, Beck MA. Obesity impairs the adaptive immune response to influenza virus. Ann Am Thorac Soc 2017;14(Supplement_5):S406–9. https://doi.org/10.1513/AnnalsATS.201706-447AW.
[49] Kanneganti TD, Dixit VD. Immunological complications of obesity. Nat Immunol 2012;13(8):707–12. https://doi.org/10.1038/ni.2343.
[50] Yang H, Youm YH, Vandanmagsar B, et al. Obesity accelerates thymic aging. Blood 2009;114(18):3803–12. https://doi.org/10.1182/blood-2009-03-213595.
[51] Stout MB, Justice JN, Nicklas BJ, Kirkland JL. Physiological aging: links among adipose tissue dysfunction, diabetes, and frailty. Physiology (Bethesda) 2017;32(1):9–19. https://doi.org/10.1152/physiol.00012.2016.
[52] Spalding KL, Arner E, Westermark PO, et al. Dynamics of fat cell turnover in humans. Nature 2008;453(7196):783–7. https://doi.org/10.1038/nature06902.
[53] Guillermier C, Fazeli PK, Kim S, et al. Imaging mass spectrometry demonstrates age-related decline in human adipose plasticity. JCI Insight 2017;2(5). https://doi.org/10.1172/jci.insight.90349, e90349.
[54] Lakowa N, Trieu N, Flehmig G, et al. Telomere length differences between subcutaneous and visceral adipose tissue in humans. Biochem Biophys Res Commun 2015;457(3):426–32. https://doi.org/10.1016/j.bbrc.2014.12.122.
[55] Preis SR, Massaro JM, Robins SJ, et al. Abdominal subcutaneous and visceral adipose tissue and insulin resistance in the Framingham heart study. Obesity (Silver Spring) 2010;18(11):2191–8. https://doi.org/10.1038/oby.2010.59.
[56] Palmer AK, Kirkland JL. Aging and adipose tissue: potential interventions for diabetes and regenerative medicine. Exp Gerontol 2016;86:97–105. https://doi.org/10.1016/j.exger.2016.02.013.
[57] Kim SM, Lun M, Wang M, et al. Loss of white adipose hyperplastic potential is associated with enhanced susceptibility to insulin resistance. Cell Metab 2014;20(6):1049–58. https://doi.org/10.1016/j.cmet.2014.10.010.

[58] Bays H, Mandarino L, DeFronzo RA. Role of the adipocyte, free fatty acids, and ectopic fat in pathogenesis of type 2 diabetes mellitus: peroxisomal proliferator-activated receptor agonists provide a rational therapeutic approach. J Clin Endocrinol Metab 2004;89(2):463–78. https://doi.org/10.1210/jc.2003-030723.

[59] Galkina E, Ley K. Immune and inflammatory mechanisms of atherosclerosis (*). Annu Rev Immunol 2009;27:165–97. https://doi.org/10.1146/annurev.immunol.021908.132620.

[60] Wang JC, Bennett M. Aging and atherosclerosis: mechanisms, functional consequences, and potential therapeutics for cellular senescence. Circ Res 2012;111(2):245–59. https://doi.org/10.1161/CIRCRESAHA.111.261388.

[61] Rocha VZ, Libby P. Obesity, inflammation, and atherosclerosis. Nat Rev Cardiol 2009;6(6):399–409. https://doi.org/10.1038/nrcardio.2009.55.

[62] Wentzel JJ, Chatzizisis YS, Gijsen FJ, Giannoglou GD, Feldman CL, Stone PH. Endothelial shear stress in the evolution of coronary atherosclerotic plaque and vascular remodelling: current understanding and remaining questions. Cardiovasc Res 2012;96(2):234–43. https://doi.org/10.1093/cvr/cvs217.

[63] Gimbrone Jr MA, Garcia-Cardena G. Endothelial cell dysfunction and the pathobiology of atherosclerosis. Circ Res 2016;118(4):620–36. https://doi.org/10.1161/CIRCRESAHA.115.306301.

[64] Girard PR, Nerem RM. Shear stress modulates endothelial cell morphology and F-actin organization through the regulation of focal adhesion-associated proteins. J Cell Physiol 1995;163(1):179–93. https://doi.org/10.1002/jcp.1041630121.

[65] Uematsu M, Ohara Y, Navas JP, et al. Regulation of endothelial cell nitric oxide synthase mRNA expression by shear stress. Am J Physiol 1995;269(6 Pt 1):C1371–8. https://doi.org/10.1152/ajpcell.1995.269.6.C1371.

[66] Walpola PL, Gotlieb AI, Cybulsky MI, Langille BL. Expression of ICAM-1 and VCAM-1 and monocyte adherence in arteries exposed to altered shear stress. Arterioscler Thromb Vasc Biol 1995;15(1):2–10. https://doi.org/10.1161/01.atv.15.1.2.

[67] Chatzizisis YS, Coskun AU, Jonas M, Edelman ER, Feldman CL, Stone PH. Role of endothelial shear stress in the natural history of coronary atherosclerosis and vascular remodeling: molecular, cellular, and vascular behavior. J Am Coll Cardiol 2007;49(25):2379–93. https://doi.org/10.1016/j.jacc.2007.02.059.

[68] Back M, Yurdagul Jr A, Tabas I, Oorni K, Kovanen PT. Inflammation and its resolution in atherosclerosis: mediators and therapeutic opportunities. Nat Rev Cardiol 2019;16(7):389–406. https://doi.org/10.1038/s41569-019-0169-2.

[69] Paone S, Baxter AA, Hulett MD, Poon IKH. Endothelial cell apoptosis and the role of endothelial cell-derived extracellular vesicles in the progression of atherosclerosis. Cell Mol Life Sci 2019;76(6):1093–106. https://doi.org/10.1007/s00018-018-2983-9.

[70] King RJ, Ajjan RA. Vascular risk in obesity: facts, misconceptions and the unknown. Diab Vasc Dis Res 2017;14(1):2–13. https://doi.org/10.1177/1479164116675488.

[71] Jia G, Aroor AR, Jia C, Sowers JR. Endothelial cell senescence in aging-related vascular dysfunction. Biochim Biophys Acta Mol Basis Dis 2019;1865(7):1802–9. https://doi.org/10.1016/j.bbadis.2018.08.008.

[72] Tyrrell DJ, Goldstein DR. Ageing and atherosclerosis: vascular intrinsic and extrinsic factors and potential role of IL-6. Nat Rev Cardiol 2021;18(1):58–68. https://doi.org/10.1038/s41569-020-0431-7.

[73] Selkoe DJ. Cell biology of protein misfolding: the examples of Alzheimer's and Parkinson's diseases. Nat Cell Biol 2004;6(11):1054–61. https://doi.org/10.1038/ncb1104-1054.

[74] Guzman-Martinez L, Maccioni RB, Andrade V, Navarrete LP, Pastor MG, Ramos-Escobar N. Neuroinflammation as a common feature of neurodegenerative disorders. Front Pharmacol 2019;10:1008. https://doi.org/10.3389/fphar.2019.01008.

[75] Amor S, Peferoen LA, Vogel DY, et al. Inflammation in neurodegenerative diseases—an update. Immunology 2014;142(2):151–66. https://doi.org/10.1111/imm.12233.

[76] Heneka MT, Carson MJ, El Khoury J, et al. Neuroinflammation in Alzheimer's disease. Lancet Neurol 2015;14(4):388–405. https://doi.org/10.1016/S1474-4422(15)70016-5.

[77] Angelova DM, Brown DR. Microglia and the aging brain: are senescent microglia the key to neurodegeneration? J Neurochem 2019;151(6):676–88. https://doi.org/10.1111/jnc.14860.

[78] Alford S, Patel D, Perakakis N, Mantzoros CS. Obesity as a risk factor for Alzheimer's disease: weighing the evidence. Obes Rev 2018;19(2):269–80. https://doi.org/10.1111/obr.12629.

[79] Miller AA, Spencer SJ. Obesity and neuroinflammation: a pathway to cognitive impairment. Brain Behav Immun 2014;42:10–21. https://doi.org/10.1016/j.bbi.2014.04.001.

[80] Minciullo PL, Catalano A, Mandraffino G, et al. Inflammaging and anti-inflammaging: the role of cytokines in extreme longevity. Arch Immunol Ther Exp (Warsz) 2016;64(2):111–26. https://doi.org/10.1007/s00005-015-0377-3.

[81] Opal SM, DePalo VA. Anti-inflammatory cytokines. Chest 2000;117(4):1162–72. https://doi.org/10.1378/chest.117.4.1162.

[82] Lio D, Candore G, Crivello A, et al. Opposite effects of interleukin 10 common gene polymorphisms in cardiovascular diseases and in successful ageing: genetic background of male centenarians is protective against coronary heart disease. J Med Genet 2004;41(10):790–4. https://doi.org/10.1136/jmg.2004.019885.

[83] Xuan Y, Wang L, Zhi H, Li X, Wei P. Association between 3 IL-10 gene polymorphisms and cardiovascular disease risk: systematic review with meta-analysis and trial sequential analysis. Medicine (Baltimore) 2016;95(6):e 2846. https://doi.org/10.1097/MD.0000000000002846.

[84] Dagdeviren S, Jung DY, Friedline RH, et al. IL-10 prevents aging-associated inflammation and insulin resistance in skeletal muscle. FASEB J 2017;31(2):701–10. https://doi.org/10.1096/fj.201600832R.

[85] Almanan M, Raynor J, Ogunsulire I, et al. IL-10-producing Tfh cells accumulate with age and link inflammation with age-related immune suppression. Sci Adv 2020;6(31):eabb 0806. https://doi.org/10.1126/sciadv.abb0806.

[86] Pollack RM, Donath MY, LeRoith D, Leibowitz G. Anti-inflammatory agents in the treatment of diabetes and its vascular complications. Diabetes Care 2016;39(Suppl. 2):S244–52. https://doi.org/10.2337/dcS15-3015.

[87] Cameron AR, Morrison VL, Levin D, et al. Anti-inflammatory effects of metformin irrespective of diabetes status. Circ Res 2016;119(5):652–65. https://doi.org/10.1161/CIRCRESAHA.116.308445.

[88] Esterson YB, Zhang K, Koppaka S, et al. Insulin sensitizing and anti-inflammatory effects of thiazolidinediones are heightened in obese patients. J Invest Med 2013;61(8):1152–60. https://doi.org/10.2310/JIM.0000000000000017.

[89] Ceriello A. Thiazolidinediones as anti-inflammatory and anti-atherogenic agents. Diabetes Metab Res Rev 2008;24(1):14–26. https://doi.org/10.1002/dmrr.790.

[90] Geldmacher DS, Fritsch T, McClendon MJ, Landreth G. A randomized pilot clinical trial of the safety of pioglitazone in treatment of patients with Alzheimer disease. Arch Neurol 2011;68(1):45–50. https://doi.org/10.1001/archneurol.2010.229.

[91] Seneviratne A, Cave L, Hyde G, et al. Metformin directly suppresses atherosclerosis in normoglycaemic mice via haematopoietic adenosine monophosphate-activated protein kinase. Cardiovasc Res 2020. https://doi.org/10.1093/cvr/cvaa171.

[92] Koenig AM, Mechanic-Hamilton D, Xie SX, et al. Effects of the insulin sensitizer metformin in Alzheimer disease: pilot data from a randomized placebo-controlled crossover study. Alzheimer Dis Assoc Disord 2017;31(2):107–13. https://doi.org/10.1097/WAD.0000000000000202.

[93] Charo IF, Taub R. Anti-inflammatory therapeutics for the treatment of atherosclerosis. Nat Rev Drug Discov 2011;10(5):365–76. https://doi.org/10.1038/nrd3444.

[94] Gyengesi E, Munch G. In search of an anti-inflammatory drug for Alzheimer disease. Nat Rev Neurol 2020;16(3):131–2. https://doi.org/10.1038/s41582-019-0307-9.
[95] Imbimbo BP, Solfrizzi V, Panza F. Are NSAIDs useful to treat Alzheimer's disease or mild cognitive impairment? Front Aging Neurosci 2010;2. https://doi.org/10.3389/fnagi.2010.00019.
[96] Howard R, Zubko O, Bradley R, et al. Minocycline at 2 different dosages vs placebo for patients with mild Alzheimer disease: a randomized clinical trial. JAMA Neurol 2020;77(2):164–74. https://doi.org/10.1001/jamaneurol.2019.3762.
[97] Venigalla M, Sonego S, Gyengesi E, Sharman MJ, Munch G. Novel promising therapeutics against chronic neuroinflammation and neurodegeneration in Alzheimer's disease. Neurochem Int 2016;95:63–74. https://doi.org/10.1016/j.neuint.2015.10.011.

CHAPTER 8

Obesity, inflammation, and diseases of the gastrointestinal tract

Anastasia C. Tillman[a] and Marcoandrea Giorgi[b]
[a]Warren Alpert Medical School, Brown University, Providence, RI, United States
[b]Surgery, Brown University, Providence, RI, United States

Introduction and epidemiology

Obesity is a global issue. One of the more recent and extensive analyses estimates that approximately 500 million adults, more than 10% of the global adult population, fall into the obese category (BMI $\geq$ 30 kg/m^2) [1]. Obesity was once thought of as a problem unique to wealthier countries; however, in the last few decades, obesity has become an increasing burden in developing countries, perhaps attributed to a nutritional shift to a more Westernized diet [2].

While the global pandemic of obesity is a more recent phenomenon, at least in the scientific literature, the obesity epidemic in the United States has been a consistent, albeit controversial, topic of discussion in public health for the last half century. Despite an increase in awareness and understanding of obesity, the obesity epidemic in the United States continues to pose a threat to individuals and the healthcare system. It is estimated that 35% of American men and 40% of women are considered obese [3]. Moreover, projections show that by 2030 that approximately 50% of adults will have obesity, with one in four US adults predicted to have severe obesity (BMI $\geq$ 35 kg/m^2) [4].

These predictions are concerning from both a nutritional and public health standpoint.

At first glance, upward trends in obesity are often tackled by changing diet and exercise; however, the damage of obesity extends well beyond the immediate obvious impacts. Obesity is a chronic health condition that is associated with a number of comorbidities, such as type 2 diabetes mellitus, cardiovascular disease, and psychiatric disorders, and can result in a decreased life span [5]. This affects not only the individual and those around them but can also place a large financial and resource strain on healthcare systems. In 2008 alone, it was estimated that obesity-related medical care expenses, not including the indirect costs of obesity such as those relating to employment loss, in the United States were estimated at $147 billion [6]. For context, according to the National Cancer Institute, the approximated medical care cost of cancer survivors in the United States in 2010 was $137.4 billion. If the obesity epidemic persists and multiplies as the trends predict, the costs will only rise.

Limitations of BMI in obesity definition

It is important to note that the current definition of obesity is limited. Obesity is defined as body mass index (BMI), calculated as weight in kilograms divided by the square of height meters, (BMI) $\geq 30\,kg/m^2$. By definition, BMI measures weight not fat. It also fails to account for certain healthy variations in body type, such as higher muscle mass or different distributions. BMI was designed in the early 19th century based on white males by a mathematician and was later brought into popularity again by an American physiologist who advocated for its use on a population level rather than an individual level [7]. Given its origins, BMI alone has limited uses, especially for nonwhite and nonmale individuals. Furthermore, it must be acknowledged that there is an "obesity paradox" that exists in the literature illustrating that among groups of lower fitness, those who are obese or overweight with cardiovascular diseases have a better prognosis than their counterparts with a BMI < 25 kg/m^2 [8].

Despite these limitations and complexities of BMI, it is still widely used as a marker of obesity and physical health. It is noninvasive and relatively easy to obtain in most clinical settings. Most research uses BMI as a surrogate for obesity, and this chapter will do so as well; however, it must be noted that BMI does not always equate to obesity and/or worse health outcomes and must be contextualized within the entire clinical picture.

Obesity incidence in certain groups
Pediatric populations

Most of the obesity research focuses on adult populations. While weight gain can occur at any age, there has been an increasing incidence of obesity in the pediatric population. According to the NEJM, given the trends in the obesity epidemic, the majority of children today will be obese by the age of 35 [9]. Similar to the adult trends, not only are the rates of obesity increasing in the pediatric population but also the severity of the obesity class. The prevalence of severe obesity in the pediatric population (BMI ≥ 120% above the 95th percentile or ≥ 35 kg/m^2) has increased from 4% in 2000 to 6% in 2016 [10].

Since obesity predisposes individuals to certain comorbidities and reduced longevity, the increasing prevalence in the pediatric population is very concerning. Furthermore, children are especially vulnerable to learning maladaptive behaviors, in correspondence with their neurological and psychological development. It can be especially hard for obese children to lose weight and reverse behavioral patterns. The World Health Organization states that childhood obesity is associated with a higher chance of premature death and disability in adulthood. Obese, and even overweight, children are more likely to have obesity as adults [11]. They are also at an increased risk of developing type 2 diabetes and cardiovascular diseases at a younger age and with a greater severity when compared with those who were nonobese in childhood [12].

Socioeconomic, racial, and equitable healthcare

Obesity disproportionately affects lower those from a lower socioeconomic background. One longitudinal study demonstrated an overall improvement in the average American diet; however, it also showed that this did not hold true for all Americans. In fact, it highlighted an increase in nutritional and dietary disparities based on race, income level, and education [13]. Individuals experiencing food insecurity or living in food deserts often do not have the option of choosing healthy, less processed foods. This, in combination with various other societal factors, leads to increased BMI.

In 2017–18, according to the CDC, the prevalence of obesity in US adults was 42.4%; however, the prevalence among Black adults (49.6%) and Latinx (44.8%) adults was shown a disproportionate effect. Analogous to the pediatric population trends, the trends for minority groups and lower-income adults are increasing in class severity as well as simply prevalence. Severe obesity is predicted to become the most common BMI category in the United States for non-Latinx Black adults, women, and those of a lower socioeconomic class by 2030 [4]. These trends are driven by social determinants of health, such as housing situations, access to health services, and structural racism, which reinforce health inequities. One recent study found a significant association between structural racism and higher BMI among Black adults, especially among those identifying as Black women [14].

It is imperative that the medical and healthcare community engages in discussions around social determinants of health in order to mitigate these concerning trends that otherwise will continue to disproportionately burden minority groups and underrepresented individuals.

Etiology

The pathogenesis of obesity is multifactorial. It is best hypothesized as a complex interaction among multiple genes, environmental factors, and societal influences. The latter two of the etiological triad have been highlighted in the prior sections, yet the role of genetics in obesity proves a constantly evolving area of research.

Genetics

Until the last few years, multifactorial and polygenic obesity was distinguished from the much rarer monogenic obesity (~5% globally), which was often more severe and presented earlier [15]. Recent studies, however, have found that certain genes previously solely attributed to monogenic obesity, most of which are involved in the leptin–melanocortin signaling pathway, actually have variants with significant effects in the general population [16]. Thus, monogenic variants, such as *MC4R* (melanocortin 4 receptor) and *LEPR* (leptin receptor), contribute to the much more common obesity that is behind the epidemic.

Another controversy behind genetics as a cause of obesity is the rate of the obesity epidemic. Some researchers and clinicians argue that the rate of the modern obesity epidemic is too exponential for genes to be a primary driver of obesity; however, genetics and epigenetics must remain a part of the obesity etiology discussion [17]. While there is clearly no single gene that causes obesity (shown by a meta-analysis of 37 genome scans for 31,000 individuals), there has been continued genetics research that has the potential to identify, with other factors, those who may be at a higher risk of obesity and revolutionize targeted treatments [15]. For instance, genome-wide association studies have implicated the cyclin-dependent kinase inhibitor *(CDKN)2a* locus (known as *INK4a/ARF*) in type 2 diabetes and other metabolic diseases. Recently, the upregulation of INK4a/ARF has been observed in dysregulated adipose tissue (AT), which opens up potential new therapies for metabolic disorders, including obesity and its consequential comorbidities [18].

Moreover, the genes that have been linked to obesity are linked to specific biochemical signaling pathways, which have helped to further understanding of the underlying inflammation, often involving these pathways, seen in obesity.

The connection between obesity and inflammation

Obesity is a chronic condition associated with a constant, low-grade inflammatory state. At baseline, obese individuals with no comorbidities have higher plasma levels of inflammatory cytokines and other reactant proteins, including C-reactive protein (CRP) and erythrocyte sedimentation rate (ESR) [19]. This can impact interpretation of standard lab values from a routine PCP office visit to research trials. Since it has been demonstrated that BMI has a positive linear correlation with white blood count (WBC), neutrophil count, and platelet count, certain studies have even proposed a different set of lab reference values for patients with obesity [20,21].

Pathogenesis

The evolution of obesity-induced inflammation is contextualized as a dysfunction in AT and adipocytes. According to one article, there is an "ominous triad" that contributes to the pathogenesis of dysfunctional AT in obesity: inappropriate extracellular matrix (ECM) remodeling (resulting in fibrosis), impaired angiogenesis, and unresolved inflammation [22]. These three factors independently drive the continued hypertrophy of AT; however, they also feed-forward and have multiplicative effects on one another in driving inappropriate or "unhealthy" AT expansion. This is in contrast to "healthy" AT cells including adipocytes, immune cells such as macrophages, fibroblasts, and endothelial cells, which normally coordinate a response to transient nutritional stress and rapidly remodel the AT for a short period of time.

The inflammatory state in obesity is also somewhat unique in that it involves tonic activation of the innate and adaptive immune systems, which impacts metabolic homeostasis on multiple levels from adipose tissue to the pancreas, skeletal muscle, and the CNS (central nervous system) [23]. While many of the proposed inflammatory mechanisms in obesity likely extend to these other organs, the main target of research is AT.

The primary resident immune cell of AT is the macrophage, which in nonobese individuals serves vital roles in maintaining "healthy" AT through regulation of the triad and controlling differentiation of adipocyte precursors [24]. Macrophages are often characterized as "polarized" as either proinflammatory or antiinflammatory. In nonobese individuals, macrophages are generally preserved in an M2-polarized state and secrete more antiinflammatory cytokines, such as IL-10, which help maintain insulin sensitivity [23,25]. In contrast, one of the hallmarks of obesity-induced inflammation is the phenotypic switch of the AT macrophage to a more M1-polarized or "metabolically activated" type [26]. These "metabolically activated" macrophages secrete proinflammatory cytokines, such as TNF-a and IL-6, which can also, in turn, recruit an increasing number of macrophages [23]. AT macrophages in obesity also trigger the adaptive immune system to favor Th1 cell activation over T regulatory cells (Tregs), which further promotes a proinflammatory state [27–29]. Over time, the chronic activation and accumulation of AT macrophages and resulting signaling of other inflammatory pathways are associated with insulin resistance and other metabolic consequences of obesity.

Although there is a consensus in the literature that obesity is linked to a proinflammatory phenotype, the upstream triggers that initiate these innate and adaptive immune pathways are not as well understood. A few of the theories have been discussed earlier; however, beyond the interplay of ECM remodeling and angiogenesis with inflammation, there are other proposed mechanisms of obesity-induced inflammation. For instance, increased circulating levels of lipopolysaccharides (LPSs) are increased in type 2 diabetes, which could be explained by increased intestinal permeability in obesity and the resulting intestinal-derived LPS initiation of an inflammatory cascade [23,30,31]. In fact, obese pregnant females had twice the level of endotoxins, or LPS, and increased expression of proinflammatory cytokines, including IL-6 and TNF-a, in AT than those who were nonobese [32]. It is also possible, however, that LPS is just another amplifier, like the other proinflammatory cytokines aforementioned, of systemic inflammation.

The actual content of an individual's diet plays a role in triggering inflammatory signaling. Free fatty acids (FFAs), especially those that are saturated (SFAs), are associated with metabolic syndromes, but they also have been shown to trigger immune responses. SFAs act as ligands and indirectly bind to pattern recognition receptors, in particular toll-like receptors TLR2 and TLR4, which activate NF-κB and JNK1 [31]. This initiates the proinflammatory cascade through secretion of monocyte chemoattractant protein-1 (MCP1) from adipocytes and recruits AT macrophages [23]. Thus, in states of chronic caloric excess, such as obesity, diets high in SFAs further contribute to adipocyte dysfunction. There are other proposed triggers for chronic inflammation, including adipocyte necrosis and hypoxia related to AT hypertrophy, and undoubtedly more mechanisms will be uncovered in the next few years [23]. Regardless of the precise origin, which is likely a combination of multiple triggers, it is clear that chronic overnutrition results in AT dysfunction, tonic inflammation, and immune system dysregulation.

Acute disease processes

The overall disruption in metabolic homeostasis in obesity and the skewed balance of the immune mediators and cells to a proinflammatory state has consequences for acute disease processes in obese individuals. While obese individuals with no other comorbidities have higher plasma levels of inflammatory cytokines at baseline, they also have a more intense inflammatory response when challenged with an infectious inoculum [33]. This heightened response is mediated by the tonically activated inflammatory cascades discussed above; however, it is also influenced by the leptin receptor. Leptin receptors are found on almost all immune cells, and leptin binding increases secretion and production of proinflammatory cytokines [19]. Although leptin inhibits hunger and diminishes fat storage in adipocytes, its effects are apparent in "healthy" obese individuals, it becomes critical in the setting of acute disease processes, such as bacterial or viral infections [34]. In infectious states, inflammatory markers such as CRP are even further elevated, and recent studies have indicated that CRP can compete with leptin for binding to the leptin receptor, potentially resulting in leptin resistance [35]. Leptin resistance and increased leptin levels are linked to obesity, and therein lies a vicious cycle of inflammation and obesity.

Individuals with obesity have both an increased risk of infection and an increased likelihood of an adverse outcome with an established infection [19,36]. Obesity exacerbates the degree and intensity of "cytokine storms" in certain disease processes [19]. For instance, there is an enhanced virulence and worsened outcome of SARS-CoV-2 in patients with obesity in part due to the predisposition to cytokine storms, which are a classic feature of COVID-19 [37]. Although the outcomes and increased risk are impacted by the social determinants of health, the enhanced virulence in obese individuals has been attributed to underlying biochemical and inflammatory pathways. Aside from cytokine storms, another proposed pathophysiological mechanism is that AT acts as a reservoir for SARS-CoV-2 as AT has increased expression of ACE-II (angiotensin-converting enzyme II), an enzyme that has been implicated in the pathogenesis COVID-19 infection [37]. Since there is dysfunction and hypertrophy of AT in obese individuals, it follows that the storage of SARS-CoV-2 in this AT would increase its virulence.

Chronic diseases processes

Obesity is a chronic disease; and therefore, it makes sense that the chronic state of low-grade inflammation would have long-term consequences for chronic inflammatory disease processes. The baseline proinflammatory state in obese individuals has been linked to an increased risk in cancer, diabetes, and other chronic systemic diseases [19,38]. In parallel to CRP, IL-1RA, an antiinflammatory member of the IL-1 (interleukin-1) family, has been shown to be elevated in obesity and has potential effects on leptin levels [39]. One study and subsequent article proposed that leptin could promote the secretion of IL-1RA from monocytes further increasing baseline elevation of circulating IL-1RA levels in obesity to compensate for the chronic proinflammatory state [19,40]. Since IL-1RA also appears to be elevated in autoimmune and chronic inflammatory diseases, likely as a compensatory mechanism, it is conceivable that there is a synergistic effect in obese individuals leading to higher rates of these diseases [41]. Similarly, ghrelin, the opposer of leptin, has been linked to an antiinflammatory state via inhibition of proinflammatory cytokines, such as TNF-a [42]. Ghrelin levels are dysregulated in obesity and have an inverse relationship with weight gain and insulin resistance [43]. Thus, individuals with obesity lose this inhibition of inflammation, which may contribute to obese individuals' increased risk for autoimmune diseases and other inflammatory-related disease processes.

Obesity and gastrointestinal diseases

The relationship between obesity and gastrointestinal diseases is multifaceted. Obesity can directly cause certain GI (gastrointestinal) and hepatic diseases, such as NAFLD (nonalcoholic fatty liver disease); however, obesity can also greatly increase the risk of developing other GI diseases, such as GERD (gastroesophageal reflux disease) and gallstones [44]. While some of these GI consequences are related to body habitus and access to medical care, they are also influenced by the chronic low-grade inflammatory state of obesity and its effects of downstream signaling and even the microbiome of the GI tract [45,46]. There are many GI complications of obesity (Table 1), which can be divided based on the various organs and locations targeted. For the purposes of this discussion, the focus will not include GI cancers or the pancreas, including diabetes.

Table 1 GI complications in adults with obesity [44].

Gastrointestinal disease	Obesity as a risk factor Risk: OR or RR	95% CI
Esophagus		
GERD	OR, 1.94	1.46–2.57
Erosive esophagitis	OR, 1.87	1.51–2.31
Barrett's esophagus	OR, 4.0	1.4–11.1
Esophageal adenocarcinoma	Men: OR, 2.4	1.9–3.2
	Women: OR, 2.1	1.4–3.2
	RR, 4.8	3.0–7.7
Stomach		
Erosive gastritis	OR, 2.23	1.59–3.11
Gastric cancer	OR, 1.55	1.31–1.84
	RR (cardia), 1.8	1.3–2.5
Small intestine		
Diarrhea	OR, 2.7	1.10–6.8
Colon and rectum		
Diverticular disease	RR, 1.78	1.08–2.94
Polyps	OR, 1.44	1.23–1.70
Colorectal cancer	Men: RR, 1.95	1.59–2.39
	Women: RR, 1.15	1.06–1.24
	RR, 1.3	1.3–1.4
Clostridium difficile infection	OR, 1.196 per 1 kg/m^2 increase in BMI	1.12–1.27
Anorectum		
Dyssynergic defecation	OR, 1.64	1.09–2.47
Liver		
NAFLD	RR, 4.6	2.5–110
Cirrhosis	RR, 4.1	1.4–11.4
Hepatocellular carcinoma	RR, 1.89	1.51–2.36
	RR, 1.8	1.6–2.1
Gallbladder		
Gallstone disease	Men: RR, 2.51	2.16–2.91
	Women: RR, 2.32	1.17–4.57
Gallbladder cancer	RR, 1.3	1.2–1.4
Pancreas		
Acute pancreatitis	RR, 2.20	1.82–2.66
Pancreatic cancer	Men: RR, 1.10	1.04–1.22
	Women: RR, 1.13	1.05–1.18
	RR, 1.5	1.2–1.8

Upper GI tract

Esophageal dysmotility is common in individuals with obesity. Dysmotility is not always symptomatic, and in cases of morbid obesity, asymptomatic cases found on manometer seem to be even more common than symptomatic GERD [47]. Thus, it is difficult to approximate the incidence of esophageal dysmotility in both the general and obese populations. Multiple studies have shown a positive association between BMI and GERD; however, independent of BMI, central adiposity has also been linked to consequences of GERD, including Barrett's esophagus [48–50]. Thus, it is clear that increased abdominal girth plays a significant role in the development of GERD likely by elevating intra-abdominal pressure and lowering lower esophageal sphincter pressure [44]. The dysfunction and hypertrophy of adipose tissue seem to contribute to the pathogenesis of reflux-related disorders. In this excess WAT (white adipose tissue), there are higher levels of leptin, and decreased levels of adiponectin, which regulates energy metabolism and protects against chronic inflammation [44,51]. Furthermore, there is an increased proinflammatory cytokines, such as IL-6 and TNF-a, produced by signaling cascades triggered by LPS, TLR4, and NF-κB, at baseline in obesity as previously discussed, which has been implicated in dysmotility. LPS also upregulates nitric oxide synthase, which has been shown to further decrease the lower esophageal sphincter and increase risk and severity of reflux [52].

There is a complex relationship of leptin and ghrelin with GERD and Barrett's esophagus [44]. Ghrelin helps to stimulate GI motility and contraction [53]. It is not surprising, therefore, that higher levels of ghrelin are associated with increased risk of Barrett's esophagus; however, interestingly, this does not hold true for ghrelin and GERD [54]. Conversely, higher levels of leptin are associated with symptomatic GERD but inversely associated with risk of developing Barrett's esophagus [54]. Moreover, while ghrelin and leptin levels are skewed in obese individuals, the study found no data implicating the ghrelin/leptin mechanism in obesity and Barrett's esophagus [54,55]. Thus, it is likely that the tonically activated inflammatory cascades in the dysfunctional WAT are the primary driver of the biochemical pathogenesis behind the prevalence of esophageal dysmotility in obesity. While there does not seem to be a clear link between ghrelin/leptin and the progression of GERD to Barrett's in obesity, there is a direct implication of this mechanism in the progression of Barrett's to adenocarcinoma in obesity [56]. Obese individuals, in similar pattern to acute infectious agents, are at an increased risk of the complications of GERD and its spectrum in comparison with the general population.

Hepatobiliary

Obesity is a risk factor for benign and malignant diseases of the gallbladder. Obese individuals have a higher incidence of cholelithiasis, cholecystitis, and cholecystosteatosis (fatty gallbladder) in comparison to nonobese individuals [57,58]. Increased fat accumulation in the gall bladder, as a result of high carbohydrate diet and obesity, causes organ damage and chronic inflammation [57,59]. At baseline, individuals with obesity have chronic inflammation. The inflammatory effects of cholecystosteatosis further exacerbate this leading to decreased contractility, increased wall gallbladder wall thickness, and reduced biliary emptying [57,60].

The theme of fatty infiltration from obesity exacerbating obesity-induced inflammation also applies to the liver. NAFLD is the accumulation of fat in the liver without any external causes, such as alcohol. NAFL (nonalcoholic fatty liver) exists on a spectrum with NASH (nonalcoholic steatohepatitis), with the latter having an increased degree of hepatic inflammation; both are on the rise globally and in the United States [61]. NAFLD can have fatal consequences: NAFLD is the third leading cause of HCC (hepatocellular carcinoma) in the United States, and 20% of individuals with NASH develop cirrhosis [62,63]. Obese individuals have a fourfold increased risk of developing NAFLD compared with nonobese individuals [64]. One study examined morbidly obese individuals (mean BMI 48 kg/m^2) who underwent bariatric surgery and found NAFLD on 73% of liver biopsies [65]. Moreover, obesity has an adverse effect on grade and severity of NAFLD in every aspect of the disease [66]. For instance, there is a significant association between obesity and hospitalization or death due to cirrhosis consequences [67]. There are various proposed mechanisms for this, including the altered GI microbiome in obese individuals. The disruption in intestinal microbiota caused by the chronic inflammatory state in obesity potentiates the catalysis of choline into hepato-toxic methylamines [68,69]. This is compounded by the further upregulation of proinflammatory cytokines from LPS and TLR4, both from the baseline obese and fatty liver states, which serve to increase permeability and inflammation with deleterious effects to the liver [68]. More exploration and better understanding of the biochemical and immunological pathways behind obesity and NAFLD are critical as the prevalence of both continues to rise.

Small intestine and colon

Despite a general consensus that obesity affects the physiology of the small intestine, with the incidence of diarrhea significantly increased in the obese population, there is some controversy in the literature in the association of irritable bowel disease (IBD) with obesity [44,70]. The innate immunity implications of obesity-induced inflammation in relation to autoimmune diseases, such as IBD, have already been briefly discussed in the section on chronic diseases processes; however, there are also contributions from the GI microbiome. Altered intestinal microbiota in obesity, similar to NAFLD, also disrupts intestinal epithelium [45]. For instance, the interaction between intestinal microbiota and TLR5 activates inflammatory cascades and increased transcription of proinflammatory cytokines and mediators, such as NFκB [71,72]. Intestinal barrier dysfunction, in turn, worsens the baseline proinflammatory pathways in obese individuals, which eventually disrupts tight junction proteins and further increases intestinal permeability [45].

The effects of chronic, low-grade inflammation in obesity are also seen in the large intestine and diverticular disease. Diverticulosis, outpouchings in the wall of the large intestine, is seen in ~65% of individuals ≥65 years old; however, it is uncommon in the younger population, with ~5% incidence in those less than 40 years old [73]. These figures correspond to the general population, yet in the obese population, the incidence of diverticulosis is significantly higher [74]. Moreover, obese individuals were significantly more likely to experience increased diverticular bleeding and recurrent diverticulitis, which is the inflammation or infection of these outpouchings, in comparison to their nonobese counterparts [75]. The proinflammatory phenotype of obesity likely potentiates the inflammatory processes of diverticular diseases [76]. Interestingly, obesity was not found to be associated with asymptomatic diverticulosis [75]. It is likely that the inflammatory pathways and even the synergistic effects of the altered microbiome lead to worsened outcomes in obese populations with diverticular diseases.

Interventions

The prevalence of GI diseases has increased both globally and in the United States, which some researchers and physicians attribute to the obesity epidemic [44]. Previously, there was a greater focus on diabetes, cardiovascular diseases, and cancer in the obese population. Given the increased incidence and adverse outcomes of GI diseases in individuals with obesity, however, there is increased exploration into medical and nonmedical intervention in this population.

Management

The fundamentals of obesity-related comorbidity reduction are weight loss, physical activity, and diet. Similarly, the management of many of these GI diseases includes elements of this triad. For instance, guidelines developed by the American College of Gastroenterology recommend physical activity and weight loss, with at least 3%–5% total loss improving steatosis of the liver [77]. Weight loss can not only improve disease processes but in some cases, can lead to their resolution. One study found that after a 6-month structured weight loss program for individuals with a mean BMI of 35 kg/m^2, 65% had complete resolution of their GERD [78]. An even greater reduction in symptoms and favorable outcome in GERD treatment are seen in bariatric surgery, especially after Roux-en-Y gastric bypass surgery [79,80]. Bariatric surgery, unlike many lifestyle changes, alters the anatomical and biochemical pathways in the body. As such, it is possible that bariatric surgery can have a stronger and more immediate effect of the inflammation cascades and dysfunctional immune response seen in obesity.

Prevention

While there are some effective management strategies in place for GI diseases and obesity, it is incredibly more beneficial to both the individual and the healthcare system to prevent the need for these interventions. Bariatric surgery is invasive and expensive; and therefore, not all patients may qualify for or elect to have these procedures. Furthermore, although some of these GI consequences are reversible or treatable, there are others that have progressed too far. For example, NAFLD can be halted or partially reversed; its downstream effects of HCC or end-stage cirrhosis cannot.

Healthcare providers must look far upstream and address social determinants of health as the best intervention for obesity and GI diseases. There needs to be increased access to medical care, reduced judgment around higher BMI in the healthcare profession, food and housing security, and an understanding of the effects of systemic racism on obesity [81]. Moreover, among communities with higher rates of obesity, there needs to more education and intervention on GI comorbidities. There needs to be emphasis on the importance of colonoscopies, treatment of GERD, and the burden of infections in individuals with obesity. Healthcare providers must also be aware of the underlying proinflammatory phenotype of obesity and its potential impacts on risk and outcome of disease processes.

References

[1] Abd El-Sayed, E.S., El-Sakhawy, M., El-Sakhawy, M.A.M., 2020. Non-wood fibres as raw material for pulp and paper industry. Nord. Pulp Pap. Res. J. 35 (2), 215–230.

[2] Abhilash, P.C., Tripathi, V., Edrisi, S.A., Dubey, R.K., Bakshi, M., Dubey, P.K., Singh, H.B., Ebbs, S.D., 2016. Sustainability of crop production from polluted lands. Energy Ecol. Environ. 1 (1), 54–65.

[3] Abtahi, H., Parhamfar, M., Saeedi, R., Villasenor, J., Sartaj, M., Kumar, V., Coulon, F., Parhamfar, M., Didehdar, M., Koolivand, A., 2020. Effect of competition between petroleum-degrading bacteria and indigenous compost microorganisms on the efficiency of petroleum sludge bioremediation: Field application of mineral-based culture in the composting process. J. Environ. Manag. 258, 110013.

[4] Agbor, V., Zurzolo, F., Blunt, W., Dartiailh, C., Cicek, N., Sparling, R., Levin, D.B., 2014. Single-step fermentation of agricultural hemp residues for hydrogen and ethanol production. Biomass Bioenergy 64, 62–69.

[5] Ahkami, A.H., White III, R.A., Handakumbura, P.P., Jansson, C., 2017. Rhizosphere engineering: enhancing sustainable plant ecosystem productivity. Rhizosphere 3, 233–243.

[6] Ahmad, M., Ullah, K., Khan, M.A., Zafar, M., Tariq, M., Ali, S., Sultana, S., 2011. Physicochemical analysis of hemp oil biodiesel: a promising non edible new source for bioenergy. Energy Sources, Part A 33 (14), 1365–1374.

[7] Akil, H., Omar, M.F., Mazuki, A.M., Safiee, S.Z.A.M., Ishak, Z.M., Bakar, A.A., 2011. Kenaf fibre reinforced composites: a review. Mater. Des. 32 (8–9), 4107–4121.

[8] Akubueze, E.U., Ezeanyanaso, C.S., Muniru, S.O., Igwe, C.C., Nwauzor, G.O., Ugoh, U., Nwaze, I.O., Mafe, O., Nwaeche, F.C., 2019. Reinforcement of plaster of Paris (POP) for suspended ceilings applications using kenaf bast fibre. Curr. J. Appl. Sci. Technol., 1–6.

[9] Albrecht, W., Fuchs, H., Kittelmann, W. (Eds.), 2006. Nonwoven Fabrics: Raw Materials, Manufacture, Applications, Characteristics, Testing Processes. John Wiley & Sons.

[10] Ali, I., Jayaraman, K., Bhattacharyya, D., 2014. Effects of resin and moisture content on the properties of medium density fibreboards made from kenaf bast fibres. Ind. Crop. Prod. 52, 191–198.

[11] Allesina, G., Pedrazzi, S., Allegretti, F., Morselli, N., Puglia, M., Santunione, G., Tartarini, P., 2018. Gasification of cotton crop residues for combined power and biochar production in Mozambique. Appl. Therm. Eng. 139, 387–394.

[12] Alotaibi, F., Bamagoos, A.A., Ismaeil, F.M., Zhang, W., Abou-Elwafa, S.F., 2021. Application of beet sugar byproducts improves sugar beet biofortification in saline soils and reduces sugar losses in beet sugar processing. Environ. Sci. Pollut. Res., 1–9.

[13] Álvarez-Mozos, J., Abad, E., Giménez, R., Campo, M.A., Goñi, M., Arive, M., Casalí, J., Díez, J., Diego, I., 2014. Evaluation of erosion control geotextiles on steep slopes. Part 1: effects on runoff and soil loss. Catena 118, 168–178.

[14] An, Y., Wang, Z., Wu, Z., Yang, D., Zhou, Q., 2009. Characterization of membrane foulants in an anaerobic non-woven fabric membrane bioreactor for municipal wastewater treatment. Chem. Eng. J. 155 (3), 709–715.

[15] Anandjiwala, R.D., Blouw, S., 2007. Composites from bast fibres-prospects and potential in the changing market environment. J. Nat. Fibers 4 (2), 91–109.

[16] Angelova, V., Ivanova, R., Delibaltova, V., Ivanov, K., 2004. Bio-accumulation and distribution of heavy metals in fibre crops (flax, cotton and hemp). Ind. Crop. Prod. 19 (3), 197–205.

[17] Ardente, F., Beccali, M., Cellura, M., Mistretta, M., 2008. Building energy performance: a LCA case study of kenaf-fibres insulation board. Energy Build. 40, 1–10.

[18] Asokan, M.A., Prabu, S.S., Prathiba, S., Akhil, V.S., Abishai, L.D., Surejlal, M.E., 2021. Emission and performance behaviour of flax seed oil biodiesel/diesel blends in DI diesel engine. Mater. Today: Proc. 17, 8148–8152.

[19] Bajpai, P., 2012. Biotechnology for Pulp and Paper Processing. Springer, New York, pp. 7–13.

[20] Bajpai, P., 2021. Nonwood Plant Fibres for Pulp and Paper. Elsevier.
[21] Balda, S., Sharma, A., Capalash, N., Sharma, P., 2021. Banana fibre: a natural and sustainable bioresource for eco-friendly applications. Clean Techn. Environ. Policy, 1–13.
[22] Barbi, S., Taurino, C., La China, S., Anguluri, K., Gullo, M., Montorsi, M., 2021. Mechanical and structural properties of environmental green composites based on functionalized bacterial cellulose. Cellulose 28 (3), 1431–1442.
[23] Barbosa, S., Castillo, L., 2020. Biodegradable pots for seedlings. In: Al-Ahmed (Ed.), Advanced Applications of Bio-degradable Green Composites. vol. 68. Materials Research Forum LLC, p. 104.
[24] Barbosa, B., Fernando, A.L., Mendes, B., 2012. Wastewater reuse in the irrigation of kenaf (Hibiscus cannabinus L) as a strategy for combating desertification. In: Proceedings of the World Forum on Soil Bioengineering and Land Management New Challenges.
[25] Barbosa, B., Costa, J., Fernando, A.L., Papazoglou, E.G., 2015. Wastewater reuse for fibre crops cultivation as a strategy to mitigate desertification. Ind. Crop. Prod. 68, 17–23.
[26] Beddu, S., Basri, A., Muda, Z.C., Farahlina, F., Mohamad, D., Itam, Z., Kamal, N.L.M., Sabariah, T., 2021, May. Comparison of thermomechanical properties of cement mortar with kenaf and polypropylene fibres. In: IOP Conference Series: Materials Science and Engineering. vol. 1144. IOP Publishing, p. 012036. No. 1.
[27] Berezovsky, Y., Kuzmina, T., Lialina, N., Yedynovych, M., Lobov, O., 2020. Technical and technological solutions for producing fibre from bast crops. INMATEH-Agric. Eng. 60 (1).
[28] Bhattacharyya, R., Smets, T., Fullen, M.A., Poesen, J., Booth, C.A., 2010. Effectiveness of geotextiles in reducing runoff and soil loss: a synthesis. Catena 81 (3), 184–195.
[29] Bidin, N., Zakaria, M.H., Bujang, J.S., Abdul Aziz, N.A., 2015. Suitability of aquatic plant fibres for handmade papermaking. Int. J. Polym. Sci. 2015.
[30] Biewinga, E.E., Van der Bijl, G., 1996. Sustainability of Energy in Europe. A Methodology Developed and Applied. Centre for Agriculture and Environment CLM, Utrecht, Netherlands.
[31] Bizkarra, K., Barrio, V.L., Gartzia-Rivero, L., Bañuelos, J., López-Arbeloa, I., Cambra, J.F., 2019. Hydrogen production from a model bio-oil/bio-glycerol mixture through steam reforming using Zeolite L supported catalysts. Int. J. Hydrog. Energy 44 (3), 1492–1504.
[32] Bjelková, M., Genčurová, V., Griga, M., 2011. Accumulation of cadmium by flax and linseed cultivars in field-simulated conditions: a potential for phytoremediation of Cd-contaminated soils. Ind. Crop. Prod. 33 (3), 761–774.
[33] Bolton, J., 1995. The potential of plant fibres as crops for industrial use. Outlook Agric. 24 (2), 85–89.
[34] Booth, J.E., 1968. Principal of Textile Testing. vol. 203 Newness Butter Worth, London, p. 315.
[35] Brite, E.B., Marston, J.M., 2013. Environmental change, agricultural innovation, and the spread of cotton agriculture in the Old World. J. Anthropol. Archaeol. 32 (1), 39–53.
[36] Brosius, D., 2006. Natural fibre composites slowly take root. Compos. Technol. 12 (1), 32–37.
[37] Cheng, C.L., Lo, Y.C., Lee, K.S., Lee, D.J., Lin, C.Y., Chang, J.S., 2011. Biohydrogen production from lignocellulosic feedstock. Bioresour. Technol. 102 (18), 8514–8523.
[38] Cherney, J.H., Small, E., 2016. Industrial hemp in North America: production, politics and potential. Agronomy 6 (4), 58.
[39] Chernova, T.E., Gorshkova, T.A., 2007. Biogenesis of plant fibres. Russ. J. Dev. Biol. 38 (4), 221–232.
[40] Chernova, T.E., Mikshina, P.V., Salnikov, V.V., Ibragimova, N.N., Sautkina, O.V., Gorshkova, T.A., 2018. Development of distinct cell wall layers both in primary and secondary phloem fibres of hemp (Cannabis sativa L.). Ind. Crop. Prod. 117, 97–109.

[41] Cherubini, F., Bird, N.D., Cowie, A., Jungmeier, G., Schlamadinger, B., Woess-Gallasch, S., 2009. Energy- and greenhouse gas-based LCA of biofuel and bioenergy systems: key issues, ranges and recommendations. Resour. Conserv. Recycl. 53, 434–447.
[42] Cheung, H.Y., Ho, M.P., Lau, K.T., Cardona, F., Hui, D., 2009. Natural fibre-reinforced composites for bioengineering and environmental engineering applications. Compos. Part B 40 (7), 655–663.
[43] Choi, H.S., Zhao, Y., Dou, H., Cai, X., Gu, M., Yu, F., 2018. Effects of biochar mixtures with pine-bark based substrates on growth and development of horticultural crops. Hortic. Environ. Biotechnol. 59 (3), 345–354.
[44] Crini, G., Lichtfouse, E., Chanet, G., Morin-Crini, N., 2020. Applications of hemp in textiles, paper industry, insulation and building materials, horticulture, animal nutrition, food and beverages, nutraceuticals, cosmetics and hygiene, medicine, agrochemistry, energy production and environment: a review. Environ. Chem. Lett. 18, 1451–1476.
[45] Danalatos, N.G., Archontoulis, S.V., 2010. Growth and biomass productivity of kenaf (Hibiscus cannabinus, L.) under different agricultural inputs and management practices in central Greece. Ind. Crop. Prod. 32 (3), 231–240.
[46] Danielewicz, D., Surma-Ślusarska, S., 2017. Properties and fibre characterisation of bleached hemp, birch and pine pulps: a comparison. Cellulose 24 (11), 5173–5186.
[47] Danish, M., Ahmad, T., Ayoub, M., Geremew, B., Adeloju, S., 2020. Conversion of flax-seed oil into biodiesel using KOH catalyst: optimization and characterization dataset. Data Brief 29, 105225.
[48] Deng, Y., Guo, Y., Wu, P., Ingarao, G., 2019. Optimal design of flax fibre reinforced polymer composite as a lightweight component for automobiles from a life cycle assessment perspective. J. Ind. Ecol. 23 (4), 986–997.
[49] Dimitrijević, V.D., Krstić, N.S., Stanković, M.N., Arsić, I., Nikolić, R.S., 2016. Biometal and heavy metal content in the soil-nettle (Urtica dioica L.): system from different localities in Serbia. Adv. Technol. 5 (1), 17–22.
[50] Du, Z., Zhang, S., Zhou, Q., Yuen, K.F., Wong, Y.D., 2018. Hazardous materials analysis and disposal procedures during ship recycling. Resour. Conserv. Recycl. 131, 158–171.
[51] Elsaid, A., Dawood, M., Seracino, R., Bobko, C., 2011. Mechanical properties of kenaf fibre reinforced concrete. Constr. Build. Mater. 25 (4), 1991–2001.
[52] Emerging Textiles, 2020. Price Reports—Emerging Textiles—Textile Market Information. https://emergingtextiles.com/. (Accessed 23 June 2021).
[53] FAO, 2019. Statistics Division, Food and Agriculture Organization of the United Nations, Viale delle Terme di Caracalla, 00153 Rome, Italy. http://www.fao.org/faostat/en/#home.
[54] Ferdous, S., Hossain, M.S., 2017. Natural fibre composite (NFC): new gateway for jute, kenaf and ALLIED fibres in automobiles and infrastructure sector. World J. Res. Rev. 5 (3), 35–42.
[55] Fernando, A.L., 2013. Environmental aspects of kenaf production and use. In: Kenaf: A Multi-Purpose Crop for Several Industrial Applications. Springer, London, pp. 83–104.
[56] Fernando, A.L., Duarte, M.P., Almeida, J., Boléo, S., Mendes, B., 2010. Environmental impact assessment of energy crops cultivation in Europe. Biofuels Bioprod. Biorefin. 4 (6), 594–604.
[57] Fernando, A.L., Duarte, M.P., Vatsanidou, A., Alexopoulou, E., 2015. Environmental aspects of fibre crops cultivation and use. Ind. Crop. Prod. 68, 105–115.
[58] Fike, J., 2016. Industrial hemp: renewed opportunities for an ancient crop. Crit. Rev. Plant Sci. 35 (5–6), 406–424.
[59] Fuller, D.Q., 2008. The spread of textile production and textile crops in India beyond the Harappan zone: an aspect of the emergence of craft specialization and systematic trade. In: Osada, T., Useugi, A. (Eds.), Linguistics, Archaeology and the Human Past. homepages.ucl.ac.uk, pp. 1–26.

[60] Gajjar, C.R., King, M.W., 2014. Biotextiles: fibre to fabric for medical applications. In: Resorbable Fibre-Forming Polymers for Biotextile Applications. Springer, Cham, pp. 11–22.
[61] Garnett, T., Appleby, M.C., Balmford, A., Bateman, I.J., Benton, T.G., Bloomer, P., Burlingame, B., Dawkins, M., Dolan, L., Fraser, D., Herrero, M., 2013. Sustainable intensification in agriculture: premises and policies. Science 341 (6141), 33–34.
[62] Gassan, J., Chate, A., Bledzki, A.K., 2001. Calculation of elastic properties of natural fibers. J. Mater. Sci. 36 (15), 3715–3720.
[63] George, M., Bressler, D.C., 2017. Comparative evaluation of the environmental impact of chemical methods used to enhance natural fibres for composite applications and glass fibre based composites. J. Clean. Prod. 149, 491–501.
[64] Ghosh, M., Choudhury, P.K., Sanyal, T., 2009. Suitability of natural fibres in geotextile applications. IGC Geotide, 497–501.
[65] Gogna, E., Kumar, R., Sahoo, A.K., Panda, A., 2019. A comprehensive review on jute fibre reinforced composites. Adv. Ind. Prod. Eng., 459–467.
[66] Gomez-Campos, A., Vialle, C., Rouilly, A., Sablayrolles, C., Hamelin, L., 2021. Flax fibre for technical textile: a life cycle inventory. J. Clean. Prod. 281, 125177.
[67] González-García, S., Hospido, A., Moreira, M.T., Feijoo, G., 2007. Life cycle environmental analysis of hemp production for non-wood pulp. In: 3rd International Conference on Life Cycle Management, 1. vol. 6.
[68] González-García, S., Hospido, A., Feijoo, G., Moreira, M.T., 2010. Life cycle assessment of raw materials for non-wood pulp mills: Hemp and flax. Resour. Conserv. Recycl. 54 (11), 923–930.
[69] González-García, S., Luo, L., Moreira, M.T., Feijoo, G., Huppes, G., 2012. Life cycle assessment of hemp hurds use in second generation ethanol production. Biomass Bioenergy 36, 268–279.
[70] Gordon, S., Hsieh, Y.L. (Eds.), 2006. Cotton: Science and Technology. Woodhead Publishing.
[71] Gorshkova, T., Chernova, T., Mokshina, N., Ageeva, M., Mikshina, P., 2018. Plant 'muscles': fibres with a tertiary cell wall. New Phytol. 218 (1), 66–72.
[72] Goudenhooft, C., Bourmaud, A., Baley, C., 2019. Flax (Linum usitatissimum L.) fibres for composite reinforcement: exploring the link between plant growth, cell walls development, and fibre properties. Front. Plant Sci. 10, 411.
[73] Gowda, B., 2007. Fibres, rubber, firewood, timber and bamboo. In: Economic Botany. University of Agricultural Sciences, Bangalore, India.
[74] Griga, M., Bjelková, M., 2013. Flax (Linum usitatissimum L.) and Hemp (Cannabis sativa L.) as fibre crops for phytoextraction of heavy metals: biological, agrotechnological and economical point of view. In: Plant-Based Remediation Processes. Springer, Berlin, Heidelberg, pp. 199–237.
[75] Gurunathan, T., Mohanty, S., Nayak, S.K., 2015. A review of the recent developments in biocomposites based on natural fibres and their application perspectives. Compos. A: Appl. Sci. Manuf. 77, 1–25.
[76] Hearle, J.W., Morton, W.E., 2008. Physical Properties of Textile Fibres. Elsevier.
[77] Hon, D.N.S., 2017. Cellulose and its derivatives: structures, reactions, and medical uses. In: Polysaccharides in Medicinal Applications. Routledge, pp. 87–105.
[78] Hosman, M.E., El-Feky, S.S., Elshahawy, M.I., Shaker, E.M., 2017. Mechanism of phytoremediation potential of flax (Linum usitatissimum L.) to Pb, Cd and Zn. Asian J. Plant Sci. Res. 7 (4), 30–40.
[79] Hou, D., O'Connor, D., Igalavithana, A.D., Alessi, D.S., Luo, J., Tsang, D.C., Sparks, D.L., Yamauchi, Y., Rinklebe, J., Ok, Y.S., 2020. Metal contamination and bioremediation of agricultural soils for food safety and sustainability. Nat. Rev. Earth Environ. 1 (7), 366–381.

[80] Houben, D., Pircar, J., Sonnet, P., 2012. Heavy metal immobilization by cost-effective amendments in a contaminated soil: effects on metal leaching and phytoavailability. J. Geochem. Explor. 123, 87–94.
[81] Houfani, A.A., Anders, N., Spiess, A.C., Baldrian, P., Benallaoua, S., 2020. Insights from enzymatic degradation of cellulose and hemicellulose to fermentable sugars–a review. Biomass Bioenergy 134, 105481.

CHAPTER 9

Obesity, inflammation, and cardiovascular disorders

Afshin Ehsan
Division of Cardiothoracic Surgery, Rhode Island Hospital, Brown University, Providence, RI, United States

Introduction

The epidemic of obesity has been a dominant health crisis in developed Western societies for several decades and is now becoming a growing problem in developing countries as well [1,2]. The World Health Organization estimates that approximately 40% the global population above 18 years of age is overweight and of those 13% are obese [3]. There are numerous studies that have demonstrated connections between obesity and cardiovascular disorders such as coronary artery disease, heart failure, arrhythmias, valvular heart disease, and aneurysms. Obesity has also been shown to increase the morbidity and mortality associated with cardiovascular disorders. The interplay between visceral ectopic fat, the metabolic syndrome, and chronic inflammation is felt to be the critical factor driving the pathophysiologic derangements that contribute to cardiovascular disease [4]. Although the prevention of obesity should be the central focus of reducing the deleterious effects of this health crisis, therapeutic strategies aimed at limiting the negative impact of this condition have been introduced with varying degrees of success. This chapter will review the current understanding of how obesity promotes cardiovascular disorders and the state of treatment options aimed at limiting its negative impact.

Atherosclerosis and coronary artery disease

Atherosclerosis and obesity have long been thought of as lipid storage disorders with accumulation of cholesterol esters in atherosclerotic plaques and triglycerides in fatty tissues. More recent findings indicate that atherosclerosis and obesity are also chronic inflammatory conditions, whereby the activation of both nonspecific and adaptive immune processes plays a significant role [5,6]. The pathogenesis of both atherosclerosis and obesity shares several common factors. Lipids, oxidized low-density lipoprotein (LDL) particles, and free fatty acids are known to activate the inflammatory process. Visceral obesity has also been shown to result in increased recruitment of macrophages to the hypertrophied adipocytes. These macrophages then act to increase the release of proinflammatory adipocytokines such as tumor necrosis factor (TNF)-α, interleukin (IL)-6, macrophage chemoattractant protein (MCP)-1, leptin, and resistin while reducing the antiinflammatory cytokines adiponectin and adipokine. This imbalance of pro- versus antiinflammatory cytokines leads to insulin resistance, endothelial dysfunction, hypercoagulability, and systemic inflammation and in turn promotes atherosclerotic plaque formation. IL-6 is also known to be a key driver in the release of C-reactive protein (CRP) from the liver and acts in concert with the proinflammatory conditions that arise from visceral obesity to contribute to the development of atherosclerosis. Moreover, increased levels of CRP are associated with an increased risk of myocardial infarction, peripheral vascular disease, and diabetes [7–16].

The progression of atherosclerotic disease to clinically significant coronary artery stenosis has also been shown to be accelerated by obesity. A report by McGill and colleagues [17] demonstrated that atherosclerosis begins in young individuals several decades before progressing to relevant coronary artery disease. More importantly, they demonstrated that patients with higher body mass indices (BMI) more frequently have atherosclerotic plaque that is also more advanced when compared with those with normal BMIs [17]. Longitudinal studies have demonstrated that at least two decades of obesity is an independent risk factor of coronary artery disease [18,19]. In the case of non-ST segment elevation myocardial infarction (NSTEMI), excess weight has been shown to result in the earlier manifestation of this clinical endpoint and is considered to be the most important risk factor ahead of smoking [20]. Similarly, this relationship has also been demonstrated in patients with ST elevation myocardial infarction (STEMI) as well [21,22]. Collectively there is solid evidence that demonstrates the contribution of obesity and inflammation to atherosclerosis and coronary artery disease.

Heart failure

The prevalence of heart failure in developed and developing countries continues to increase and with that it remains a major cause of global mortality. Obese and overweight patients are known to develop heart failure 10 years earlier than patients with a normal BMI. The duration of morbid obesity is closely correlated to the development of heart failure as well. After 20 and 30 years of obesity, the prevalence of heart failure grows by 70% and 90%, respectively [23]. Several studies have demonstrated this correlation between heart failure and obesity. In one report, 32%–49% of patients suffering from heart failure were found to be obese and 31%–40% were overweight. The Framingham Heart Study demonstrated an increased risk of heart failure by 5% in men and 7% in women with a rise of BMI by just $1\,kg/m^2$ [24]. Obesity is believed to lead to heart failure through several direct and indirect mechanisms. The structural and functional changes of the heart observed in obesity alone contribute to deterioration in myocardial function, which is often referred to as "obesity cardiomyopathy." [25] Excess weight is known to lead to hemodynamic changes in the form of a rise in both cardiac output and blood pressure [26]. This rise in blood pressure has been shown to be the result of activation of the renin-angiotensin-aldosterone system and to the increased activity of the sympathetic nervous system [27,28]. Hypertension increases left ventricular afterload, which results in structural and electrical myocardial remodeling ultimately leading to left ventricular hypertrophy and to diastolic and later to systolic ventricular dysfunction [29]. Fat cells have been shown to produce angiotensinogen, which is then converted to the potent vasoconstrictor angiotensin II. In addition to its potential to increase blood pressure, angiotensin II prevents the differentiation of preadipocytes into well-differentiated mature adipocytes resulting in fat cell hypertrophy, a phenomenon known to promote the release of proinflammatory adipocytokines [30]. Additionally, the hypertrophied adipocytes are known to by hyperlipolytic resulting in the secretion of more angiotensinogen resulting in a viscous cycle of inflammation and hypertension [31]. Obesity also increases aldosterone levels and the expression of the mineralocorticoid receptor, which in turn promotes interstitial cardiac fibrosis, platelet aggregation, and endothelial dysfunction. The above findings are supported by the results of the EMPHASISHF trial. Treatment with eplerenone, an aldosterone antagonist, in patients with heart failure with reduced ejection fraction showed a greater benefit to those with abdominal obesity as compared with those that were not obese [32,33]. Increased blood volume facilitates enhanced ventricular preload, causing increased ventricular wall tension and ultimately leading to ventricular dilatation.

The systemic proinflammatory state caused by obesity and metabolic stress has been shown to be a major determinant in the pathophysiology of heart failure as well. Endomyocardial biopsies have demonstrated the recruitment of inflammatory cells in patients with heart failure [34]. Microvascular endothelial inflammation has been shown to impair nitric oxide production, thus triggering cardiomyocyte dysfunction [35,36]. Inflammatory cytokines such as TNF-α and IL-6, whose production is increased in obesity, also play an important role in the development of heart failure [37,38]. Inflammatory mediators and acute-phase proteins in circulation have been shown to cause myocardial fibrosis, which increases myocardial stiffness that can lead to diastolic and later systolic dysfunction [39]. Leptin and adiponectin contribute directly to myocardial transformation through their effect on metabolism, tissue structure, and the extracellular matrix. Triglyceride accumulation in the cardiac muscle facilitates the generation of toxic metabolites in obese patients, thus enhancing the apoptosis of cardiomyocytes [40,41]. Moreover, obesity has been shown to increase the chances of heart failure not only by itself but also through the associated medical comorbidities that arise from this systemic physiologic state. Insulin resistance reduces the contractility of the myocardium [42], while it enhances the activity of the renin-angiotensin-aldosterone system and the deleterious effects noted earlier [43]. Obesity's role in atherosclerosis and the formation of coronary artery disease as detailed earlier increases the risk of ischemic cardiomyopathy and subsequent development of heart failure. Myocardial lipid accumulation and enhanced fibrosis can also play a pathogenic role in the genesis of various cardiac arrhythmias, which may contribute to the development of heart failure.

Arrhythmias

The role of obesity and inflammation in the development of arrhythmias has also been documented. Epicardial fat is a highly active visceral tissue producing a host of pro- and antiinflammatory adipocytokines, metabolic and growth factors that can directly diffuse into the myocardium. The paracrine effect of epicardial fat has been shown to contribute to the development of atrial interstitial fibrosis. This in conjunction with the infiltration of fat into the myocardium results in a heterogeneous atrial pulse conduction, which subsequently contributes to endocardial and epicardial electrical dissociation [44,45]. Collectively, these pathologic changes facilitate the development of ectopic atrial reentry circuits that ultimately lead to atrial fibrillation. Various studies have proven the relationship between obesity and atrial fibrillation. In a report published by Foy and colleagues, using a cohort of 67,238 patients derived from a database of healthcare claims in the United States, obesity was associated with new onset atrial fibrillation independent of age, diabetes, hypertension, and gender [46]. The occurrence of atrial fibrillation has also been shown to be 1.52 times higher in obese patients as compared with the normal weight population. An increase in BMI by just one unit can increase the frequency of newly developed atrial fibrillation by 4%. Left atrial enlargement and subsequent dysfunction are known to occur in patients with obesity [47]. An increase in 5 mm of the cross-sectional diameter of the left atrium increases the chance of paroxysmal atrial fibrillation. The inflammatory derangements associated with obesity are also believed to contribute to the development of arrhythmias. TNF-α has been shown to increase the local arrhythmic vulnerability of the pulmonary veins ultimately leading to atrial fibrillation while leptin lengthens the duration of the action potential, which is believed to have a proarrhythmic effect [48,49]. In coronary artery bypass surgery patients, where atrial fibrillation is a common postoperative complication, high levels of proinflammatory cytokines including TNF-α and IL-6 were observed in the epicardial fat compared with subcutaneous adipose tissue samples [50]. In patients that experienced atrial fibrillation after undergoing valve surgery, there were higher levels of right atrial nuclear factor-kappa beta (NF-kappa beta), which is a key regulator of the immune response. Additionally, TNF-α and IL-6 levels were higher in the presence of increased atrial fibrosis and severe lympho-monocyte infiltration [51]. In the end, local inflammation mediated by a locally driven immune cell and cytokine response appears to play a key role in the development of atrial fibrillation and is likely to underpin its relationship to epicardial fat.

Aortic stenosis

The pathogenesis of aortic valve stenosis is not completely understood but links to atherosclerotic risk factors such as hypertension, dyslipidemia, and diabetes have been demonstrated. The role of obesity in the development of aortic stenosis, however, has been a source of controversy. Studies have ranged from those showing an inverse relationship between measures of BMI and aortic stenosis to those demonstrating no association and others that have demonstrated a positive association [52–54]. A report by Larsson and colleagues, where two large population-based prospective cohorts were used to examine the relationship between obesity and aortic stenosis, demonstrated that obese patients were at increased risk of developing aortic stenosis. Specifically, BMI and waist circumference (WC) were positively associated with the incidence of aortic stenosis, and individuals with a BMI of $\geq 30\,kg/m^2$ had an approximately 80% increased risk of aortic stenosis compared with lean individuals. These differences persisted when the analysis was restricted to patients without hypertension, hypercholesterolemia, and diabetes. Additionally, approximately one-third of the patients with aortic stenosis underwent aortic valve replacement, with both BMI and WC being positively associated with the need for surgery. The prospective nature and size of this study population (71,817) give these findings significant weight relative to previous reports and strongly argue in favor of a causal relationship between obesity and aortic stenosis [55].

The metabolic profile of viscerally obese patients demonstrates a high quantity of small and dense LDL particles. These small and dense particles are transformed into oxidized LDLs at higher rates and have been shown to penetrate the arterial wall more easily than their larger counterparts. Histologic analysis of explanted stenotic aortic valves has demonstrated similarities between calcific aortic stenosis and vascular atherosclerosis, such as the presence of oxidized LDL and inflammatory cells as well as some receptors involved in the formation of vascular plaques [56,57]. The reduction in adiponectin levels associated with obesity has also been linked to the progression of aortic stenosis. In a report by Mohty and colleagues, lower adiponectin levels were a predictor of disease progression along with greater valvular inflammatory activity, thus supporting the concept that adiponectin may serve to protect the aortic valve from the inflammatory and calcifying processes that lead to aortic stenosis [58]. These collective findings offer evidence that aortic stenosis is at least in part related to the metabolic derangements associated with obesity and its associated proatherosclerotic processes.

Aneurysmal disease

The development of aortic dilatation and the contribution of obesity to this condition remain somewhat uncertain. Aneurysm formation is believed to have a different pathophysiology than occlusive arterial disease while also being associated with some but not all the risk factors associated with atherosclerosis [59]. While insulin resistance is known to be one of the central mechanisms by which obesity promotes atherosclerotic disease, population-based studies have demonstrated a negative association between diabetes and the development of abdominal aortic aneurysms (AAA) [60,61]. On the other hand, the adipocytokines that are known to promote the inflammatory processes associated with obesity have also been shown to be integral to the pathogenesis of AAA in experimental models [62].

The method by which obesity is measured or quantified has resulted in different associations with AAA. The use of BMI as a measure of obesity has been criticized given that it measures general obesity and can also be erroneous in its quantification of fat mass. Specifically, patients with increased BMI may not have increased fat mass as seen in athletes while having a normal BMI does not preclude individuals from having increased fat mass. On the other hand, visceral abdominal obesity, as quantified by waist circumference or waist-to-hip ratio, is believed to drive the pathophysiologic derangements that are associated with obesity and therefore more relevant to quantify and subsequently correlate to disease states. To this end, studies have failed to demonstrate a connection between BMI and aneurysm formation while increased abdominal visceral obesity has been shown to have an independent association with AAA formation [63]. This association has also been shown to be strongest with aneurysms that are ≥ 40 mm and not influenced by patient height [64]. Further evidence suggests that increased waist circumference results in a 30% higher risk of AAA as compared with those with normal waist size and a 15% increased risk per 5 cm increments up to a level of 100 cm for men and 88 cm for women. Even in patients without cardiovascular disorders, the positive association between waist circumference and AAA has been shown to persist [65].

Although a direct mechanism by which obesity leads to AAA formation has not been clearly elucidated, there is evidence to suggest that aortic inflammation leads to weakening of the vessel wall and subsequent dilatation. Circulating levels of the adipocytokines resitin and adiponectin have been shown to be independently associated with AAA formation [64]. Visceral adipose tissue has been proposed as a driver of periaortic inflammation through angiogenesis and matrix remodeling [62]. Histologic examination of aortic tissue has demonstrated close proximity of adipocytes producing IL-8 and MCP-1 to smooth muscle cells of the media and endothelial cells of the vasa vasorum with these chemokines having the ability to induce change in the smooth muscle cell phenotype [66]. Perivascular adipose tissue has also been shown to secrete chemokines at higher concentrations than subcutaneous adipose tissue. In a mouse model for AAA, cytokine expression and macrophage infiltration have been shown to be increased while weight loss has been reported to limit the progression of AAA expansion [67]. Alternatively, others have argued that visceral adiposity is not the driver of AAA progression, rather a phenotypic change related to underlying lifestyle habits, with the real diver being poor diet and little exercise. Although not definitive, there is adequate evidence to suggest that obesity as characterized by anthropometric measures, in addition to the anatomic, physiologic, and histologic measures of obesity-related inflammation, demonstrates a link between AAA formation and obesity.

The obesity paradox

Despite the demonstrated pathophysiologic derangements associated with obesity and its contribution to cardiovascular disorders, there remains the controversial phenomenon of the "obesity paradox." First described by Horwich and colleagues, the paradox is the result of findings that demonstrate favorable outcomes as it relates to all-cause mortality and cardiovascular mortality in overweight and obese patients. The mechanisms underlying these findings are not completely understood. One theory to explain this observation is centered on the limitations that come from using BMI as a measure of obesity. As previously stated, patients with increased BMI may not have increased fat mass as seen in athletes while having a normal BMI does not preclude individuals from having increased fat mass. Alternatively, adiposity measurements such as waist-to-hip ratio and waist circumference are associated with cardiac events, even after adjustment for other risk factors. In the end, a more accurate measure of body composition that better defines components of body weight may more accurately reflect a patient's fat mass and its subsequent contribution to clinical outcomes. Another explanation centers on the presence of increased levels of serum lipoproteins and their potential to neutralize bacterial toxins and circulating cytokines [68]. The earlier diagnosis of cardiovascular disorders in obese patients and their subsequent treatment as compared with nonobese patients have also been proposed as an explanation for these findings.

References

[1] Swinburn BA, Sacks G, Hall KD, McPherson K, Finegood DT, Moodie ML, Gortmaker SL. The global obesity pandemic: shaped by global drivers and local environments. Lancet 2011;378(9793):804–14.
[2] Ng M, Fleming T, Robinson M, et al. Global, regional, and national prevalence of overweight and obesity in children and adults during 1980-2013: a systematic analysis for the Global Burden of Disease Study 2013. Lancet 2014;384(9945):766–81.
[3] Poirier P, Giles TD, Bray GA, Hong Y, Stern JS, Pi-Sunyer FX, Eckel RH, American Heart Association, Obesity Committee of the Council on Nutrition, Physical Activity, and Metabolism. Obesity and cardiovascular disease: pathophysiology, evaluation, and effect of weight loss: an update of the 1997 American heart association Scientific

Statement on Obesity and Heart Disease from the Obesity committee of the council on Nutrition, Physical Activity, and Metabolism. Circulation 2006;113(6):898–918.
[4] Mathieu P, Pibarot P, Larose E, Poirier P, Marette A, Després JP. Visceral obesity and the heart. Int J Biochem Cell Biol 2008;40(5):821–36.
[5] Rocha VZ, Libby P. Obesity, inflammation, and atherosclerosis. Nat Rev Cardiol 2009;6(6):399–409.
[6] Ross R. Atherosclerosis—an inflammatory disease. N Engl J Med 1999;340(2):115–26.
[7] Després JP. Inflammation and cardiovascular disease: is abdominal obesity the missing link? Int J Obes Relat Metab Disord 2003;27(Suppl 3):S22–4.
[8] Cartier A, Lemieux I, Alméras N, Tremblay A, Bergeron J, Després JP. Visceral obesity and plasma glucose-insulin homeostasis: contributions of interleukin-6 and tumor necrosis factor-alpha in men. J Clin Endocrinol Metab 2008;93(5):1931–8.
[9] Blackburn P, Després JP, Lamarche B, Tremblay A, Bergeron J, Lemieux I, Couillard C. Postprandial variations of plasma inflammatory markers in abdominally obese men. Obesity (Silver Spring) 2006;14(10):1747–54.
[10] Spalding KL, et al. Dynamics of fat cell turnover in humans. Nature 2008;453:783–7.
[11] Gustafson B, Gogg S, Hedjazifar S, Jenndahl L, Hammarstedt A, Smith U. Inflammation and impaired adipogenesis in hypertrophic obesity in man. Am J Physiol Endocrinol Metab 2009;297(5):E999–E1003.
[12] Matsuzawa Y. The metabolic syndrome and adipocytokines. FEBS Lett 2006;580:2917–21.
[13] Andersson CX, Gustafson B, Hammarstedt A, Hedjazifar S, Smith U. Inflamed adipose tissue, insulin resistance and vascular injury. Diabetes Metab Res Rev 2008;24:595–603.
[14] Mathieu P, Pibarot P, Després JP. Metabolic syndrome: the danger signal in atherosclerosis. Vasc Health Risk Manag 2006;2:285–302.
[15] Nguyen MT, et al. A subpopulation of macrophages infiltrates hypertrophic adipose tissue and is activated by free fatty acids via toll-like receptors 2 and 4 and JNK-dependent pathways. J Biol Chem 2007;282:35279–92.
[16] Lyngsø D, Simonsen L, Bülow J. Metabolic effects of interleukin-6 in human splanchnic and adipose tissue. J Physiol 2002;543(Pt 1):379–86.
[17] McGill HC, McMahan CA, Herderick EE, et al. Obesity accelerates the progression of coronary atherosclerosis in young men. Circulation 2002;105(23):2712–8.
[18] Manson JAE, Colditz GA, Stampfer MJ, et al. A prospective study of obesity and risk of coronary heart disease in women. N Engl J Med 1990;322(13):882–9.
[19] Wilson PWF, D'Agostino RB, Sullivan L, Parise H, Kannel WB. Overweight and obesity as determinants of cardiovascular risk: the Framingham experience. Arch Intern Med 2002;162(16):1867–72.
[20] Madala MC, Franklin BA, Chen AY, et al. Obesity and age of first non-ST-segment elevation myocardial infarction. J Am Coll Cardiol 2008;52(12):979–85.
[21] Das SR, Alexander KP, Chen AY, et al. Impact of body weight and extreme obesity on the presentation, treatment and in-hospital outcomes of 50,149 patients with ST segment elevation myocardial infarction results from the NCDR (National Cardiovascular Data Registry). J Am Coll Cardiol 2011;58(25):2642–50.
[22] Jamil G, Jamil M, Alkhazraji H, et al. Risk factor assessment of young patients with acute myocardial infarction. Am J Cardiovasc Dis 2013;3(3):170–4.
[23] Alpert MA, Terry BE, Mulekar M, et al. Cardiac morphology and left ventricular function in normotensive morbidly obese patients with and without congestive heart failure, and effect of weight loss. Am J Cardiol 1997;80(6):736–40.
[24] Kenchaiah S, Evans JC, Levy D, et al. Obesity and the risk of heart failure. N Engl J Med 2002;347(5):305–13.
[25] Alpert MA, Omran J, Bostick BP. Effects of obesity on cardiovascular hemodynamics, cardiac morphology, and ventricular function. Curr Obes Rep 2016;5(4):424–34.

[26] Schmieder RE, Messerli FH. Does obesity influence early target organ damage in hypertensive patients? Circulation 1993;87(5):1482–8.
[27] Ebong IA, Goff Jr DC, Rodriguez CJ, Chen H, Bertoni AG. Mechanisms of heart failure in obesity. Obes Res Clin Pract 2014;8(6):e540–8.
[28] Rabbia F, Silke B, Conterno A, et al. Assessment of cardiac autonomic modulation during adolescent obesity. Obes Res 2003;11(4):541–8.
[29] de Simone G, Palmieri V, Bella JN, et al. Association of left ventricular hypertrophy with metabolic risk factors: the HyperGEN study. J Hypertens 2002;20(2):323–31.
[30] Mathieu P, Poirier P, Pibarot P, Lemieux I, Després JP. Visceral obesity: the link among inflammation, hypertension, and cardiovascular disease. Hypertension 2009;53:577–84.
[31] Mazzolai L, et al. Endogenous angiotensin II induces atherosclerotic plaque vulnerability and elicits a Th1 response in ApoE−/− mice. Hypertension 2004;44:277–82.
[32] Ahmed A, Blackman MR, White M, Anker SD. Emphasis on abdominal obesity as a modifier of eplerenone effect in heart failure: hypothesis-generating signals from EMPHASIS-HF. Eur J Heart Fail 2017;19(9):1198–200.
[33] Olivier A, Pitt B, Girerd N, et al. Effect of eplerenone in patients with heart failure and reduced ejection fraction: potential effect modification by abdominal obesity. Insight from the EMPHASIS-HF trial. Eur J Heart Fail 2017;19(9):1186–97.
[34] Westermann D, Lindner D, Kasner M, et al. Cardiac inflammation contributes to changes in the extracellular matrix in patients with heart failure and normal ejection fraction. Circ Heart Fail 2011;4:44–52.
[35] Paulus WJ, Tschope C. A novel paradigm for heart failure with preserved ejection fraction: comorbidities drive myocardial dysfunction and remodeling through coronary microvascular endothelial inflammation. J Am Coll Cardiol 2013;62:263–71.
[36] van Heerebeek L, Hamdani N, Falcao-Pires I, et al. Low myocardial protein kinase G activity in heart failure with preserved ejection fraction. Circulation 2012;126:830–9.
[37] Levine B, Kalman J, Mayer L, Fillit HM, Packer M. Elevated circulating levels of tumor necrosis factor in severe chronic heart failure. N Engl J Med 1990;323(4):236–41.
[38] Torre-Amione G, Kapadia S, Benedict C, Oral H, Young JB, Mann DL. Proinflammatory cytokine levels in patients with depressed left ventricular ejection fraction: a report from the studies of left ventricular dysfunction (SOLVD). J Am Coll Cardiol 1996;27(5):1201–6.
[39] Cavalera M, Wang JH, Frangogiannis NG. Obesity, metabolic dysfunction, and cardiac fibrosis: pathophysiological pathways, molecular mechanisms, and therapeutic opportunities. Transl Res 2014;164(4):323–35.
[40] Karmazyn M, Purdham DM, Rajapurohitam V, Zeidan A. Signalling mechanisms underlying the metabolic and other effects of adipokines on the heart. Cardiovasc Res 2008;79(2):279–86.
[41] Schram K, Sweeney G. Implications of myocardial matrix remodeling by adipokines in obesity-related heart failure. Trends Cardiovasc Med 2008;18(6):199–205.
[42] Horwich TB, Fonarow GC. Glucose, obesity, metabolic syndrome, and diabetes relevance to incidence of heart failure. J Am Coll Cardiol 2010;55(4):283–93.
[43] Cozzolino D, Grandone A, Cittadini A, et al. Subclinical myocardial dysfunction and cardiac autonomic dysregulation are closely associated in obese children and adolescents: the potential role of insulin resistance. PLoS ONE 2015;10(4), e0123916.
[44] Zlochiver S, Munoz V, Vikstrom KL, Taffet SM, Berenfeld O, Jalife J. Electrotonic myofibroblast-tomyocyte coupling increases propensity to reentrant arrhythmias in two-dimensional cardiac monolayers. Biophys J 2008;95(9):4469–80.
[45] Maesen B, Zeemering S, Afonso C, et al. Rearrangement of atrial bundle architecture and consequent changes in anisotropy of conduction constitute the 3-dimensional substrate for atrial fibrillation. Circ Arrhythm Electrophysiol 2013;6(5):967–75.

[46] Foy AJ, Mandrola J, Liu G, Naccarelli GV. Relation of obesity to new-onset atrial fibrillation and atrial flutter in adults. Am J Cardiol 2018;121(9):1072–5.
[47] Wang TJ, Parise H, Levy D, et al. Obesity and the risk of new-onset atrial fibrillation. JAMA 2004;292(20):2471–7.
[48] Lee SH, Chen YC, Chen YJ, et al. Tumor necrosis factor-α alters calcium handling and increases arrhythmogenesis of pulmonary vein cardiomyocytes. Life Sci 2007;80(19):1806–15.
[49] Mohamed-Ali V, Goodrick S, Bulmer K, Holly JMP, Yudkin JS, Coppack SW. Production of soluble tumor necrosis factor receptors by human subcutaneous adipose tissue in vivo. Am J Physiol Endocrinol Metab 1999;277(6):E971–5.
[50] Mazurek T, Zhang L, Zalewski A, et al. Human epicardial adipose tissue is a source of inflammatory mediators. Circulation 2003;108:2460–6.
[51] Qu YC, Du YM, Wu SL, et al. Activated nuclear factor-kappaB and increased tumor necrosis factor-alpha in atrial tissue of atrial fibrillation. Scand Cardiovasc J 2009;43:292–7.
[52] Lindroos M, Kupari M, Valvanne J, Strandberg T, Heikkila J, Tilvis R. Factors associated with calcific aortic valve degeneration in the elderly. Eur Heart J 1994;15:865–70.
[53] Stewart BF, Siscovick D, Lind BK, Gardin JM, Gottdiener JS, Smith VE, Kitzman DW, Otto CM. Clinical factors associated with calcific aortic valve disease. Cardiovascular health study. J Am Coll Cardiol 1997;29:630–4.
[54] Peltier M, Trojette F, Sarano ME, Grigioni F, Slama MA, Tribouilloy CM. Relation between cardiovascular risk factors and nonrheumatic severe calcific aortic stenosis among patients with a three-cuspid aortic valve. Am J Cardiol 2003;91:97–9.
[55] Larsson SC, Wolk A, Hakansson N, Back M. Overall and abdominal obesity and incident aortic valve stenosis: two prospective cohort studies. Eur Heart J 2017;38:2192–7.
[56] Olsson M, Thyberg J, Nilsson J. Presence of oxidized low density lipoprotein in nonrheumatic stenotic aortic valves. Arterioscler Thromb Vasc Biol 1999;19:1218–22.
[57] Otto CM, Kuusisto J, Reichenbach DD, et al. Characterization of the early lesion of degenerative valvular aortic stenosis. Histological and immunohistochemical studies. Circulation 1994;90:844–53.
[58] Mohty D, Cartier A, Pibarot P, et al. Hypoadiponectemia is associated with aortic valve inflammation and faster disease progression in patients with aortic stenosis. Circulation 2006;114:II657 [Abst].
[59] Golledge J, Norman PE. Atherosclerosis and abdominal aortic aneurysm: cause, response, or common risk factors? [editorial]. Arterioscler Thromb Vasc Biol 2010;30(6):1075–7.
[60] Lederle FA, Johnson GR, Wilson SE, et al. Prevalence and associations of abdominal aortic aneurysm detected through screening. Aneurysm detection and management (ADAM) veterans affairs cooperative study group. Ann Intern Med 1997;126(6):441–9.
[61] Pleumeekers HJ, Hoes AW, van der Does E, et al. Aneurysms of the abdominal aorta in older adults. The Rotterdam study. Am J Epidemiol 1995;142(12):1291–9.
[62] Police SB, Thatcher SE, Charnigo R, Daugherty A, Cassis LA. Obesity promotes inflammation in periaortic adipose tissue and angiotensin II-induced abdominal aortic aneurysm formation. Arterioscler Thromb Vasc Biol 2009;29:1458–64.
[63] Lederle FA, Johnson GR, Wilson SE, et al. The aneurysm detection and management study screening program: validation cohort and final results. Arch Intern Med 2000;160(10):1425–30.
[64] Golledge J, Clancy P, Jamrozik K, Norman PE. Obesity, adipokines, and abdominal aortic aneurysm: health in men study. Circulation 2007;116(20):2275–9.
[65] Stackelberg O, Bjorck M, Sadr-Azodi O, Larsson SC, Orsini N, Wolk A. Obesity and abdominal aortic aneurysm. Br J Surg 2013;100:360–6.
[66] Henrichot E, Juge-Aubry CE, Pernin A, et al. Production of chemokines by perivascular adipose tissue: a role in the pathogenesis of atherosclerosis? Arterioscler Thromb Vasc Biol 2005;25(12):2594–9.

[67] Police SB, Putnam K, Thatcher S, Batifoulier-Yiannikouris F, Daugherty A, Cassis LA. Weight loss in obese C57BL/6 mice limits adventitial expansion of established angiotensin II-induced abdominal aortic aneurysms. Am J Physiol Heart Circ Physiol 2010;298(6):H1932–8.

[68] Lavie CJ, Ventura HO. Weighing in on obesity and the obesity paradox in heart failure. J Card Fail 2011;17(5):381–3.

CHAPTER 10

Obesity, inflammation, and CNS disorders

Sheel Shah[a], Justin Lee[a], and Michael Gong-Ruey Ho[b]

[a]Department of Neurosurgery, David Geffen School of Medicine at UCLA, Los Angeles, CA, United States
[b]Department of Neurology, David Geffen School of Medicine at UCLA, Los Angeles, CA, United States

Introduction

The growing prevalence of obesity has reached pandemic proportions with WHO estimates showing that globally over 2 billion people are likely overweight with roughly 700 million of those people estimated to be obese. These numbers are projected to roughly double in the next 20–25 years [1]. In 2008, the CDC estimated the medical cost of the obesity epidemic at $147 billion dollars in the United States alone [2].

Growing preponderance of evidence suggests that the health sequela of obesity extends to almost every organ system leading to the significantly increased morbidity and mortality in this population. While the cardiovascular and cerebrovascular risks of obesity are well publicized, more incipient data point to systemic deleterious effects of obesity particularly as it relates to diseases of the central nervous system (CNS) and their progression. Central to these effects is the complex interactions of the increased burden of adipose tissue in obese patients and the resulting low-grade chronic inflammatory state [3–5]. This milieu of chronic inflammation has the effect of potentiating diseases of the central nervous system that have already taken hold in this patient population along with inviting new indolent processes to begin.

While once thought to be a simple storage device of excess energy and source of thermoregulation, the current research points to adipose tissue to be an organ system unto itself with important endocrine and metabolic functions involved in energy homeostasis. This organ is not only made up of adipocytes but rather relies on the complex interactions between adipocytes, fibroblasts, endothelial cells, and immune cells [6]. The endocrine functions of adipocytes have only now begun to be fully appreciated with discoveries of various adipokines such as adiponectin, leptin, and resistin, which play pivotal roles in satiety, insulin sensitivity, and maintaining the balance between proinflammatory and antiinflammatory states [7–9]. In fact, an excess burden of adipocytes, particularly visceral fat, has been found to lead to the secretion of proinflammatory cytokines, particularly Interluekin-6 (IL-6), Interleukin-1 (IL-1), leptin, and tumor necrosis factor alpha (TNF-α) [10]. Furthermore, antiinflammatory adipokines are downregulated and chemo-attracting adipokines, such as monocyte chemoattractant protein 1, are upregulated causing inflammation in adipose tissue by recruiting leukocytes locally [11]. These activated leukocytes in the adipose tissue further release inflammatory cytokines systemically, resulting in a systemic inflammatory state [12]. Systemic inflammation in turn leads to increased insulin resistance mediated by TNF-α causing a positive feedback loop of increasing systemic inflammation [13]. While the exact mechanisms underlying obesity and the resulting proinflammatory state are not fully understood yet, the infiltration of immune cells into adipose tissue is thought to be the more important step toward the development of a proinflammatory state (Fig. 1).

Long-standing obesity leads to a chronic inflammatory state as the body is unable to remove the persistent inflammatory stimulus due to the steady production of inflammatory cytokines and reactive oxygen species. This chronic low-grade proinflammatory state is now being referred to as chronic low-grade sterile inflammation or meta-inflammation, which is characterized by a slight increase in circulating proinflammatory markers, but a lack of overt clinical signs of inflammation [14]. The systemic adverse effects of meta-inflammation are now also being appreciated with evidence showing resulting dysregulation in almost every organ system, particularly the CNS [15]. Obesity has been associated with various neurological disorders including various dementias, multiple sclerosis (MS), idiopathic intracranial hypertension, vasculitis, and neurological sequela of systemic lupus erythematosus.

CNS disorders associated with obesity
Idiopathic intracranial hypertension

Idiopathic intracranial hypertension (IIH), also known as pseudotumor cerebri, is characterized by increased intracranial pressure of unclear etiology. IIH is a rare entity that tends to afflict primary young, overweight women of reproductive age. These patients typically present with headache, nausea, and vomiting, but the hallmark symptoms tend to be visual in nature

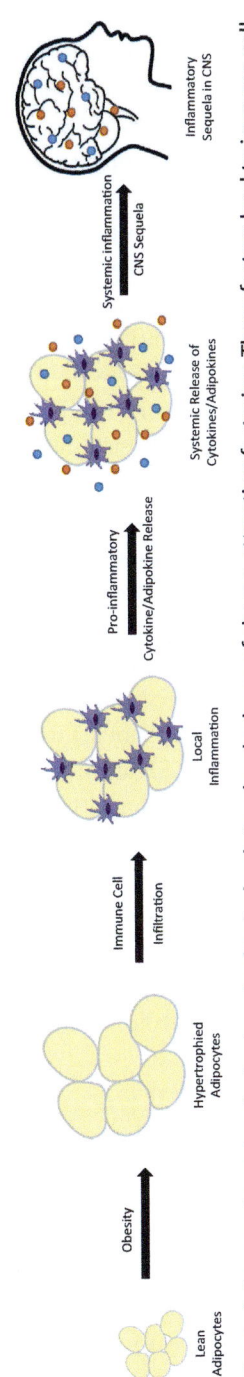

Fig. 1 Adipocyte hypertrophy in chronic obesity leads to a local release of chemo-attracting factoring. These factors lead to immune cell infiltration of adipose tissue. These activated immune cells then release cytokines, which exacerbates the local inflammation. This inflammation then causes systemic release of proinflammatory cytokines and adipokines leading to a systemic proinflammatory state.

including photopsias, diplopia, eye pain, and at times, visual impairment and blindness. In fact, up to 30% of patients may suffer from some level of blindness due to this disease [16]. Fundoscopic exam is central to obtaining the diagnosis as papilledema with an increased opening pressure on lumbar puncture in the presence of no mass occupying lesions or other causes of intracranial hypertension makes the diagnosis [17].

The association between IIH and obesity has been established by many studies over the last several decades. In fact, more than 10 independent studies have shown that obesity rates in patients with IIH tend to be 10-fold greater than the general population [18–27]. Of further interest is the fact that along with baseline weight, recent weight gain also seems to be an important factor in the development of IIH in patients. Daniels et al. show that a cohort of 34 newly diagnosed IIH patients showed a greater degree of weight gain over the previous year when compared with controls [28]. These studies bear out that even a modest weight gain of about 5%–15% is enough to increase a patient's risk of developing IIH [29].

Many mechanisms have been proposed including increased CSF production, increased brain volume from edema, increased cerebral arterial pressure, decreased venous drainage, and poor CSF absorption [30]. While current opinion tends to lean toward a combination of impaired absorption of CSF along with decrease brain compliance, further research is needed to elucidate the mechanisms involved. CSF absorption abnormalities may be due to decreased absorption by the arachnoid villi or venous hypertension. In fact, manometry has found increased pressure in the venous sinuses in patients with IIH [31]. However, it is unclear whether IIH is the cause of venous hypertension or if venous hypertension causes IIH. Secondary IIH has also been described due to the effects of various medications, dysregulation of the hypothalamic-pituitary-adrenal axis as seen in Addison's disease or Cushing's disease, abrupt corticosteroid withdrawal, and hypervitaminosis A [32,33].

Most recent theories as to the underlying etiology of IIH seem to focus around the neuroendocrine functions of the mineralocorticoid receptors (MRs) [34]. MRs have been found to be abundant in the choroid plexus, and their activation stimulates CSF secretion resulting in CSF imbalances and increased intracranial pressure. Obesity plays a central role in this model of IIH as adipose tissue secretes mineralocorticoid and corticosteroid-releasing factors. Given that corticosteroids can also have a high affinity for mineralocorticoid receptors, the resulting corticosteroid and mineralocorticoid excess caused by obesity can lead to increased CSF production in the choroid plexus causing IIH [35]. Furthermore, studies have shown that vitamin A can induce the production of neurosteroids in the glial cell lines, which may be the cause of vitamin-A-induced IIH.

Controversy exists regarding whether the degree of obesity affects the disease burden of IIH and outcomes. A relatively recent study has shown that patients with BMI > 40 were more likely to present with advanced symptoms such as severe papilledema and that for every 10-point increased in BMI, the chances of severe vision loss increased by 40% [36]. Also, numerous studies have tried to identify obesity markers that may predict the onset of IIH or prognosis for patient. These studies show that estrogenic fat distribution (i.e., increased lower body fat versus central obesity) is highly prevalent in patients with IIH vs. controls [37]. This finding along with the prevalence of IIH in younger reproductive age females supports the role of estrogen in the possible mechanisms to the development of IIH.

Leptin as an obesity marker and its contribution to the pathophysiology of IIH have also been extensively studied although the findings have been mixed. Lampl et al. found significantly higher serum leptin levels in IIH patients compared with controls, and Ball et al. found significantly higher CSF leptin levels in IIH patients compared with controls [38]. However, a study by Behbehani et al. found no association between serum and CSF leptin levels when the data were adjusted for age and BMI [39]. Similarly, insulin levels and ghrelin levels have also been studied with no significant association found.

Management of patients with IIH has revolved around three major tenets: remove possible medication causes, weight loss, and intracranial pressure management with medications and possible surgical interventions. Weight reduction with a low-sodium diet has been recommended for all obese patients with IIH. Weight loss has been shown to be a predictor of disease progression and outcomes. Studies have shown that even a modest reduction of weight of around 6% can result in reduction of symptoms [40]. More interest has shifted these days toward the role of bariatric surgery in the management of IIH. A metaanalysis of 11 studies that looked at bariatric surgery in IIH patients found that 92% of patients with IIH reported resolution of symptoms and 97% demonstrated resolution of papilledema [41]. Furthermore, bariatric surgery was also found to be superior to CSF shunting and acetazolamide monotherapy [42,43]. Bariatric surgery also has the added benefit of reducing other systemic deleterious effects of obesity, such as joint disease, metabolic syndrome, and other CNS complications.

Besides weight loss, acetazolamide has been the mainstay of medical management as it reduces the rate of CSF production due to its activity as a carbonic anhydrase inhibitor. Topiramate also inhibits carbonic anhydrase activity and has been used in IIH. Topiramate is particularly gaining favor as it also has been associated with weight loss and has shown similar efficacy when compared with acetazolamide [44]. Furosemide may also be used in conjunction with acetazolamide to help potentiate its action. Smaller studies have advocated for the use of indomethacin as it can reduce cerebral blood flow and has shown modest efficacy [45].

Surgical management other than bariatric surgery has involved either CSF shunting or venous sinus stenting. While studies have shown improvement of symptoms with CSF shunting, the resulting complications of shunting have caused shunting to have fallen out of favor. In some studies, shunt revision rates have been as high as 40%–60% [46]. Venous sinus stenting is a newer treatment option that requires more study at this stage. A literature review on data of 143 patients showed that 88% of patients reported improved headaches and 87% of patients had improved visual symptoms [47].

Obesity and stroke

Stroke is one of the major causes of disability and the second most common cause of death worldwide. While ultimately the cause of stroke is multifactorial, obesity and the resulting metabolic derangements and systemic inflammatory state have been shown to lead to cerebrovascular remodeling and definitely contribute to stroke risk. Several studies have outlined the increase risk of stroke in obese patient populations. A comprehensive meta-analysis published in 2010 by Strazzullo et al. included 25 studies with over 2 million participants and found that the ischemic stroke risk was 22% higher in overweight individuals and 64% higher in obese individuals. Interestingly, hemorrhagic stroke risk was not elevated for overweight or obese individuals [48]. Further investigation has showed that BMI is an independent risk factor apart from diabetes, hypertension, and hyperlipidemia [49]. Metabolic syndrome has also been found to be an independent risk factor for stroke with patients with insulin resistance showing a twofold increase in stroke risk.

Cerebrovascular effects of obesity and resulting systemic inflammation may be a key factor in the pathophysiology of stroke in obese patients. While human studies are rare for obvious reasons, animal models have shown significant cerebrovascular remodeling in the setting of obesity. Diet-induced obesity has been studied in a rat model by feeding the rats a high-fat diet from 3 weeks of age. By week 13, these rats all developed abdominal obesity, hypertension, and insulin resistance. The middle cerebral arteries (MCAs) from these rats were harvested along with age-matched controls. When compared, the MCA from high-fat-diet rats were found to have a markedly reduced lumen diameter and outer wall diameter and increased wall thickness and wall-to-lumen ratio resulting in increased vessel stiffness [50]. This decrease in vessel size is thought to lead to an increased risk of ischemic stroke in obese patients. While the molecular mechanism leading to this vessel remodeling remains unelucidated, inflammation is thought to play at least a small roll in vessel remodeling.

The nitric oxide (NO) synthesis pathway, which is involved in arterial dilation, has also been found to be impaired in rat models of obesity. The upregulation of inflammatory pathways has also been implicated in the dysregulation of the NO pathway in the cerebral vasculature. In obese rat models, the NO-mediated vascular dilation has been found to be impaired. However, exogenous NO administration results in appropriate dilation of the vessels suggesting that NO bioavailability or production is decreased in obese rats. Further investigation revealed that NO bioavailability is reduced due to the increased presence of reactive oxygen species (ROS) [51]. ROS are a key end effector in the inflammatory pathway, and the increase in ROS and resulting decreased bioavailability of NO may at least in part be due to the systemic inflammatory state mediated by obesity.

Increased oxidative stress due to systemic inflammation not only affects the NO pathways but has also been found to result in potassium channel dysregulation and further impairment of normal cerebrovascular physiology. The normal function of potassium channels is central in the appropriate dilation of the vessel walls due to smooth muscle activity. The increased ROS in cerebral blood vessels in the setting of obesity leads to dysregulation of the potassium channels and impaired vessel dilation [52]. This effect has been studied in the cardiovascular system and found to lead to increased infarct size following ischemia; however, this effect has not been specifically investigated in the cerebrovascular system [53].

Finally, a novel function of insulin as a cerebral artery dilator has recently emerged. Insulin has been found to increase blood flow in the cerebral cortex. This function seems to be mediated by the activity of insulin on endothelin receptor type B. However, in the setting of obesity and resulting insulin resistance, the endothelin nitrous oxide synthase (eNOS) becomes decoupled from the receptor and uncoupled eNOS produces more ROS [54].

Taken as a whole, these mechanisms that lead from obesity, inflammation, to stroke are mediated by cerebrovascular changes. This remodeling has significant ramification for not only stroke risk but also stroke severity. In these same rat models, infarct area was found to be significantly larger in the obese models as the collateral circulation is less able to dilate and compensate for the lack of perfusion [55]. Furthermore, obese animal models were found to exhibit more inflammation poststroke, possibly from the baseline inflammatory state of obesity. Terao et al. have reported that after 30 min of ischemia and 4 h of reperfusion in their model, they found an increase in the number of leukocytes and platelets adhered to the surrounding vasculature as compared with nonobese controls. In addition, in the obese model they found increased breakdown of the blood-brain barrier, increased edema, and increased inflammatory cytokines [56]. In fact, a study found that antibodies toward MCP-1 actually reduced the severity of the stroke [57].

Lifestyle changes have long been a cornerstone in stroke prevention and management. Weight loss has been recommended for primary and secondary prevention of stroke for obese patients by the American Stroke Association [58]. A metaanalysis has found that weight loss of about 5 kg can lead to almost a 4–5-point reduction in systolic blood pressure [59]. Therefore, weight loss along with aggressive hypertension management is pivot for stroke prevention. Finally, aspirin and statin therapies are also vital to the secondary prevention of stroke. These medical therapies become even more vital in the obese patient as the systemic inflammatory state caused by obesity also leads to a prothrombotic state. Statins have been shown to reduce inflammation in the vasculature, and aspirin therapy can further help mitigate the risk of a prothrombotic state.

While much more investigation needs to be pursued in this area, the link between chronic obesity and cerebrovascular remodeling has been well established. This has been best studied in the context of stroke, but further research is needed as to the affect that this remodeling for other pathologies such as aneurysms, vasculitis, cerebral atherosclerosis, cerebral venous thrombosis, and Moyamoya disease.

Autoimmune CNS disorders and obesity

Over the last decade, as the scientific community has begun to appreciate the link between obesity and inflammation, there has been a keen interest in studying the mechanistic relationship between obesity and autoimmune diseases. Indeed, clinical and basic science data have established a strong relationship between obesity and various autoimmune diseases, such as

MS, rheumatoid arthritis, systemic lupus erythematosus, and inflammatory bowel disease, among others. The dysregulation of adipokines, including increase in leptin, resistin, and visfatin secretion and decrease in adiponectin secretion, has been found to lead to a persistent proinflammatory state that potentiates the effects of existing autoimmune disease and increases the vulnerability to developing autoimmune diseases [5].

MS is the most common primary autoimmune condition affecting the central nervous system. This disease entity is characterized by white matter inflammatory plaques resulting in demyelination leading to axonal loss and gliosis in the central nervous system. Patients typically present with varied neurological symptoms that are localized to varied regions of that brain and change over time. Diagnosis is made through clinical history, CSF studies, and MRI findings based on the McDonald criteria. This disease afflicts about 2.8 million people worldwide, and studies show that the prevalence has been increasing [60]. The developed nations tend to have a higher prevalence of MS than developing nations and a higher prevalence, by 2–3 times, in women than men. Patients also typically present in their 20s or 30s. The etiology of MS is still unknown; however, data suggest that genetic, environmental, and immune factors all play a role [61].

The rise in the incidence of MS in the developed world coincides with the rise of obesity in the developed world. This correlation has led to many studies investigating the link between childhood obesity and risk of developing MS. Two of the largest studies, one American and one Swedish, both report a roughly twofold increase in the lifetime risk of developing MS in obese patients [62,63]. The association between BMI and the severity of disease has also been investigated with mixed results as some studies have found no correlation and others shows a positive correlation of BMI with disease severity [64–66].

An active area of research in the field of MS is trying to elucidate the complex mechanistic link between obesity and MS. Adding to the complexity is the large number of confounding variables, such as sun exposure, smoking status, and Epstein-Barr virus exposure. These complexities notwithstanding, evidence is mounting that there exists at least some degree of causal relationship between obesity and MS. Current research and theories posit a central role for leptin in the causal link between MS and obesity. Leptin has been found to have proinflammatory effects by prompting the proliferation and upregulating the activity of monocytes, macrophages, T cells, B cells, and neutrophils [67]. Leptin receptor was found to be upregulated in patients having an acute MS flare as compared with stable MS patients and healthy controls [68]. The expression of leptin itself was found to be elevated in MS lesions, CSF, and serum of patients who were actively being treated with interferon therapy for MS relapse [69]. Conversely, caloric restriction, which reduces leptin levels in the body, in animal models of MS has found to be beneficial in reducing the severity of the disease burden and increased the survival of the animal models [70].

Another important molecule in the pathway leading from obesity to a proinflammatory state to MS is adiponectin. Adiponectin has an overall antiinflammatory effect as it reduces secretion of inflammatory cytokines and decreases B and T cell activity [71]. In animal models of MS, lack of adiponectin was found to be associated with greater disease severity; however, when these animals were given exogenous adiponectin, disease progression was limited [72]. Similar roles have been posited for visfatin and resistin, which both have been found to have a proinflammatory effect.

Alternative hypothesis linking obesity, inflammation, and MS is also being actively investigated. One such theory looks at the direct immunological activity of adipose tissue as opposed to the secreted adipokines. Recent evidence shows that adipose tissue can activate T cells and natural killer cells while also recruiting monocytes [73]. These recruited immune cells then begin producing proinflammatory cytokines, such as TNF, IL-1, IL-6 [74]. The increased circulating levels of these cytokines themselves lead to activation of several proinflammatory signaling pathways in many organs including the brain along with increasing insulin resistance systemically. Insulin resistance itself further potentiates the proinflammatory pathways.

Finally, there also may be a role for neuropeptide Y (NPY) in modulating the interaction between energy balance and the immune system. NPY is a neurotransmitter that plays a major role in regulating feeding drives in the hypothalamus, and recently, NPY receptors have even been found in immune cells. In animal models, the administration of NPY was found to reduce the severity of symptoms in a dose-dependent fashion [75]. Further study showed that NPY administration led to a decrease in the circulating IFN-γ and reduced CNS penetration of T cells and macrophages [76]. Given these findings, NPY and its role in neuroimmunomodulation are becoming a very active field of research and may provide more insight into the mechanistic link between energy homeostasis, obesity, and autoimmune disease.

Currently, MS treatment revolves around disease-modifying drugs, which altered the immune response. For example, one of the drugs involves interferon-β (IFN-β). The mechanism of action of IFN-β is not fully known, data show that IFN-β inhibits T cell activation and proliferation, promotes autoreactive T cells apoptosis, induction of Treg cells, and lowers the concentration of proinflammatory cytokines. Similarly, another MS disease-modifying drug glatiramer exerts its effect by promoting the secretion of antiinflammatory cytokines, decreasing the amount of Th17 cells and increasing Treg cells. Given these mechanisms of action and the proinflammatory state induced by obesity, the assumption would be that the efficacy of these drugs would be decreased in obese patients; however, no study has found an association between the two. In fact, the only MS drug found to have a link to obesity is with a dimethyl-fumarate (DMF). DMF has been shown to inhibit the differentiation of preadipocytes by downregulating the expression of adipogenic transcription factors [77]. More clinical research is needed in looking at the interaction of DMF and other MS drugs and obesity to further characterize the effect of obesity on drug efficacy. Interestingly, statin therapy has also been studied in the setting of MS and found to have benefit in the secondary progressive phase; however, whether this salutary effect is due to antiinflammatory properties, anticholesterol properties, or some heretofore undiscovered neuroprotective function is unknown.

Obesity, inflammation, and cognition

Evidence has been accumulating that obesity negatively impacts cognitive function and increases the lifetime risk of dementia. Mild cognitive impairment is generally the precursor to dementia, and many studies have shown that obesity increases the risk of mild cognitive impairment even when the data are adjusted for age [78–80]. While there is some controversy in the field [81], the greater preponderance of evidence shows a like between increased BMI and decline or dysfunction in various cognitive measures, including attention deficit disorder, poor executive function, and decreased memory function.

Various meta-analyses have shown a strong association between obesity and dementia, particularly Alzheimer's disease. These data show that obesity nearly doubles the risk of Alzheimer's disease when compared with individuals with a healthy BMI [82]. Also, obesity in midlife has been shown to confer greater risk in developing dementias later in life [83]. With regard to Alzheimer's disease specifically, postmortem studies have found that patients with morbid obesity tend to have higher concentrations of amyloid-beta deposits and tau plaques than nonobese patients.

Increased BMI has also been associated with structural changes in the brain, which may be central in the underlying pathophysiology linking obesity to decline in cognitive function. These structural changes tend to center on the temporal lobe and particularly the hippocampus—a brain structure found in the temporal lobe that is vital for learning and memory formation. In fact, Alzheimer's disease is generally characterized by temporal lobe atrophy and particularly hippocampus dysfunction. Hippocampus dysfunction of any level is also a major cause of general cognitive decline. CT-based volumetric analysis has shown that increased BMI is an independent predictor for temporal lobe atrophy [84]. Further MRI studies have also shown that BMI and brain volume are generally inversely correlated [85]. Additionally, increased BMI has been independently associated with decreased general neuronal viability [86] and increased gliosis particularly in the hypothalamus [87]. Further structural changes in the brain have been by morphology studies, where analysis has shown increased BMI to be negatively correlated with the global amount of gray matter in the brain with particularly decreased gray matter volume in the midbrain, cerebellum, and frontal, temporal, and occipital lobes. Various lines of evident particularly link obesity to atrophy in the hippocampus, thalamus, anterior cingulate gyrus, and frontal lobes [88,89].

This volume loss in various areas of the brain has not only been observed in the elderly population, but also has been seen the pediatric population. Children and adolescents with elevated BMI have been found to have atrophy of the frontal lobes and hippocampus also as compared with healthy BMI controls [90]. These areas of the brain are vital to memory and executive functions, and their atrophy can lead to significant detrimental effects in the development of these children.

The mechanisms underlying these structural changes in the brain that are associated with obesity are not fully understood, but various studies in animal models point to possible mechanistic links. Many of these mechanistic links endorse a role for general inflammation in the pathophysiological link between obesity and cognitive decline. Two independent studies have shown that long-term potentiation, a process by which synaptic connections in the brain are strengthened after repeated use, is impaired in mice fed with a high-fat diet [91,92]. A high-fat diet in this animal model was also associated with decreased neurogenesis and plasticity [93,94].

The sentinel event in these various derangements in the normal functioning of neurons in the brain has been found to be inflammation of the hypothalamus [95]. The hypothalamus has various roles from controlling hormones to regulating body temperatures. In relation to obesity, the hypothalamus is also heavily involved in regulating feeding habits and energy homeostasis in general. Through the median eminence, the hypothalamus senses the nutrient content in the circulation and can coordinate the efforts of the neuroendocrine system and autonomic nervous system to mediate satiety based on nutritional status [96]. However, as the median eminence needs direct access to the central circulation, it is not protected by the blood-brain barrier making it venerable to the net inflammatory effects of the various adipokines secreted in obesity.

Immediately adjacent to the median eminence is a collection of neurons that make up the arcuate nucleus. These neurons produce neuropeptide Y and when activated produce increased hunger. Leptin, insulin, and peptide YY inhibit these neurons, and ghrelin has a strong activating function. In animal models of obesity, high concentrations of TNF-α and microglial activation were found in the arcuate nucleus [97]. In fact, after only 1 day of high-fat diet feeding, inflammatory markers were found in this region of the hypothalamus [98]. Furthermore, inflammatory markers were present in the hypothalamus even before they could be detected in the adipose tissue or even peripheral blood [99]. Microglial activation is thought to be the essential first step in hypothalamic inflammation as they express toll-like receptor 4 (TLR4), which is sensitive to long-chain fatty acids [100]. This activation of microglia and TLR4 leads to an inflammatory cascade mediated by TNFα, interleukin 1β, and interleukin 6 [101]. In addition, stress pathways in the endoplasmic reticulum, the c-jun pathways, and NF-κB pathways are activated leading to further gliosis of the hypothalamus [102]. These inflammatory changes ultimately lead to apoptosis of neurons in the hypothalamus impairing appetite control. First, leptin-based satiety signaling in the hypothalamus is blunted, then the loss of proopiomelanocortin neurons, which reduce appetite and increase energy expenditure, leads to hyperphagia and further weight gain.

This positive feedback loop eventually leads to damage and dysregulation in various other regions of the brain, particularly the hippocampus. The activation of microglia by proinflammatory adipokines and the resulting glial cytokine production cause a breakdown of the blood-brain barrier surrounding the hippocampus allowing reactive lymphocytes to cause neuroinflammation in the region [103]. In addition, triglycerides and fatty acids have been shown to directly lead to hippocampus dysfunction in both animal models and humans [104,105]. The feed-forward loop initiated by hypothalamic inflammation leads to further destruction of the blood-brain barrier in the hippocampus and other regions of the brain leading to global cognitive decline and eventually increasing the lifetime risk of dementia.

Obesity however is a reversible condition. Exercise itself independent of weight loss has been shown to increase neurogenesis and synaptic density, which improves learning and memory function, along with suppressing inflammation in the hippocampus of animal models [106–108]. Similarly, caloric restriction through dieting or intermittent fasting has also shown to reduce markers of oxidative stress and inflammation in the brain [109]. Intermittent fasting particularly has been associated with increased neurogenesis in the hippocampus and neuronal preservation in Alzheimer's disease, Parkinson's disease, and Huntington's disease models. While the mechanisms underlying the neuronal protection effects of caloric restriction and intermittent fasting need further study, BDNF and FGF2 production has been found as possible avenue [110]. In human subjects particularly, higher level of aerobic fitness was associated with increased hippocampal volume and better memory [108]. A study that looked as exercise intervention for 6 months found that the intervention group had improved memory function and increased gray matter in the cingulate gyrus and prefrontal cortex. Finally, an MR spectroscopy study found that endurance athletes tended to have higher levels of N-acetyl-aspartate and choline [111]. Further studies elucidating the underlying mechanisms in cognitive enhancement from weight loss, exercise, and caloric restriction have great promise in producing both novel pharmacological and interventional treatment paradigms to combat cognitive decline and dementia.

Conclusions

As our scientific understanding of adipose tissue expands, the scientific community is better appreciating that adipose tissue is more than just a passive storage site. Adipose tissue is rather a dispersed complex organ that has wide-ranging endocrine properties and affects the function of almost every other organ system. As more research is done, the systemic effects of adipokine secretion are being better understood. The scientific and medical communities are also beginning to appreciate the role of obesity independent of other risk factors in the progression of various disease entities.

Both obesity and neurodegeneration have been on the rise in the developing world, and combating these diseases will be one of the greatest challenges of the 21st century. The deleterious effects of obesity on the CNS have been extensively documented, and almost all studies show that the general proinflammatory state mediated by obesity is one of the central effectors in this process. While weight loss for obese patients is advisable for any number of reasons, much more work needs to be done to further understand the effects of weight loss treatment. Particularly, large-scale studies are needed in comparing weight loss paradigms (i.e., pharmacological versus surgical versus lifestyle modification) and the resulting improvement in CNS disease processes.

While this text has focused on dementia, stroke, MS, and idiopathic intracranial hypertension as specific examples of the effect of obesity on the CNS, the severity of almost all CNS diseases is potentiated by obesity. While obesity prevention through lifestyle management is the best course of action, many studies have shown that weight loss can at least to some measure reduce the severity of the diseases. A deeper understanding of this connection at the mechanistic level however needs to be pursued as this understanding will invariably lead to novel new treatment methods. Understanding the molecular pathways at play in the progression from obesity to inflammation to CNS disorder will likely lead to new translational insights in the form of possible drug targets and new surgical indications for bariatric surgery. These future interventions have the potential in turning the tide in the battle against obesity and its harmful effects on the diseases of the CNS.

References

[1] World Health Organization. Obesity and Overweight. World Health Organization; April 1, 2021. https://www.who.int/news-room/fact-sheets/detail/obesity-and-overweight.
[2] Center for Disease Control and Prevention. Adult Obesity Facts. Centers for Disease Control and Prevention; June 29, 2020. https://www.cdc.gov/obesity/data/adult.html.
[3] O'Brien PD, Hinder LM, Callaghan BC, Feldman EL. Neurological consequences of obesity. Lancet Neurol 2017;16(6):465–77.
[4] Palavra F, Almeida L, Ambrósio AF, Reis F. Obesity and brain inflammation: a focus on multiple sclerosis. Obes Rev 2016;17(3):211–24.
[5] Versini M, Jeandel PY, Rosenthal E, Shoenfeld Y. Obesity in autoimmune diseases: not a passive bystander. Autoimmun Rev 2014;13(9):981–1000.
[6] Bartness TJ, Shrestha YB, Vaughan CH, Schwartz GJ, Song CK. Sensory and sympathetic nervous system control of white adipose tissue lipolysis. Mol Cell Endocrinol 2010;318:34–43.
[7] Kloting N, Bluher M. Adipocyte dysfunction, inflammation and metabolic syndrome. Rev Endocr Metab Disord 2014;15:277–87.
[8] Tchoukalova YD, Votruba SB, Tchkonia T, Giorgadze N, Kirkland JL, Jensen MD. Regional differences in cellular mechanisms of adipose tissue gain with overfeeding. Proc Natl Acad Sci U S A 2010;107:18226–31.

[9] Cildir G, Akincilar SC, Tergaonkar V. Chronic adipose tissue inflammation: all immune cells on the stage. Trends Mol Med 2013;19:487–500.
[10] Blüher M. Adipose tissue dysfunction in obesity. Exp Clin Endocrinol Diabetes 2009;117:241–50.
[11] Booth A, Magnuson A, Fouts J, Foster M. Adipose tissue, obesity and adipokines: role in cancer promotion. Horm Mol Biol Clin Investig 2015;21:57–74.
[12] Roda JM, Eubank TD. The cellular component of chronic inflammation. In: Roy S, Bagchi D, Raychaudhuri SP, editors. Chronic Inflammation: Molecular Pathophysiology, Nutritional and Therapeutic Interventions. USA: CRC Press, Taylor & Francis Group; 2013. p. 21–33 [Chapter 2].
[13] Hotamisligil GS, Shargill NS, Spiegelman BM. Adipose expression of tumor necrosis factor-alpha: direct role in obesity-linked insulin resistance. Science 1993;259:87–91.
[14] Anderson EK, Gutierrez DA, Hasty AH. Adipose tissue recruitment of leukocytes. Curr Opin Lipidol 2010;21:172–7.
[15] Whitmer RA, Gustafson DR, Barrett-Connor E, Haan MN, Gunderson EP, Yaffe K. Central obesity and increased risk of dementia more than three decades later. Neurology 2008;71:1057–64.
[16] Corbett JJ, Savino PJ, Thompson HS, et al. Visual loss in pseudotumor cerebri. Follow-up of 57 patients from five to 41 years and a profile of 14 patients with permanent severe visual loss. Arch Neurol 1982;39(461).
[17] Smith JL. Whence pseudotumor cerebri? J Clin Neuroophthalmol 1985;5:55.
[18] Durcan FJ, Corbett JJ, Wall M. The incidence of pseudotumor cerebri: population studies in Iowa and Louisiana. Arch Neurol 1988;45:875–7.
[19] Craig JJ, Mulholland DA, Gibson JM. Idiopathic intracranial hypertension: incidence, presenting features and outcome in Northern Ireland (1991–1995). Ulster Med J 2001;70:31–5.
[20] Carta A, Bertuzzi F, Cologno D, Giorgi C, Montanari E, Tedesco S. Idiopathic intracranial hypertension (*Pseudotumor cerebri*): descriptive epidemiology, clinical features, and visual outcome in Parma, Italy, 1990 to 1999. Eur J Ophthalmol 2004;14:48–54.
[21] Kesler A, Gadoth N. Epidemiology of idiopathic intracranial hypertension in Israel. J Neuroophthalmol 2001;21:12–4.
[22] Yabe I, Moriwaka F, Notoya A, Ohtaki M, Tashiro K. Incidence of idiopathic intracranial hypertension in Hokkaido, the northernmost island of Japan. J Neurol 2000;247:474–5.
[23] Radhakrishnan K, Thacker AK, Bohlaga NH, Maloo JC, Gerryo SE. Epidemiology of idiopathic intracranial hypertension: a prospective and case-control study. J Neurol Sci 1993;116:18–28.
[24] Raoof N, Sharrack B, Pepper IM, Hickman SJ. The incidence and prevalence of idiopathic intracranial hypertension in Sheffield, UK. Eur J Neurol 2011;18:1266–8.
[25] Kim TW, Choung HK, Khwarg SI, Hwang JM, Yang HJ. Obesity may not be a risk factor for idiopathic intracranial hypertension in Asians. Eur J Neurol 2008;15:876–9.
[26] Liu IH, Wang AG, Yen MY. Idiopathic intracranial hypertension: clinical features in Chinese patients. Jpn J Ophthalmol 2011;55:138–42.
[27] Tibussek D, Distelmaier F, von Kries R, Mayatepek E. Pseudotumor cerebri in childhood and adolescence—results of a Germany-wide ESPED-survey. Klin Padiatr 2013;225:81–5.
[28] Daniels AB, Liu GT, Volpe NJ, et al. Profiles of obesity, weight gain, and quality of life in idiopathic intracranial hypertension (*Pseudotumor cerebri*). Am J Ophthalmol 2007;143:635–41.
[29] Biousse V, Bruce BB, Newman NJ. Update on the pathophysiology and management of idiopathic intracranial hypertension. J Neurol Neurosurg Psychiatry 2012;83:488.

[30] Walker RW. Idiopathic intracranial hypertension: any light on the mechanism of the raised pressure? J Neurol Neurosurg Psychiatry 2001;71:1–5.
[31] Salpietro V, Polizzi A, Berte LF, et al. Idiopathic intracranial hypertension: a unifying neuroendocrine hypothesis through the adrenal-brain axis. Neuro Endocrinol Lett 2012;33:569–73.
[32] Friedman DI, Jacobson DM. Diagnostic criteria for idiopathic intracranial hypertension. Neurology 2002;59:1492–5.
[33] Degnan AJ, Levy LM. Pseudotumor cerebri: brief review of clinical syndrome and imaging findings. AJNR Am J Neuroradiol 2011;32:1986–93.
[34] Salpietro V, Ruggieri M, Sancetta F, et al. New insights on the relationship between pseudotumor cerebri and secondary hyperaldosteronism in children. J Hypertens 2012;30:629–30.
[35] Andrews LE, Liu GT, Ko MW. Idiopathic intracranial hypertension and obesity. Horm Res Paediatr 2014;81(4):217–25. https://doi.org/10.1159/000357730.
[36] Szewka AJ, Bruce BB, Newman NJ, Biousse V. Idiopathic intracranial hypertension: relation between obesity and visual outcomes. J Neuroophthalmol 2013;33:4–8.
[37] Baldwin MK, Lobb B, Tanne E, Egan R. Weight and visual field deficits in women with idiopathic intracranial hypertension. J Womens Health (Larchmt) 2010;19:1893–8.
[38] Lampl Y, Eshel Y, Kessler A, et al. Serum leptin level in women with idiopathic intracranial hypertension. J Neurol Neurosurg Psychiatry 2002;72:642–3.
[39] Behbehani R, Mabrook A, Abbas JM, Al-Rammah T, Mojiminiyi O, Doi SA. Is cerebrospinal fluid leptin altered in idiopathic intracranial hypertension? Clin Endocrinol (Oxf) 2010;72:851–2.
[40] Johnson LN, Krohel GB, Madsen RW, March Jr GA. The role of weight loss and acetazolamide in the treatment of idiopathic intracranial hypertension (*Pseudotumor cerebri*). Ophthalmology 1998;105:2313–7.
[41] Fridley J, Foroozan R, Sherman V, Brandt ML, Yoshor D. Bariatric surgery for the treatment of idiopathic intracranial hypertension. J Neurosurg 2011;114:34–9.
[42] Sugerman HJ, Felton 3rd WL, Sismanis A, Kellum JM, DeMaria EJ, Sugerman EL. Gastric surgery for *Pseudotumor cerebri* associated with severe obesity. Ann Surg 1999;229:634–40 [discussion 640–642].
[43] Kesler A, Kliper E, Shenkerman G, Stern N. Idiopathic intracranial hypertension is associated with lower body adiposity. Ophthalmology 2010;117:169–74.
[44] Celebisoy N, Gökçay F, Sirin H, Akyürekli O. Treatment of idiopathic intracranial hypertension: topiramate vs acetazolamide, an open-label study. Acta Neurol Scand 2007;116:322.
[45] Rasmussen M. Treatment of elevated intracranial pressure with indomethacin: friend or foe? Acta Anaesthesiol Scand 2005;49:341.
[46] Fonseca PL, Rigamonti D, Miller NR, Subramanian PS. Visual outcomes of surgical intervention for pseudotumour cerebri: optic nerve sheath fenestration versus cerebrospinal fluid diversion. Br J Ophthalmol 2014;98:1360.
[47] Puffer RC, Mustafa W, Lanzino G. Venous sinus stenting for idiopathic intracranial hypertension: a review of the literature. J Neurointerv Surg 2013;5:483.
[48] Strazzullo P, D'Elia L, Cairella G, Garbagnati F, Cappuccio FP, Scalfi L. Excess body weight and incidence of stroke: meta-analysis of prospective studies with 2 million participants. Stroke 2010;41(5):e418–26 [Epub 2010/03/20].
[49] Willeumier KC, Taylor DV, Amen DG. Elevated BMI is associated with decreased blood flow in the prefrontal cortex using SPECT imaging in healthy adults. Obesity (Silver Spring) 2011;19(5):1095–7 [Epub 2011/02/12].

[50] Smith AD, Brands MW, Wang MH, Dorrance AM. Obesity-induced hypertension develops in young rats independently of the renin-angiotensin-aldosterone system. Exp Biol Med (Maywood) 2006;231(3):282–7.
[51] Erdos B, Snipes JA, Miller AW, Busija DW. Cerebrovascular dysfunction in Zucker obese rats is mediated by oxidative stress and protein kinase C. Diabetes 2004;53(5):1352–9 [Epub 2004/04/28].
[52] Katakam PV, Wappler EA, Katz PS, et al. Depolarization of mitochondria in endothelial cells promotes cerebral artery vasodilation by activation of nitric oxide synthase. Arterioscler Thromb Vasc Biol 2013;33(4):752–9 [Epub 2013/01/19].
[53] Katakam PV, Jordan JE, Snipes JA, Tulbert CD, Miller AW, Busija DW. Myocardial preconditioning against ischemia-reperfusion injury is abolished in Zucker obese rats with insulin resistance. Am J Physiol Regul Integr Comp Physiol 2007;292(2):R920–6 [Epub 2006/09/30].
[54] Katakam PV, Domoki F, Lenti L, et al. Cerebrovascular responses to insulin in rats. J Cereb Blood Flow Metab 2009;29(12):1955–67 [Epub 2009/09/03].
[55] Razinia T, Saver JL, Liebeskind DS, Ali LK, Buck B, Ovbiagele B. Body mass index and hospital discharge outcomes after ischemic stroke. Arch Neurol 2007;64(3):388–91.
[56] Dell'Omo G, Penno G, Pucci L, Mariani M, Del Prato S, Pedrinelli R. Abnormal capillary permeability and endothelial dysfunction in hypertension with comorbid metabolic syndrome. Atherosclerosis 2004;172(2):383–9 [Epub 2004/03/17].
[57] Terao S, Yilmaz G, Stokes KY, Ishikawa M, Kawase T, Granger DN. Inflammatory and injury responses to ischemic stroke in obese mice. Stroke 2008;39(3):943–50.
[58] Meschia JF, et al. Guidelines for the primary prevention of stroke: a statement for healthcare professionals from the American Heart Association/American Stroke Association. Stroke 2014;45(12):3754–832. https://doi.org/10.1161/STR.0000000000000046.
[59] Neter JE, Stam BE, Kok FJ, Grobbee DE, Geleijnse JM. Influence of weight reduction on blood pressure: a meta-analysis of randomized controlled trials. Hypertension 2003;42:878–84.
[60] World Health Organization. Atlas of multiple sclerosis. Multiple Sclerosis International Federation (MSIF); 2013.
[61] Milo R, Kahana E. Multiple sclerosis: geoepidemiology, genetics and the environment. Autoimmun Rev 2010;9(5):A387–94.
[62] Munger KL, Chitnis T, Ascherio A. Body size and risk of MS in two cohorts of US women. Neurology 2009;73(19):1543–50.
[63] Hedström AK, Olsson T, Alfredsson L. High body index before age 20 is associated with increased risk for multiple sclerosis men and women. Mult Scler J 2012;18(9):1334–6.
[64] Munger KL, Bentzen J, Laursen B, Stenager E, Koch-henriksen N, Sørensen TIA. Childhood body mass index and multiple sclerosis risk: a long-term cohort study. Mult Scler J 2013;19(10):1323–9.
[65] Langer-gould A, Beaber BE. Childhood obesity and risk of pediatric multiple sclerosis and clinically isolated syndrome. Neurology 2013;80(6):548–52.
[66] Hedström AK, Lima Bomfim I, Barcellos L, Gianfrancesco M, Schaefer C, Kockum I, et al. Interaction between adolescent obesity and HLA risk genes in the etiology of multiple sclerosis. Neurology 2014;82(10):865–72.
[67] Matarese G, Di Giacomo A, Sanna V, Lord GM, Howard JK, Di Tuoro A, et al. Requirement for leptin in the induction and progression of autoimmune encephalomyelitis. J Immunol 2001;166(10):5909–16.
[68] Sanna V, Di Giacomo A, La Cava A, Lechler RI, Fontana S, Zappacosta S, et al. Leptin surge precedes onset of autoimmune encephalomyelitis and correlates with development of pathogenic T cell responses. J Clin Invest 2003;111(2):241–50.

[69] Matarese G, Carrieri PB, La Cava A, Perna F, Sanna V, De Rosa V, et al. Leptin increase In multiple sclerosis associates with reduced number of CD4(+) CD25+regulatory T cells. Proc Natl Acad Sci U S A 2005;102(14):5150–5.
[70] MatareseG CPB, Montella S, DeRosa V, La Cava A. Leptin as a metabolic link to multiple sclerosis. Nat Rev Neurol 2010;6(8):455–61.
[71] Mikita J, Dubourdieu-Cassagno N, Deloire MS, Vekris A, Biran M, Raffard G, et al. Altered M1/M2 activation patterns of monocytes in severe relapsing experimental rat model of multiple sclerosis. Amelioration of clinical status by M2 activated monocyte administration. Mult Scler 2011;17(1):2–15.
[72] Kraszula L, Jasińska A, Eusebio M-O, Kuna P, Głąbiński A, Pietruczuk M. Evaluation of the relationship between leptin, resistin, adiponectin and natural regulatory T cells in relapsing-remitting multiple sclerosis. Neurol Neurochir Pol 2012;46(1):22–8.
[73] Olefsky JM, Glass CK. Macrophages, inflammation, and insulin resistance. Annu Rev Physiol 2010;72:219–46.
[74] Odegaard JI, Chawla A. The immune system as a sensor of the metabolic state. Immunity 2013;38:644–54.
[75] Simpson KA, Martin NM, Bloom SR. Hypothalamic regulation of food intake and clinical therapeutic applications. Arq Bras Endocrinol Metab 2009;53:120–8.
[76] Xapelli S, Agasse F, Ferreira R, Silva AP, Malva JO. Neuropeptide Y as an endogenous antiepileptic, neuroprotective and pro-neurogenic peptide. Recent Pat CNS Drug Discov 2006;1:315–24.
[77] Stoof TJ, Flier J, Sampat S, Nieboer C, Tensen CP, Boorsma DM. The antipsoriatic drug dimethylfumarate strongly suppresses chemokine production in human keratinocytes and peripheral blood mononuclear cells. Br J Dermatol 2001;144:1114–20.
[78] Jeong SK, Nam HS, Son MH, Son EJ, Cho KH. Interactive effect of obesity indexes on cognition. Dement Geriatr Cogn Disord 2005;19:91–6.
[79] Yaffe K, Haan MN, Blackwell T, Cherkasova E, Whitmer RA, West N. Metabolic syndrome and cognitive decline in elderly latinos: findings from the SALSA study. J Am Geriatr Soc 2007;55:758–62.
[80] Taylor VH, MacQueen GM. Cognitive dysfunction associated with metabolic syndrome. Obes Rev 2007;8:409–18.
[81] Bruce-Keller AJ, Keller JN, Morrison CD. Obesity and vulnerability of the CNS. In: Biochimica et Biophysica Acta—Molecular Basis of Disease, vol. 1792 (5). Elsevier; 2009. p. 395–400.
[82] Awada R, Parimisetty A, Lefebvre dHellencourt C. Influence of obesity on neurodegenerative diseases. In: Neurodegenerative Diseases. InTech; 2013.
[83] Qiu C, De Ronchi D, Ratiglioni L. The epidemiology of the dementias: an update. Curr Opin Psychiatry 2007;4:380–5.
[84] Debette S, Beiser A, Hoffmann U, Decarli C, O'Donnell CJ, Massaro JM, Au R, Himali JJ, Wolf PA, Fox CS, Seshadri S. Visceral fat is associated with lower brain volume in healthy middle-aged adults. Ann Neurol 2010;68(2):136–44.
[85] Pannacciulli N, Del Parigi A, Chen K, Le DS, Reiman EM, Tataranni PA. Brain abnormalities in human obesity: a voxel-based morphometric study. Neuroimage 2006;31(4):1419–25.
[86] Walther K, Birdsill AC, Glisky EL, Ryan L. Structural brain differences and cognitive functioning related to body mass index in older females. Hum Brain Mapp 2010;31(7):1052–64.
[87] Raji CA, Ho AJ, Parikshak NN, Becker JT, Lopez OL, Kuller LH, Hua X, Leow AD, Toga AW, Thompson PM. Brain structure and obesity. Hum Brain Mapp 2010;31(3):353–64.
[88] Ho AJ, Stein JL, Hua X, Lee S, Hibar DP, Leow AD, Dinov ID, Toga AW, Saykin AJ, Shen L, Foroud T, Pankratz N, Huentelman MJ, Craig DW, Gerber JD, Allen AN,

Corneveaux JJ, Stephan DA, DeCarli CS, DeChairo BM, Potkin SG, Jack Jr CR, Weiner MW, Raji CA, Lopez OL, Becker JT, Carmichael OT, Thompson PM. A commonly carried allele of the obesity-related FTO gene is associated with reduced brain volume in the healthy elderly. Proc Natl Acad Sci U S A 2010;107(18):8404–9.
[89] Gustafson D, Lissner L, Bengtsson C, Bjorkelund C, Skoog I. A 24-year follow-up of body mass index and cerebral atrophy. Neurology 2004;63(10):1876–81.
[90] Mei Z, Grummer-Strawn LM, Pietrobelli A, Goulding A, Goran MI, Dietz WH. Validity of body mass index compared with other body-composition screening indexes for the assessment of body fatness in children and adolescents. Am J Clin Nutr 2002;75:978–85.
[91] Wayner MJ, Armstrong DL, Phelix CF, Oomura Y. Orexin-A (Hypocretin-1) and leptin enhance LTP in the dentate gyrus of rats in vivo. Peptides 2004;25:991–6.
[92] Oomura Y, Hori N, Shiraishi T, Fukunaga K, Takeda H, Tsuji M, Matsumiya T, Ishibashi M, Aou S, Li X, Kohno D, Uramura K, Sougawa H, Yada T, Wayner M, Sasaki K. Leptin facilitates learning and memory performance and enhances hippocampal CA1 long-term potentiation and CaMK II phosphorylation in rats. Peptides 2006;11:2738–49.
[93] Stangl D, Thuret S. Impact of diet on adult hippocampal neurogenesis. Genes Nutr 2009;4(4):271–82.
[94] Harry GJ, McPherson CA, Wine RN, Atkinson K, Lefebvre d'Hellencourt C. Tri- methyltin-induced neurogenesis in the murine hippocampus. Neurotox Res 2004;5(8):623–7.
[95] Thaler JP, Yi CX, Schur EA, Guyenet SJ, Hwang BH, Dietrich MO, Zhao X, Sarruf DA, Izgur V, Maravilla KR, Nguyen HT, Fischer JD, Matsen ME, Wisse BE, Morton GJ, Horvath TL, Baskin DG, Tschop MH, Schwartz MW. Obesity is associated with hypothalamic injury in rodents and humans. J Clin Invest 2012;122(1):153–62.
[96] Kokoeva MV, Yin H, Flier JS. Neurogenesis in the hypothalamus of adult mice: potential role in energy balance. Science 2005;310(5748):679–83.
[97] McNay DE, Briancon N, Kokoeva MV, Maratos-Flier E, Flier JS. Remodeling of the arcuate nucleus energy-balance circuit is inhibited in obese mice. J Clin Invest 2012;122(1):142–52.
[98] Kalmijn S. Fatty acid intake and the risk of dementia and cognitive decline: a review of clinical and epidemiological studies. J Nutr Health Aging 2000;4(4):202–7.
[99] Bouret SG, Gorski JN, Patterson CM, Chen S, Levin BE, Simerly RB. Hypothalamic neural projections are permanently disrupted in diet-induced obese rats. Cell Metab 2008;7(2):179–85. https://doi.org/10.1016/j.cmet.2007.12.001.
[100] Shi H, Kokoeva MV, Inouye K, Tzameli I, Yin H, Flier JS. TLR4 links innate immunity and fatty acid-induced insulin resistance. J Clin Invest 2006;116(11):3015–25.
[101] Drake C, Boutin H, Jones MS, Denes A, McColl BW, Selvarajah JR, Hulme S, Georgiou RF, Hinz R, Gerhard A, Vail A, Prenant C, Julyan P, Maroy R, Brown G, Smigova A, Herholz K, Kassiou M, Crossman D, Francis S, Proctor SD, Russell JC, Hopkins SJ, Tyrrell PJ, Rothwell NJ, Allan SM. Brain inflammation is induced by co-morbidities and risk factors for stroke. Brain Behav Immun 2011;25(6):1113–22.
[102] Lee EB, Mattson MP. The neuropathology of obesity: insights from human disease. In: Acta Neuropathologica, vol. 127 (1). NIH Public Access; 2014. p. 3–28.
[103] Lee J, Duan W, Mattson MP. Evidence that brain-derived neurotrophic factor is required for basal neurogenesis and mediates, in part, the enhancement of neurogenesis by dietary restriction in the hippocampus of adult mice. J Neurochem 2002;82(6):1367–75.
[104] Lee J, Lim E, Kim Y, Li E, Park S. Ghrelin attenuates kainic acid-induced neuronal cell death in the mouse hippocampus. J Endocrinol 2010;205(3):263–70. https://doi.org/10.1677/JOE-10-0040.

[105] Stranahan AM, Lee K, Martin B, Maudsley S, Golden E, Cutler RG, Mattson MP. Voluntary exercise and caloric restriction enhance hippocampal dendritic spine density and BDNF levels in diabetic mice. Hippocampus 2009;19(10):951–61. https://doi.org/10.1002/hipo.20577.

[106] Erickson KI, Prakash RS, Voss MW, Chaddock L, Hu L, Morris KS, White SM, Wojcicki TR, McAuley E, Kramer AF. Aerobic fitness is associated with hippocampal volume in elderly humans. Hippocampus 2009;19(10):1030–9. https://doi.org/10.1002/hipo.20547.

[107] Erickson KI, Voss MW, Prakash RS, Basak C, Szabo A, Chaddock L, Kim JS, Heo S, Alves H, White SM, Wojcicki TR, Mailey E, Vieira VJ, Martin SA, Pence BD, Woods JA, McAuley E, Kramer AF. Exercise training increases size of hippocampus and improves memory. Proc Natl Acad Sci U S A 2011;108(7):3017–22. https://doi.org/10.1073/pnas.1015950108.

[108] Ewers M, Schmitz S, Hansson O, Walsh C, Fitzpatrick A, Bennett D, Minthon L, Trojanowski JQ, Shaw LM, Faluyi YO, Vellas B, Dubois B, Blennow K, Buerger K, Teipel SJ, Weiner M, Hampel H. Body mass index is associated with biological CSF markers of core brain pathology of Alzheimer's disease. Neurobiol Aging 2012;33(8):1599–608. https://doi.org/10.1016/j.neurobiolaging.2011.05.005.

[109] Libert S, Pletcher SD. Modulation of longevity by environmental sensing. Cell 2007;131:1231–4.

[110] Swift DL, Johannsen NM, Myers VH, Earnest CP, Smits JA, Blair SN, Church TS. The effect of exercise training modality on serum brain derived neurotrophic factor levels in individuals with type 2 diabetes. PLoS ONE 2012;7(8). https://doi.org/10.1371/journal.pone.0042785, e42785.

[111] Gonzales MM, Tarumi T, Kaur S, Nualnim N, Fallow BA, Pyron M, Tanaka H, Haley AP. Aerobic fitness and the brain: increased N-acetyl-aspartate and choline concentrations in endurance-trained middle-aged adults. Brain Topogr 2013;26(1):126–34. https://doi.org/10.1007/s10548-012-0248-8.

CHAPTER 11

Obesity, inflammation and muscle weakness

Per-Olof Hasselgren[a,b]
[a]Department of Surgery, Beth Israel Deaconess Medical Center, Boston, MA, United States
[b]George H.A. Clowes Distinguished Professor of Surgery, Harvard Medical School, Boston, MA, United States

Introduction

Obesity and skeletal muscle are related in several ways. Excess body weight in itself may initially result in increased absolute muscle mass and strength secondary to the "training effect" caused by carrying a heavy body. Ultimately, however, this increase in muscle mass and strength may become insufficient to compensate for the enhanced workload caused by excess body weight. This discrepancy will result in "relative muscle weakness" (reduced muscle strength normalized to body mass).

In the elderly, an age-related loss of muscle mass is common. If this condition (sarcopenia) is coupled with obesity, it is frequently referred to as "sarcopenic obesity."

Both these obesity-related muscle impairments will be discussed in this chapter. We will review some aspects of definitions, mechanisms, clinical consequences, diagnostic criteria, and prevention/treatment.

Obesity and relative muscle weakness

Although sarcopenic obesity may be the most significant aspect of obesity-related changes in muscle mass and function, the influence of excess body mass alone (in the absence of sarcopenia) on muscle strength is also important.

Multiple studies have provided evidence for increased absolute muscle mass and function in obesity [1]. When the condition of excess body weight worsens, the increase in muscle weight and strength does not keep up with the upregulated demands, resulting in "relative muscle weakness" [2].

Mechanisms

The increase in absolute muscle mass and function seen in obese individuals mainly reflects the stimulated workload on the antigravity muscles of the lower extremities and can be compared with the effects of exercise and training. This effect of training elicited in skeletal muscle is similar to the increase in lower extremity muscle strength induced experimentally in individuals wearing weighted vests, mimicking the weight of excess body (fat) mass [3]. The notion that the absolute increase in muscle strength in obesity reflects a training effect in lower extremity muscle groups is supported by studies showing unchanged handgrip strength in obese individuals having exercise-induce increased strength of knee extensor muscles [4].

The training effect of obesity is observed in different age groups, ranging from adolescent individuals [5] to young and old adults [4]. Importantly, the obesity-induced increase in absolute muscle strength tapers off with increasing age [6].

When the compensatory muscle hypertrophy in obesity is outpaced by an accelerated increase in excess body weight, muscle mass and function become insufficient to meet the demands of the body weight. The outcome of these changes is reduced muscle mass and strength related to body mass (relative muscle weakness).

Of note, the relative muscle weakness in obesity may not only be the result of a simple mismatch between a continuous increase in body weight and the ability of muscle to respond, but may also, at least in part, reflect intrinsic changes in skeletal muscle induced by obesity. Thus, obesity is associated with multiple metabolic, hormonal, and inflammatory changes that may affect muscle mass and strength and that may ultimately override the compensatory increase in muscle strength seen in obesity [1]. For example, the infiltration of skeletal muscle of adipose tissue, both inter- and intracellularly, documented to occur in obesity, may contribute to the inability of muscle strength to keep up with the increased workload caused by excess body mass [7]. Recent studies revealing the importance of fat tissue surrounding muscles (perimuscular adipose tissue, PMAT) may offer an additional mechanism by which muscles develop weakness in obesity [8].

The role of adipose tissue in the regulation of circulating levels of hormones and proinflammatory cytokines is becoming increasingly recognized, in part reflecting the endocrine and inflammatory properties of fat tissue [9]. Several of these factors may play a role in declining muscle strength in obese individuals even without actual loss of muscle mass but become even more important in sarcopenic obesity.

Clinical consequences of relative muscle weakness in obesity

Notwithstanding that sarcopenic obesity is accompanied by particularly severe clinical consequences, the relative muscle weakness seen in obese individuals without muscle wasting is also associated with impairment of physical activities. Supporting that notion, Rolland et al. [10] described self-reported difficulties with physical activities (walking, climbing stairs, and rising from a chair) in four groups of women 75 years old or older (healthy, purely sarcopenic, purely obese, or sarcopenic obese). Women being purely obese had an approximately 40%–80% higher probability of experiencing physical difficulties than women in the healthy group. This observation probably at least in part reflected obesity-related relative muscle weakness. Somewhat surprisingly, the purely sarcopenic women had no increased odds of having impaired physical activities, whereas when sarcopenia coexisted with obesity, the likelihood of having difficulties walking, climbing stairs, and rising from a chair was 2.6 times greater than in healthy women. The observations reported by Rolland et al. [10] are important because they confirm that obesity alone may give rise to physical difficulties, at least in elderly individuals. The results also suggest that obesity and sarcopenia act in a synergistic fashion, dramatically increasing the risk of physical disability.

In addition to difficulties walking, climbing stairs, and rising from a chair, obese individuals with reduced relative muscle strength may experience impaired postural stability [11], which in turn increases the risk of falls, fractures, and physical impediment [12]. Studies suggest that reduced strength and function of the plantar flexor muscles may be important for the inadequate postural stability and increased risk of falls in obese persons [1,13].

Prevention and treatment

An important implication of the relative muscle weakness in obese individuals is that weight-losing programs need to be applied with caution. An exceedingly aggressive weight loss may result not only in loss of fat mass but also in muscle mass, potentially even risking induction of sarcopenia [14–16]. This "side effect" of excessive weight loss may aggravate some of the clinical consequences of obesity, at least those related to muscle weakness. For example, although bariatric surgery has proven effective in decreasing excess body weight and ameliorating many of the metabolic consequences of obesity [17], studies suggest that muscle tissue may be negatively affected. In a study by Lyytinen at al [16], bariatric surgery resulted in increased content of fat and connective tissue in skeletal muscle. Vaurs et al. [14] reported that in more than half of obese patients undergoing bariatric surgery, >15% of the initial weight loss reflected loss of muscle mass. Although these potential negative effects on skeletal muscle are probably by far outweighed by the positive influence of bariatric surgery and other weight-reducing regimens on many obesity-related conditions (including diabetes, hypertension, inflammation, and cancer), researchers and clinicians should be aware of the relationship between rapid and pronounced weight loss and the influence on muscle mass, quality, and strength.

These aspects of weight loss therapies are even more important for patients with sarcopenic obesity in whom further loss of muscle mass during weight reduction may be particularly detrimental.

Sarcopenic obesity

It is well known that the prevalence of obesity has reached epidemic levels both in this country and globally [18–20]. At the same time, longevity is increasing in many countries; recent estimates suggest that adults above the age of 65 make up 13% of the global population and presently represent the fastest-growing demographic group in the world, expected to reach 2.1 billion within the next 30 years [21,22]. As we grow older, our muscles start to undergo atrophy, resulting in age-dependent sarcopenia [21,23]. In combination, these demographic changes (increasing prevalence of obesity and growing numbers of elderly people) are creating a "perfect storm" of sarcopenic obesity.

In this segment of the chapter, we will review the current understanding of sarcopenic obesity, paying special attention to definitions, prevalence, diagnosis, mechanisms, clinical consequences, and prevention/treatment.

Definitions

Although the overall definition of sarcopenic obesity (the combination of sarcopenia and obesity) is relatively straightforward and easy to understand, numerous different definitions of both components of the condition are used by clinicians and researchers, making the field somewhat complicated. The lack of a universal definition is commonly quoted as a reason why the advancement of the understanding of the condition has been slowed and was one of the key points in a recent review by Zamboni et al. [24]: "Many definitions of sarcopenic obesity have been proposed, but a clear and decisive definition is still lacking."

Even if the term sarcopenia is most commonly used to describe loss of muscle mass and strength in elderly (>65 years) individuals [25], in the context of sarcopenic obesity, many different alternative definitions have been employed. The word sarcopenia is sometimes substituted for by muscle atrophy or muscle wasting [26,27], focusing on the loss of muscle mass in the context of sarcopenia. Because loss of muscle quality and strength are equally important in sarcopenia, the terms muscle atrophy and muscle wasting cannot fully substitute for sarcopenia. Although obesity can be associated with both sarcopenia and cachexia [28], muscle cachexia is typically described as a component of a syndrome consisting of loss of muscle mass (often severe loss of muscle mass) and body weight, loss of appetite, and reduced food intake [29].

Different definitions of the sarcopenia component of sarcopenic obesity were summarized in recent reviews [21,30]. Changes in muscle mass, strength, and function have been part of the description of sarcopenic obesity. In several reports, the muscle mass was assessed by dual-energy X-ray absorptiometry (DEXA) [25,31] and reported as "appendicular lean mass," (ALM), typically meaning lower extremity muscle mass, divided by height (in meters) square. Using this measure, cutoffs ranging from 7.23 to 8.51 kg/m^2 in men and from 5.45 to 6.29 kg/m^2 in women have been used to define sarcopenia [25,32–36]. In some studies, physical function, measured as gait speed [31] or muscle (handgrip) strength [25], was included in the definition of the sarcopenia component of sarcopenic obesity.

Even the obesity component of sarcopenic obesity is not always universally defined. Although a BMI $\geq 30\,\text{kg/m}^2$ is commonly used [37], other definitions have also been employed, including "an unhealthy excess body fat that increases the risk of medical illness and mortality" [38], body fat as percentage of body weight (> 25%–37% for men and > 38%–40% for women) [21,32,39], and waist circumference as a surrogate for abdominal fat ($\geq 102\,\text{cm}$ for men and $\geq 88\,\text{cm}$ for women) [21].

While obesity is commonly seen in the absence of sarcopenia and sarcopenia can occur without excess body and fat mass, the combination of the two conditions (sarcopenic obesity) creates particularly challenging consequences.

Prevalence

In part reflecting the lack of clear definitions of the sarcopenia and obesity components of sarcopenic obesity, a wide range of the prevalence of sarcopenic obesity has been reported. In many studies, the prevalence was higher in women than men. In a report by Stenholm et al. [30] reviewing the definition, cause, and consequences of sarcopenic obesity, the prevalence of the condition ranged from 4.4% to 9.6% in men and from 7.4% to 12.4% in women when muscle mass was used to assess sarcopenia and body fat percentage to determine obesity. Similar estimates of the prevalence of sarcopenic obesity have been reported by other investigators [32,39,40] with even wider ranges of the prevalence described by others [21].

Mechanisms

When sarcopenia and obesity occur in the same individual, the progress of the condition is influenced by interactions between fat and muscle, both at the physical and molecular levels, often creating vicious cycles worsening the consequences of sarcopenic obesity. Indeed, the consequences of sarcopenia and obesity are augmented in a synergistic fashion when present simultaneously [1,10].

There are several mechanisms that may explain why the interaction between sarcopenia and obesity results in a vicious cycle, worsening the effects of both conditions. One mechanism is centered on the reduced physical activity caused by both sarcopenia and obesity. Other mechanisms are to be found at the molecular level with influences of hormones and regulators of inflammation in both fat and muscle tissue.

Reduced physical activity

As mentioned, the sarcopenia component of sarcopenic obesity has been defined and assessed in several different ways, contributing to the confusion plaguing the research and clinical fields of the disorder [24]. Sarcopenia alone is often referred to as age-related loss of muscle mass and strength. Investigators have provided more encompassing definitions. For example, Cruz-Jentoft et al. [41] recently reported an updated European consensus on the definition and diagnosis of the condition describing sarcopenia as "a muscle disease (muscle failure) rooted in the adverse muscle changes that accrue across a life time; sarcopenia is common among adults of older age but can also occur earlier in life. Low muscle strength is a key characteristic of sarcopenia." An additional definition of sarcopenia emphasized the consequences of the condition: "A progressive and generalized skeletal muscle disorder involving the accelerated loss of muscle mass and function that is associated with increased adverse outcomes including falls, functional decline, frailty, and mortality" [42].

Mechanisms involved in sarcopenia were reviewed recently by Wiedmer et al. [43]. Although altered life style with lack of exercise is one of the mechanisms of sarcopenia, the condition in itself further reduces the inclination to participate in physical activity, thus creating a vicious cycle.

Other mechanisms contributing to the loss of muscle mass in elderly individuals are reduced synthesis and/or increased degradation of muscle proteins, in particular myofibrillar proteins, secondary to hormonal changes, such as age-related decreases of growth hormone, testosterone, and IGF-1, and increased circulating and tissue levels of proinflammatory cytokines (TNFα, IL-1β, and IL-6).

Decreased neuromuscular function and impaired recruitment of satellite cells are additional mechanisms contributing to sarcopenia. In addition, changes in eating habits and reduced food intake in elderly individuals, even to the level of malnutrition, may also be part of the development of sarcopenia [44].

Obesity, even without sarcopenia, is associated with reduced physical activity. Multiple factors contribute to the lack of exercise among individuals with obesity. The increased workload caused by excess body weight is an important reason why obesity hinders physical activity. Joint pain, in particular from the hips and knees, is aggravated by obesity [45,46]. A "shame factor" ("weight stigma") may contribute to the unwillingness to participate in sports and other types of physical exercise among overweight persons, further increasing the accumulation of excess body weight [47]. Poor education and an inability to realize the connection between lack of physical activity and obesity may be an additional factor why obese individuals do not exercise [48].

The central role of reduced physical activity in the vicious cycle created by the coexistence of sarcopenia and obesity is illustrated in Fig. 1.

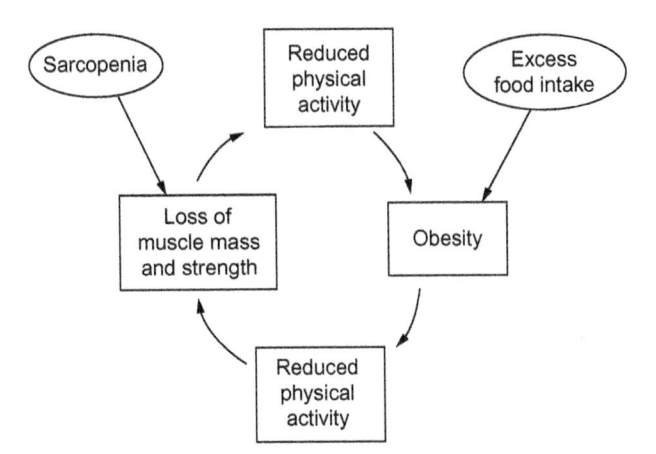

Fig. 1 Both sarcopenia and excess body weight are associated with reduced physical activity. The two conditions act together creating a vicious cycle in sarcopenic obesity.

Of note, sarcopenia may not only coexist with obesity (as in sarcopenic obesity) but may interact with and worsen other conditions as well, including liver and kidney diseases [27,49–51].

Proinflammatory cytokines

There is overwhelming evidence that obesity results in a state of inflammation. The adipose tissue becomes a source of production and release of TNFα, IL-1β, and IL-6, in part reflecting the production of the cytokines by hypertrophic and hyperplastic adipocytes [52,53] and in part reflecting the activation of proinflammatory macrophages [54].

The increased production and release of proinflammatory mediators result in elevated circulating levels of the cytokines, targeting multiple organs and tissues [55]. In skeletal muscle, proinflammatory cytokines stimulate breakdown of myofibrillar proteins, resulting in loss of muscle mass and strength [56,57]. The mechanisms regulating the catabolic effects of proinflammatory cytokines in skeletal muscle are complex and involve posttranslational modifications of various transcription factors and activation of ubiquitin-proteasome-dependent protein breakdown as well as other proteolytic pathways [58].

In addition to direct cellular and molecular catabolic effects in the myocyte, proinflammatory cytokines can also exert atrophic effects by inducing insulin resistance [59].

Of note, proinflammatory cytokines are also involved in the regulation of muscle breakdown in sarcopenia [60], in part explaining why the loss of muscle mass and strength is particularly severe in sarcopenic obesity.

Importantly, studies suggest that muscle-derived myokines and proinflammatory cytokines can influence the inflammatory response in adipose tissue, providing evidence for an intriguing cross talk between muscle and fat tissue [61–63]. For example, IL-6 released from myocytes may influence metabolism in adipose tissue, and IL-6 secreted from adipocytes can influence protein metabolism in skeletal muscle [61]. These interactions form the basis for an additional vicious cycle in sarcopenic obesity.

Adipokines (leptin and adiponectin)

Adipokines are regulatory proteins released from adipose tissue. Leptin and adiponectin are the most important adipokines with regard to obesity-associated inflammation [64–66]. The production of leptin is increased in obesity, and the adiponectin production is reduced. Leptin has pronounced proinflammatory properties, in part reflecting stimulated production of TNFα, IL-1β, and IL-6 in adipocytes and proinflammatory macrophages in adipose tissue [54,67].

Studies suggest that adipose tissue is not the sole source of adipokines. Both leptin and adiponectin are also produced by myocytes, making skeletal muscle an additional important site of adipokine production [68,69]. The production of leptin and adiponectin in both muscle and adipose tissue illustrates the importance of a complex interaction and cross talk between muscle and adipose tissue in sarcopenic obesity [61–63,68–70].

There is evidence that leptin may be involved in the development of sarcopenia in the elderly, probably reflecting increased production of the adipokine in both fat and muscle tissue [71]. The increased expression of leptin in aging skeletal muscle may at least in part originate from adipocytes accumulated in muscle (intermuscular adipose tissue) and may induce sarcopenia-like changes secondary to IL-6-mediated inflammation [72]. The increased production of leptin in both muscle and adipose tissue plays an important role in accelerating the loss of muscle mass in sarcopenic obesity [73,74].

In addition to interacting with and stimulating the production of proinflammatory cytokines, the catabolic effects of leptin may also reflect its opposing effects to insulin [8,75,76].

Importantly, obesity results in reduced production of the antiinflammatory adipokine adiponectin (in addition to the increased production of the proinflammatory leptin) both in adipose tissue and skeletal muscle [64–66,69]. The decrease in adiponectin levels worsens the obesity-induced inflammation and the muscle catabolism seen in sarcopenic obesity.

The perturbed balance between leptin and adiponectin is an important factor for the catabolic response in skeletal muscle. In addition to upregulated expression of proinflammatory cytokines, insulin resistance caused by the changes in the adipokine levels contributes to the negative protein balance seen in catabolic muscle. Thus, high leptin levels and low levels of the "insulin-sensitizer" adiponectin work together in the induction of insulin resistance [8,70,75–77].

Myokines

Myokines are regulatory peptides produced and released by myocytes. The myokines are important in the regulation of muscle metabolism but can also influence metabolism in other organs and tissues, including adipose tissue [78].

Recent research has focused on the role of muscle-adipose tissue cross talk involving myokines and adipokines in sarcopenic obesity [61–63,68–70,79].

The myokines that have been most widely studied in the regulation of muscle protein metabolism and muscle mass in the context of sarcopenic obesity include myostatin and irisin. Although, in this chapter, we will mainly review the roles of myostatin and irisin in sarcopenic obesity, it is worth noting that the family of myokines is large and keeps growing, containing other regulatory peptides, such as IL-6, IL-8, IL-15, fibroblast growth factor 21, and myonectin. The more complete role of these myokines in obesity and obesity-associated muscle weakness remains to be further explored.

Obesity is associated with increased circulating levels of myostatin [80]. Myostatin produced by myocytes influences muscle mass by autocrine and paracrine mechanisms. Myostatin released into the circulation from muscle acts as a hormone, influencing metabolism in other organs and tissues, including adipose tissue [81,82]. In general, myostatin regulates many metabolic changes seen during inflammation. In skeletal muscle, increased levels of myostatin result in loss of muscle mass, similar to sarcopenic obesity [83] and several other muscle-wasting conditions, such as cancer [84], sepsis [85], and critical illness [86].

Interestingly, myostatin contributes to the obesity-induced inflammatory response in adipose tissue, reflecting the muscle to adipose tissue cross talk [87]. Experimental work in myostatin-null mice provided evidence that myostatin is involved in the development of diet-induced obesity, fat mass accumulation, and metabolic dysfunction [81,88]. Blocking myostatin with an antimyostatin peptibody in mice with diet-induced obesity suppressed the obesity-induced increase of proinflammatory cytokines and M1 (inflammatory) macrophages in adipose tissue [89]. In the same study, inhibition of myostatin also prevented the inflammatory response in skeletal muscle, stimulated muscle growth, and improved insulin sensitivity. Taken together, results from previous studies support an important role of increased myostatin expression in the development of obesity and obesity-induced inflammatory responses in adipose tissue and muscle. The results also provide strong support for a muscle to adipose tissue cross talk involving myostatin. The observations have significant clinical implications with regard to sarcopenic obesity [83,88,90]. Indeed, myostatin has been suggested as a target for the prevention and treatment of obesity-induced metabolic changes [80].

In contrast to myostatin, the production of irisin is reduced in obesity, although some controversy exists [91]. Myostatin and irisin have several opposite biological functions, both in adipose and muscle tissue. Whereas myostatin induces an inflammatory response to obesity in adipose tissue

[81,82,87] and promotes muscle wasting [83–86], irisin reduces obesity-induced inflammation in adipose tissue [92] and is a promyogenic factor that induces skeletal muscle hypertrophy [93].

Myostatin and irisin are reversely related, not only with regard to their functions, but also with regard to their production. For example, inhibition of myostatin in obese mice resulted in increased irisin levels in both muscle and adipose tissue, and the increase in irisin levels was at least in part responsible for the beneficial effects of mysostatin inhibition [89,94].

Recent in vitro experiments shed further light on the interaction between myostatin and irisin. When cultured human muscle cells were treated with irisin, myostatin expression decreased [95]. Interestingly, in the same experiments, treatment of the muscle cells with irisin increased the production of IGF-1, providing a potential mechanism by which irisin exerts its promyogenic effects [93,95,96].

It should be noted that low irisin levels may not only be involved in obesity-associated sarcopenia but in other metabolic consequences of obesity as well, including type 2 diabetes mellitus, cardiovascular disease, and nonalcoholic fatty liver disease [97,98].

The cross talk of myokines, proinflammatory cytokines, and adipokines between muscle and adipose tissue and its role in sarcopenic obesity are illustrated in Fig. 2.

The importance of a cross talk between adipocytes and myocytes in the development of muscle wasting in sarcopenic obesity is further illustrated

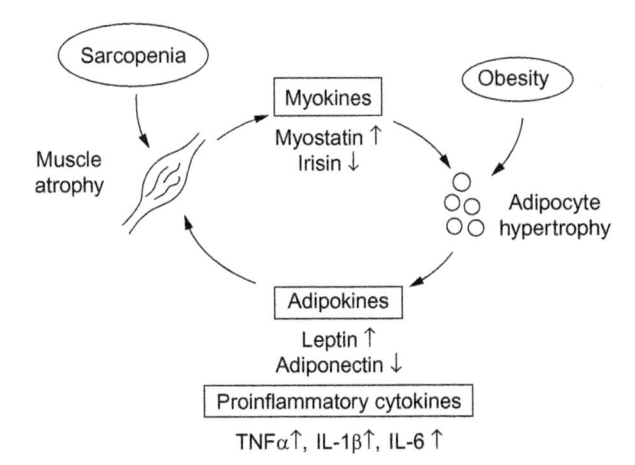

Fig. 2 The regulatory peptides released from muscle and adipose tissue interact and influence both tissues, creating another vicious cycle in sarcopenic obesity.

by the infiltration into skeletal muscle of fat cells (intramuscular adipose tissue, IMAT) [99] and the accumulation in muscle of lipid metabolic products in obesity [100].

In addition to intramuscular infiltration of fat tissue, studies suggest that elderly individuals with sarcopenia display accumulation of PMAT around atrophic muscles [8]. Recent observations provided evidence for a cross talk between PMAT and the adjacent muscles resulting in the breakdown of muscle proteins [101]. The muscle protein degradation induced by PMAT was regulated by the same molecular mechanisms that are involved in other muscle-wasting conditions, including cancer critical illness, and sepsis [84–86].

A more detailed and comprehensive review of factors involved in the cross talk between muscle and adipose tissue in sarcopenia was provided by Kablinkovich and Livshits [100].

Hormones

Hormonal changes induced by aging and obesity are additional factors involved in sarcopenic obesity. Some of the endocrine adjustments are secondary to changes in proinflammatory cytokines, adipokines, and myokines. Recent studies confirm the development of insulin resistance in patients with sarcopenic obesity [90,102,103]. Reduced insulin sensitivity results in muscle atrophy secondary to reduced synthesis and increased degradation of muscle proteins and is an important mechanism of age-related sarcopenia and the worsened loss of muscle mass in sarcopenic obesity.

Several factors contribute to insulin resistance in sarcoepnic obesity, including elevated levels of proinflammatory cytokines, in particular TNFα [104], and leptin [105]. Increased myostatin levels may be especially important for the insulin resistance in skeletal muscle in subjects with sarcopenic obesity [90].

In addition to insulin resistance, reduced levels of IGF-1 contribute to the loss of muscle mass in sarcopenic obesity [106]. Exercise, in particular resistance training, has proven beneficial on both muscle strength and IGF-1 levels in older adults with sarcopenic obesity [106].

Testosterone and growth hormone are additional anabolic hormones involved in the maintenance of muscle mass and strength. Studies suggest that reduced levels of these hormones in aging individuals are important factors for the development of sarcopenic obesity [21,107,108]. In elderly individuals, obesity is associated with depressed growth homone secretion, at least in part accounting for the loss of muscle mass [108]. In a recent report, decreased salivary levels of testosterone were proposed as a biomarker for the diagnosis of sarcopenic obesity in elderly individuals [109]. In adult women with sarcopenic obesity (mean BMI 44 kg/m^2), loss of muscle mass was associated with reduced levels of thyroid hormones, providing an additional potential hormonal mechanism of sarcopenic obesity [110].

Clinical consequences

Sarcopenic obesity is associated with multiple clinical consequences. The condition results in frailty, in part reflecting the discrepancy between the loss of muscle mass and strength and the increased demand for strength to carry excess body weight. Other clinical consequences of sarcopenic obesity are related to the interaction with coexisting diseases, both with regard to the severity and the treatment of such diseases.

Sarcopenic obesity and frailty

An important consequence of sarcopenic obesity in the elderly is the development of frailty. The loss of muscle strength severely reduces the quality of life in many respects. Individuals with sarcopenic obesity may experience difficulties climbing and descending stairs, rising up from a chair, and getting out of bed [10,33,111,112]. The difficulties negotiating stairs may also be aggravated by reduced postural stability [11]. Although loss of handgrip strength is commonly used as a diagnostic tool for muscle weakness in sarcopenic obesity, it may in itself also lead to reduced quality of life due to impaired functions when working in the kitchen or performing other household tasks [113].

A severe consequence of frailty in individuals with sarcopenic obesity is an increased risk of falls and fractures [114–116]. The increased load on the lower extremities coupled with reduced muscular strength to protect the joints may explain a more than twofold increase in the prevalence of knee osteoarthritis in sarcopenic obesity [117,118]. Studies suggest that the obesity is a more important factor than the sarcopenia component of sarcopenic obesity for the development of knee osteoarthritis [118].

Sarcopenic obesity and cancer

Sarcopenic obesity has several important implications with regard to cancer. First, individuals with sarcopenic obesity have an increased risk of various cancers, at least in part reflecting the well-documented risk of cancer in obese persons [119,120]. Second, advanced cancer is often associated with muscle wasting (cachexia) [29], which may worsen the sarcopenia component of sarcopenic obesity. Third, patients with sarcopenic obesity often do worse from their malignancies. For example, overall death rates from various types of cancer are increased in patients with sarcopenic obesity [26,121].

Finally, the treatment for cancer can be negatively affected by sarcopenic obesity. For instance, complications after surgery for gastric or pancreatic cancer are increased in patients with sarcopenic obesity [26,122–124]. It is not only the surgical care of patients with cancer that may be negatively impacted by sarcopenic obesity. Studies have shown that patients with cancer and sarcopenic obesity undergoing chemotherapy experience more toxic effects and develop dose-limiting toxicity more often than nonsarcopenic obese patients [28,125].

Sarcopenic obesity and coexisting conditions other than cancer

Sarcopenic obesity may be a complicating factor in the care of patients with coexisting conditions other than cancer. Critically ill patients cared for in the ICU are challenged by metabolic stress, muscle wasting, and need for extra nutritional support [126]. The muscle wasting in critical illness is aggravated and at least in part caused by glucocorticoids and ventilator support. The metabolic challenges and muscle wasting experienced in the ICU are magnified in patients with sarcopenic obesity by mechanisms involved in the molecular regulation of muscle protein breakdown [127]. Although much research and effort have been spent on optimizing the metabolic and nutritional care of patients in the ICU, there is still a need for a better understanding of the role of nutrition in patients with sarcopenic obesity who are treated in the ICU [127].

Other conditions that may need extra attention if associated with sarcopenic obesity include kidney failure, in particular in patients undergoing peritoneal dialysis [128–130], and liver cirrhosis in patients needing a liver transplantation [131].

Treatment

Although both the excess fat mass and the sarcopenia component need to be addressed in the treatment of sarcopenic obesity, the cross talk between muscle and adipose tissue necessitates a comprehensive approach taking both aspects of the condition into account. One important and seemingly paradoxical phenomenon, already alluded to, is that the loss of muscle mass in sarcopenic obesity may actually be worsened if the weight-reducing treatments are too aggressive [14–16].

Several studies have focused on the effects of different types of exercise in patients with sarcopenic obesity [106,132]. Chen et al. [106] reported that both resistance training and aerobic training increased muscle mass in individuals 65–75 years old who presented with sarcopenic obesity. Results in that study suggested that the beneficial effects of exercise on muscle strength may be related to an increase in IGF-1 levels. In addition, the exercise did not only improve muscle mass, but also reduced visceral fat [106].

Other studies have highlighted the importance of nutritional support, in particular protein supplementation, when individuals with sarcopenic obesity undergo exercise training [133,134].

In addition to physical exercise, pharmacological and hormonal treatments may also be beneficial in the management of sarcopenic obesity. For example, in animal experiments, resveratrol prevented high-fat diet-induced obesity and muscle atrophy in aged rodents [135]. Other studies suggested that vitamin D supplementation may improve muscle mass in "pre-sarcopenic" elderly individuals [136]. In older men with low testosterone levels and frailty, testosterone treatment increased insulin sensitivity and improved body composition, suggesting a potential role of testosterone treatment to reduce the progression of sarcopenia and frailty [107].

Summary and conclusions

Obesity and muscle strength are related in at least two different ways. In individuals without muscle atrophy, obesity initially results in muscle hypertrophy and increased strength. This effect of obesity is a result of a "training effect" caused by the increased workload on muscle related to carrying excess body weight. If the progression of obesity continues with accumulation of more excess body weight, the muscle hypertrophy and strength are not sufficient to compensate for the increased demand resulting in "relative muscle weakness."

If elderly individuals with age-related muscle atrophy and weakness (sarcopenia) also develop obesity, the combined condition is called "sarcopenic obesity." This is a serious condition with the negative effects of sarcopenia and obesity acting synergistically. The synergistic interaction between sarcopenia and obesity at least in part reflects the release of inflammatory mediators from both muscle and adipose tissue with a cross talk between the two tissues. Sarcopenic obesity is associated with multiple significant clinical consequences, including frailty, risk for falls and fractures, impairment of daily activities (such as climbing stairs and inability to perform common household activities), increased risk of diabetes, and other metabolic adverse effects. The risk of cancer is increased in individuals with sarcopenic obesity and the treatment (both surgical and nonsurgical) of malignancies is also negatively affected by sarcopenic obesity. An increased awareness of these risk factors is important when carrying for patients with sarcopenic obesity.

Different treatment strategies in the management of patients with sarcopenic obesity, in addition to inducing weight loss by reduced food intake or bariatric surgery, include various exercise regimens and hormonal and nutritional treatments. An important aspect of weight loss regimens in sarcopenic obesity is that an overly aggressive weight loss may also aggravate the sarcopenia why weight loss regimens need to be applied with caution in these patients.

References

[1] Tomlinson DJ, Erskine RM, Morse CI, Winwood K, Onambélé-Pearson G. The impact of obesity on skeletal muscle strength and structure through adolescence to old age. Biogerontology 2016;17:467–83.
[2] LaRoche DP, Kralian RJ, Millett ED. Fat mass limits lower-extremity relative strength and maximal walking performance in older women. J Electromyogr Kinesiol 2011;21:754–61.
[3] Bosco C, Rusko H, Hirvonen J. The effect of extra-load conditioning on muscle performance in athletes. Med Sci Sports Exerc 1986;18:415–9.
[4] Hulens M, Vansant G, Lysens R, Claessens AL, Muls E, Brumagne S. Study of differences in peripheral muscle strength of lean versus obese women: an allometric approach. Int J Obes Relat Metab Disord 2001;25:676–81.
[5] Blimkie CJ, Sale DG, Bar-Or O. Voluntary strength, evoked twitch contractile properties and motor unit activation of knee extensors in obese and non-obese adolescent males. Eur J Appl Physiol Occup Physiol 1990;61:313–8.
[6] Hulens M, Vansant G, Lysens R, Claessens AL, Muls E. Assessment of isokinetic muscle strength in women who are obese. J Orthop Sports Phys Ther 2002;32:347–56.
[7] Delmonico MJ, Harris TB, Visser M, et al. Longitudinal study of muscle strength, quality, and adipose tissue infiltration. Am J Clin Nutr 2009;90:1579–85.
[8] Wu H, Ballantyne CM. Skeletal muscle inflammation and insulin resistance in obesity. J Clin Invest 2017;127:43–54.
[9] Kojta I, Chacińska M, Błachnio-Zabielska A. Obesity, bioactive lipids, and adipose tissue inflammation in insulin resistance. Nutrients 2020;12:1305.
[10] Rolland Y, Lauwers-Cances V, Cristini C, et al. Difficulties with physical function associated with obesity, sarcopenia, and sarcopenic-obesity in community-dwelling elderly women: the EPIDOS (EPIDemiologie de l'OSteoporose) study. Am J Clin Nutr 2009;89:1895–900.
[11] Maffiuletti NA, Agosti F, Proietti M, et al. Postural instability of extremely obese individuals improves after a body weight reduction program entailing specific balance training. J Endocrinol Invest 2005;28:2–7.
[12] Himes CL, Reynolds SL. Effect of obesity on falls, injury, and disability. J Am Geriatr Soc 2012;60:124–9.
[13] Onambele GL, Narici MV, Maganaris CN. Calf muscle-tendon properties and postural balance in old age. J Appl Physiol 2006;100:2048–56.

[14] Vaurs C, Diméglio C, Charras L, Anduze Y, Chalret du Rieu M, Ritz P. Determinants of changes in muscle mass after bariatric surgery. Diabetes Metab 2015;41:416–21.
[15] Thibault R, Huber O, Azagury DE, Pichard C. Twelve key nutritional issues in bariatric surgery. Clin Nutr 2016;35:12–7.
[16] Lyytinen T, Liikavainio T, Pääkkönen M, Gylling H, Arokoski JP. Physical function and properties of quadriceps femoris muscle after bariatric surgery and subsequent weight loss. J Musculoskelet Neuronal Interact 2013;13:329–38.
[17] Arterburn DE, Telem DA, Kushner RF, Courcoulas AP. Benefits and risks of bariatric surgery in adults: a review. JAMA 2020;324:879–87.
[18] Barazzoni R, Bischoff S, Boirie Y, et al. Sarcopenic obesity: time to meet the challenge. Obes Facts 2018;11:294–305.
[19] NCD Risk Factor Collaboration (NCD-RisC). Trends in adult body-mass index in 200 countries from 1975 to 2014: a pooled analysis of 1698 population-based measurement studies with 19·2 million participants. Lancet 2016;387:1377–96.
[20] Global BMI Mortality Collaboration, Di Angelantonio E, Bhupathiraju S, Wormser D, et al. Body-mass index and all-cause mortality: individual-participant-data meta-analysis of 239 prospective studies in four continents. Lancet 2016;388:776–86.
[21] Batsis JA, Villareal DT. Sarcopenic obesity in older adults: aetiology, epidemiology and treatment strategies. Nat Rev Endocrinol 2018;14:513–37.
[22] Hales CM, Carroll MD, Fryar CD, Ogden CL. Prevalence of obesity and severe obesity among adults: United States, 2017–2018. NCHS Data Brief 2020;360:1–8.
[23] Sayer AA, Syddall H, Martin H, Patel H, Baylis D, Cooper C. The developmental origins of sarcopenia. J Nutr Health Aging 2008;12:427–32.
[24] Zamboni M, Rubele S, Rossi AP. Sarcopenia and obesity. Curr Opin Clin Nutr Metab Care 2019;22:13–9.
[25] Cruz-Jentoft AJ, Baeyens JP, Bauer JM, et al. Sarcopenia: European consensus on definition and diagnosis: report of the European working group on sarcopenia in older people. Age Ageing 2010;39:412–23.
[26] Baracos VE, Arribas L. Sarcopenic obesity: hidden muscle wasting and its impact for survival and complications of cancer therapy. Ann Oncol 2018;29(supplement 2):ii1–9.
[27] Guida B, Trio R, Di Maro M, et al. Prevalence of obesity and obesity-associated muscle wasting in patients on peritoneal dialysis. Nutr Metab Cardiovasc Dis 2019;29:1390–9.
[28] Prado CM, Cushen SJ, Orsso CE, Ryan AM. Sarcopenia and cachexia in the era of obesity: clinical and nutritional impact. Proc Nutr Soc 2016;75:188–98.
[29] Baracos VE, Martin L, Korc M, Guttridge DC, Fearon KCH. Cancer-associated cachexia. Nat Rev Dis Primers 2018;4:17105.
[30] Stenholm S, Harris TB, Rantanen T, Visser M, Kritchevsky SB, Ferrucci L. Sarcopenic obesity: definition, cause and consequences. Curr Opin Clin Nutr Metab Care 2008;11:693–700.
[31] Perez-Sousa MA, Venegas-Sanabria LC, Chavarro-Carvajal DA, et al. Gait speed as a mediator of the effect of sarcopenia on dependency in activities of daily living. Cachexia Sarcopenia Muscle 2019;10:1009–15.
[32] Baumgartner RN. Body composition in healthy aging. Ann N Y Acad Sci 2000;904:437–48.
[33] Janssen I, Baumgartner RN, Ross R, Rosenberg IH, Roubenoff R. Skeletal muscle cutpoints associated with elevated physical disability risk in older men and women. Am J Epidemiol 2004;159:413–21.
[34] Newman AB, Kupelian V, Visser M, et al. Sarcopenia: alternative definitions and associations with lower extremity function. J Am Geriatr Soc 2003;51:1602–9.
[35] Dent E, Morley JE, Cruz-Jentoft AJ, et al. International clinical practice guidelines for sarcopenia (ICFSR): screening, diagnosis and management. J Nutr Health Aging 2018;22:1148–61.

[36] Bouchard DR, Dionne IJ, Brochu M. Sarcopenic/obesity and physical capacity in older men and women: data from the nutrition as a determinant of successful aging (NuAge)-the Quebec longitudinal study. Obesity (Silver Spring) 2009;17:2082–8.
[37] Garvey WT, Mechanick JI, Brett EM, et al. American Association of Clinical Endocrinologists and American College of Endocrinology comprehensive clinical practice guidelines for medical care of patients with obesity. Endocr Pract 2016;22(Supplement 3):1–203.
[38] Villareal DT, Apovian CM, Kushner RF, Klein S, American Society for Nutrition; NAASO, The Obesity Society. Obesity in older adults: technical review and position statement of the American Society for Nutrition and NAASO, The Obesity Society. Am J Clin Nutr 2005;82:923–34.
[39] Davison KK, Ford ES, Cogswell ME, Dietz WH. Percentage of body fat and body mass index are associated with mobility limitations in people aged 70 and older from NHANES III. J Am Geriatr Soc 2002;50:1802–9.
[40] Zoico E, Di Francesco V, Guralnik JM, et al. Physical disability and muscular strength in relation to obesity and different body composition indexes in a sample of healthy elderly women. Int J Obes Relat Metab Disord 2004;28:234–41.
[41] Cruz-Jentoft AJ, Bahat G, Bauer J, Boirie Y, et al. Writing Group for the European Working Group on sarcopenia in older people 2 (EWGSOP2), and the extended group for EWGSOP2. Sarcopenia: revised European consensus on definition and diagnosis. Age Ageing 2019;48:16–31.
[42] Cruz-Jentoft AJ, Sayer AA. Sarcopenia. Lancet 2019;393(10191):2636–46.
[43] Wiedmer P, Jung T, Castro JP, et al. Sarcopenia—molecular mechanisms and open questions. Ageing Res Rev 2021;65, 101200.
[44] Sieber CC. Malnutrition and sarcopenia. Aging Clin Exp Res 2019;31:793–8.
[45] Li JS, Tsai TY, Clancy MM, Li G, Lewis CL, Felson DT. Weight loss changed gait kinematics in individuals with obesity and knee pain. Gait Posture 2019;68:461–5.
[46] Schwarze M, Häuser W, Schmutzer G, et al. Obesity, depression and hip pain. Musculoskeletal Care 2019;17:126–32.
[47] Puhl RM, Himmelstein MS, Pearl RL, Puhl RM, et al. Weight stigma as a psychosocial contributor to obesity. Am Psychol 2020;75:274–89.
[48] Andrei F, Nuccitelli C, Mancini G, Reggiani GM, Trombini E. Emotional intelligence, emotion regulation and affectivity in adults seeking treatment for obesity. Psychiatry Res 2018;269:191–8.
[49] Hsu CS, Kao JH. Sarcopenia and chronic liver diseases. Expert Rev Gastroenterol Hepatol 2018;12:1229–44.
[50] Moorthi RN, Avin KG. Clinical relevance of sarcopenia in chronic kidney disease. Curr Opin Nephrol Hypertens 2017;26:219–28.
[51] Watanabe H, Enoki Y, Maruyama T. Sarcopenia in chronic kidney disease: factors, mechanisms, and therapeutic interventions. Biol Pharm Bull 2019;42:1437–45.
[52] Coppack SW. Pro-inflammatory cytokines and adipose tissue. Proc Nutr Soc 2001;60:349–56.
[53] Popko K, Gorska E, Stelmaszczyk-Emmel A, et al. Proinflammatory cytokines Il-6 and TNF-α and the development of inflammation in obese subjects. Eur J Med Res 2010;15(Supplement 2):120–2.
[54] Deng T, Lyon CJ, Bergin S, Caligiuri MA, Hsueh WA. Obesity, inflammation, and cancer. Annu Rev Pathol 2016;11:421–49.
[55] Wang T, He C. Pro-inflammatory cytokines: the link between obesity and osteoarthritis. Cytokine Growth Factor Rev 2018;44:38–50.
[56] Hasselgren PO. Catabolic response to stress and injury: implications for regulation. World J Surg 2000;24:1452–9.
[57] Sharma B, Dabur R. Role of pro-inflammatory cytokines in regulation of skeletal muscle metabolism: a systematic review. Curr Med Chem 2020;27:2161–88.

[58] Hasselgren PO. Ubiquitination, phosphorylation, and acetylation—triple threat in muscle wasting. J Cell Physiol 2007;213:679–89.
[59] Bastard JP, Maachi M, Lagathu C, et al. Recent advances in the relationship between obesity, inflammation, and insulin resistance. Eur Cytokine Netw 2006;17:4–12.
[60] Fan J, Kou X, Yang Y, Chen N. MicroRNA-regulated proinflammatory cytokines in sarcopenia. Mediators Inflamm 2016;2016:1438686.
[61] Trayhurn P, Drevon CA, Eckel J. Secreted proteins from adipose tissue and skeletal muscle—adipokines, myokines and adipose/muscle cross-talk. Arch Physiol Biochem 2011;117:47–56.
[62] Raschke S, Eckel J. Adipo-myokines: two sides of the same coin—mediators of inflammation and mediators of exercise. Mediators Inflamm 2013;2013, 320724.
[63] Li F, Li Y, Duan Y, Hu CA, Tang Y, Yin Y. Myokines and adipokines: involvement in the crosstalk between skeletal muscle and adipose tissue. Cytokine Growth Factor Rev 2017;33:73–82.
[64] Ouchi N, Parker JL, Lugus JJ, Walsh K. Adipokines in inflammation and metabolic disease. Nat Rev Immunol 2011;11:85–97.
[65] Jung UJ, Choi MS. Obesity and its metabolic complications: the role of adipokines and the relationship between obesity, inflammation, insulin resistance, dyslipidemia and nonalcoholic fatty liver disease. Int J Mol Sci 2014;15:6184–223.
[66] Unamuno X, Gómez-Ambrosi J, Rodríguez A, Becerril S, Frühbeck G, Catalán V. Adipokine dysregulation and adipose tissue inflammation in human obesity. Eur J Clin Invest 2018;48, e12997.
[67] Carbone F, La Rocca C, Matarese G. Immunological functions of leptin and adiponectin. Biochimie 2012;94:2082–8.
[68] Wolsk E, Mygind H, Grøndahl TS, Pedersen BK, van Hall G. Human skeletal muscle releases leptin in vivo. Cytokine 2012;60:667–73.
[69] Krause MP, Milne KJ, Hawke TJ. Adiponectin-consideration for its role in skeletal muscle health. Int J Mol Sci 2019;20:1528.
[70] Martinez-Huenchullan SF, Tam CS, Ban LA, Ehrenfeld-Slater P, Mclennan SV, Twigg SM. Skeletal muscle adiponectin induction in obesity and exercise. Metabolism 2020;102, 154008.
[71] Hamrick MW. Role of the cytokine-like hormone leptin in muscle-bone crosstalk with aging. J Bone Metab 2017;24:1–8.
[72] Zoico E, Rossi A, Di Francesco V, et al. Adipose tissue infiltration in skeletal muscle of healthy elderly men: relationships with body composition, insulin resistance, and inflammation at the systemic and tissue level. J Gerontol A Biol Sci Med Sci 2010;65:295–9.
[73] Kohara K, Ochi M, Tabara Y, Nagai T, Igase M, Miki T. Leptin in sarcopenic visceral obesity: possible link between adipocytes and myocytes. PLoS ONE 2011;6, e24633.
[74] Rossi FE, Lira FS, Silva BSA, Freire APCF, Ramos EMC, Gobbo LA. Influence of skeletal muscle mass and fat mass on the metabolic and inflammatory profile in sarcopenic and non-sarcopenic overfat elderly. Aging Clin Exp Res 2019;31:629–35.
[75] Ceddia RB, William Jr WN, Curi R. The response of skeletal muscle to leptin. Front Biosci 2001;6:D90–7.
[76] Mitrou P, Lambadiari V, Maratou E, et al. Skeletal muscle insulin resistance in morbid obesity: the role of interleukin-6 and leptin. Exp Clin Endocrinol Diabetes 2011;119:484–9.
[77] Yadav A, Kataria MA, Saini V, Yadav A. Role of leptin and adiponectin in insulin resistance. Clin Chim Acta 2013;417:80–4.
[78] Pedersen BK, Febbraio MA. Muscles, exercise and obesity: skeletal muscle as a secretory organ. Nat Rev Endocrinol 2012;8:457–65.
[79] Leal LG, Lopes MA, Batista Jr ML. Physical exercise-induced myokines and muscle-adipose tissue crosstalk: a review of current knowledge and the implications for health and metabolic diseases. Front Physiol 2018;9:1307.

[80] Amor M, Itariu BK, Moreno-Viedma V, et al. Serum myostatin is upregulated in obesity and correlates with insulin resistance in humans. Exp Clin Endocrinol Diabetes 2019;127:550–6.
[81] Zhang C, McFarlane C, Lokireddy S, et al. Inhibition of myostatin protects against diet-induced obesity by enhancing fatty acid oxidation and promoting a brown adipose phenotype in mice. Diabetologia 2012;55:183–93.
[82] Barbalho SM, Prado Neto EV, et al. Myokines: a descriptive review. J Sports Med Phys Fitness 2020;60:1583–90.
[83] Consitt LA, Clark BC. The vicious cycle of myostatin signaling in sarcopenic obesity: myostatin role in skeletal muscle growth, insulin signaling and implications for clinical trials. J Frailty Aging 2018;7:21–7.
[84] Smith RC, Lin BK. Myostatin inhibitors as therapies for muscle wasting associated with cancer and other disorders. Curr Opin Support Palliat Care 2013;7:352–60.
[85] Kobayashi M, Kasamatsu S, Shinozaki S, Yasuhara S, Kaneki M. Myostatin deficiency not only prevents muscle wasting but also improves survival in septic mice. Am J Physiol Endocrinol Metab 2021;320:E150–9.
[86] Constantin D, McCullough J, Mahajan RP, Greenhaff PL. Novel events in the molecular regulation of muscle mass in critically ill patients. J Physiol 2011;589:3883–95.
[87] Kirk B, Feehan J, Lombardi G, Duque G. Muscle, bone, and fat crosstalk: the biological role of myokines, osteokines, and adipokines. Curr Osteoporos Rep 2020;18:388–400.
[88] Lebrasseur NK. Building muscle, browning fat and preventing obesity by inhibiting myostatin. Diabetologia 2012;55:13–7.
[89] Dong J, Dong Y, Dong Y, Chen F, Mitch WE, Zhang L. Inhibition of myostatin in mice improves insulin sensitivity via irisin-mediated cross talk between muscle and adipose tissues. Int J Obes (Lond) 2016;40:434–42.
[90] Polyzos SA, Margioris AN. Sarcopenic obesity. Hormones (Athens) 2018;17:321–31.
[91] Jia J, Yu F, Wei WP, et al. Relationship between circulating irisin levels and overweight/obesity: a meta-analysis. World J Clin Cases 2019;7:1444–55.
[92] Korta P, Pocheć E, Mazur-Biały A. Irisin as a multifunctional protein: implications for health and certain diseases. Medicina (Kaunas) 2019;55:485.
[93] Reza MM, Subramaniyam N, Sim CM, et al. Irisin is a pro-myogenic factor that induces skeletal muscle hypertrophy and rescues denervation-induced atrophy. Nat Commun 2017;8:1104.
[94] Cai C, Qian L, Jiang S, et al. Loss-of-function myostatin mutation increases insulin sensitivity and browning of white fat in Meishan pigs. Oncotarget 2017;8:34911–22.
[95] Huh JY, Dincer F, Mesfum E, Mantzoros CS. Irisin stimulates muscle growth-related genes and regulates adipocyte differentiation and metabolism in humans. Int J Obes (Lond) 2014;38:1538–44.
[96] Reza MM, Sim CM, Subramaniyam N, et al. Irisin treatment improves healing of dystrophic skeletal muscle. Oncotarget 2017;8:98553–66.
[97] Polyzos SA, Anastasilakis AD, Efstathiadou ZA, et al. Irisin in metabolic diseases. Endocrine 2018;59:260–74.
[98] Arhire LI, Mihalache L, Covasa M. Irisin: a hope in understanding and managing obesity and metabolic syndrome. Front Endocrinol (Lausanne) 2019;10:524.
[99] Biltz NK, Collins KH, Shen KC, Schwartz K, Harris CA, Meyer GA. Infiltration of intramuscular adipose tissue impairs skeletal muscle contraction. J Physiol 2020;598:2669–83.
[100] Kalinkovich A, Livshits G. Sarcopenic obesity or obese sarcopenia: a cross talk between age-associated adipose tissue and skeletal muscle inflammation as a main mechanism of the pathogenesis. Ageing Res Rev 2017;35:200–21.
[101] Zhu S, Tian Z, Torigoe D, et al. Aging- and obesity-related peri-muscular adipose tissue accelerates muscle atrophy. PLoS ONE 2019;14, e0221366.

[102] Hong SH, Choi KM. Sarcopenic obesity, insulin resistance, and their implications in cardiovascular and metabolic consequences. Int J Mol Sci 2020;21:494.
[103] Poggiogalle E, Mendes I, Ong B, et al. Sarcopenic obesity and insulin resistance: application of novel body composition models. Nutrition 2020;75-76, 110765.
[104] Michalakis K, Goulis DG, Vazaiou A, Mintziori G, Polymeris A, Abrahamian-Michalakis A. Obesity in the ageing man. Metabolism 2013;62:1341–9.
[105] Groeneveld MP, Huang-Doran I, Semple RK. Adiponectin and leptin in human severe insulin resistance—diagnostic utility and biological insights. Biochimie 2012;94:2172–9.
[106] Chen HT, Chung YC, Chen YJ, Ho SY, Wu HJ. Effects of different types of exercise on body composition, muscle strength, and IGF-1 in the elderly with sarcopenic obesity. J Am Geriatr Soc 2017;65:827–32.
[107] Saad F, Röhrig G, von Haehling S, Traish A. Testosterone deficiency and testosterone treatment in older men. Gerontology 2017;63:144–56.
[108] Waters DL, Qualls CR, Dorin RI, Veldhuis JD, Baumgartner RN. Altered growth hormone, cortisol, and leptin secretion in healthy elderly persons with sarcopenia and mixed body composition phenotypes. J Gerontol A Biol Sci Med Sci 2008;63:536–41.
[109] Diago-Galmés A, Guillamón-Escudero C, Tenías-Burillo JM, Soriano JM, Fernández-Garrido J. Salivary testosterone and cortisol as biomarkers for the diagnosis of sarcopenia and sarcopenic obesity in community-dwelling older adults. Biology (Basel) 2021;10:93.
[110] Silveira EA, Souza JD, Santos ASEAC, Canheta ABS, Pagotto V, Noll M. What are the factors associated with sarcopenia-related variables in adult women with severe obesity? Arch Public Health 2020;78:71.
[111] Levine ME, Crimmins EM. The impact of insulin resistance and inflammation on the association between sarcopenic obesity and physical functioning. Obesity (Silver Spring) 2012;20:2101–6.
[112] Dufour AB, Hannan MT, Murabito JM, Kiel DP, McLean RR. Sarcopenia definitions considering body size and fat mass are associated with mobility limitations: the Framingham study. J Gerontol A Biol Sci Med Sci 2013;68:168–74.
[113] Oliveira TM, Roriz AKC, Barreto-Medeiros JM, Ferreira AJF, Ramos L. Sarcopenic obesity in community-dwelling older women, determined by different diagnostic methods. Nutr Hosp 2019;36:1267–72.
[114] Huo YR, Suriyaarachchi P, Gomez F, et al. Phenotype of sarcopenic obesity in older individuals with a history of falling. Arch Gerontol Geriatr 2016;65:255–9.
[115] Scott D, Seibel M, Cumming R, et al. Sarcopenic obesity and its temporal associations with changes in bone mineral density, incident falls, and fractures in older men: the Concord Health and Ageing in Men Project. J Bone Miner Res 2017;32:575–83.
[116] Follis S, Cook A, Bea JW, et al. Association between sarcopenic obesity and falls in a multiethnic cohort of postmenopausal women. J Am Geriatr Soc 2018;66:2314–20.
[117] Lee S, Kim TN, Kim SH. Sarcopenic obesity is more closely associated with knee osteoarthritis than is nonsarcopenic obesity: a cross-sectional study. Arthritis Rheum 2012;64:3947–54.
[118] Misra D, Fielding RA, Felson DT, et al. Risk of knee osteoarthritis with obesity, sarcopenic obesity, and sarcopenia. Arthritis Rheumatol 2019;71:232–7.
[119] De Pergola G, Silvestris F. Obesity as a major risk factor for cancer. J Obes 2013;2013, 291546.
[120] Avgerinos KI, Spyrou N, Mantzoros CS, Dalamaga M. Obesity and cancer risk: emerging biological mechanisms and perspectives. Metabolism 2019;92:121–35.
[121] Pecorelli N, Capretti G, Sandini M, et al. Impact of sarcopenic obesity on failure to rescue from major complications following pancreaticoduodenectomy for cancer: results from a multicenter study. Ann Surg Oncol 2018;25:308–17.

[122] Nishigori T, Tsunoda S, Okabe H, et al. Impact of sarcopenic obesity on surgical site infection after laparoscopic total gastrectomy. Ann Surg Oncol 2016;23(Supplement 4):524–31.
[123] Ryu Y, Shin SH, Kim JH, et al. The effects of sarcopenia and sarcopenic obesity after pancreaticoduodenectomy in patients with pancreatic head cancer. HPB (Oxford) 2020;22:1782–92.
[124] Sandini M, Bernasconi DP, Fior D, et al. A high visceral adipose tissue-to-skeletal muscle ratio as a determinant of major complications after pancreatoduodenectomy for cancer. Nutrition 2016;32:1231–7.
[125] Anandavadivelan P, Brismar TB, Nilsson M, Johar AM, Martin L. Sarcopenic obesity: a probable risk factor for dose limiting toxicity during neo-adjuvant chemotherapy in oesophageal cancer patients. Clin Nutr 2016;35:724–30.
[126] van Gassel RJJ, Baggerman MR, van de Poll MCG. Metabolic aspects of muscle wasting during critical illness. Curr Opin Clin Nutr Metab Care 2020;23:96–101.
[127] Tieland M, van Dronkelaar C, Boirie Y. Sarcopenic obesity in the ICU. Curr Opin Clin Nutr Metab Care 2019;22:162–6.
[128] Fukuda T, Bouchi R, Asakawa M, et al. Sarcopenic obesity is associated with a faster decline in renal function in people with type 2 diabetes. Diabet Med 2020;37:105–13.
[129] Bellafronte NT, Sizoto GR, Vega-Piris L, Chiarello PG, Cuadrado GB. Bed-side measures for diagnosis of low muscle mass, sarcopenia, obesity, and sarcopenic obesity in patients with chronic kidney disease under non-dialysis-dependent, dialysis dependent and kidney transplant therapy. PLoS ONE 2020;15, e0242671.
[130] Tabibi H, As'habi A, Najafi I, Hedayati M. Prevalence of dynapenic obesity and sarcopenic obesity and their associations with cardiovascular disease risk factors in peritoneal dialysis patients. Kidney Res Clin Pract 2018;37:404–13.
[131] Carias S, Castellanos AL, Vilchez V, et al. Nonalcoholic steatohepatitis is strongly associated with sarcopenic obesity in patients with cirrhosis undergoing liver transplant evaluation. J Gastroenterol Hepatol 2016;31:628–33.
[132] Montero-Fernández N, Serra-Rexach JA. Role of exercise on sarcopenia in the elderly. Eur J Phys Rehabil Med 2013;49:131–43.
[133] Deutz NE, Bauer JM, Barazzoni R, et al. Protein intake and exercise for optimal muscle function with aging: recommendations from the ESPEN expert group. Clin Nutr 2014;33:929–36.
[134] Trouwborst I, Verreijen A, Memelink R, et al. Exercise and nutrition strategies to counteract sarcopenic obesity. Nutrients 2018;10:605.
[135] Huang Y, Zhu X, Chen K, et al. Resveratrol prevents sarcopenic obesity by reversing mitochondrial dysfunction and oxidative stress via the PKA/LKB1/AMPK pathway. Aging (Albany NY) 2019;11:2217–40.
[136] El Hajj C, Fares S, Chardigny JM, Boirie Y, Walrand S. Vitamin D supplementation and muscle strength in pre-sarcopenic elderly Lebanese people: a randomized controlled trial. Arch Osteoporos 2018;14:4.

CHAPTER 12

Resolution of inflammation

Ronald Tyszkowski[a] and Raman Mehrzad[b]

[a]Private Practice, Allied Health, Women and Infants Hospital, Providence, RI, United States
[b]Division of Plastic and Reconstructive Surgery, Rhode Island Hospital, The Warren Alpert School of Brown University, Providence, RI, United States

Resolution of inflammation

Historically, the emphasis in development of antiinflammatory drugs has been focused largely on interfering with the proinflammatory signaling cascade. Only recently has the focus shifted to augmenting naturally occurring pro-resolution responses in the host [1]. The identification of key actors in the pro-resolution process, including pro-resolving lipid mediators (SPMs) (lipoxins, resolvins, protectins, maresins), has created new avenues in the potential pharmacological management and potential resolution of inflammation [2].

Fig. 1 demonstrates the basic timeline of the acute inflammatory response with significant modulators and their roles. Inflammation begins after tissue insult and/or foreign agent presentation. Infiltration of polymorphonuclear monocytes (PMNs) occurs through the adjacent capillary wall. These initiating biochemical mediators include lipid autacoids, prostaglandins, and leukotrienes. Subsequent steps focus on the clearing of the PMNs and their exudate following activity; Resolution of inflammation has been understood for over a century to occur when neutrophils that have invaded the involved tissue leave [3]. The continued presence of the initiating mediators and/or cellular exudate may result in chronic inflammation and tissue damage. These steps include the following. Apoptosis, or programmed cell death, of PMNs is initiated, and dead cells are cleared by pro-resolving macrophages (Mϕ) via efferocytosis. Highlighted in the arrow is the "Lipid mediator class switch," in which pro-resolving lipid mediators (SPMs) are created to facilitate resolution by promoting Mϕ activity, promoting tissue regeneration, and controlling pain. Pro-resolving miRNAs and microparticles also play an important role in the pathway to resolution and offer additional novel approaches to treatment of impaired resolution of inflammation.

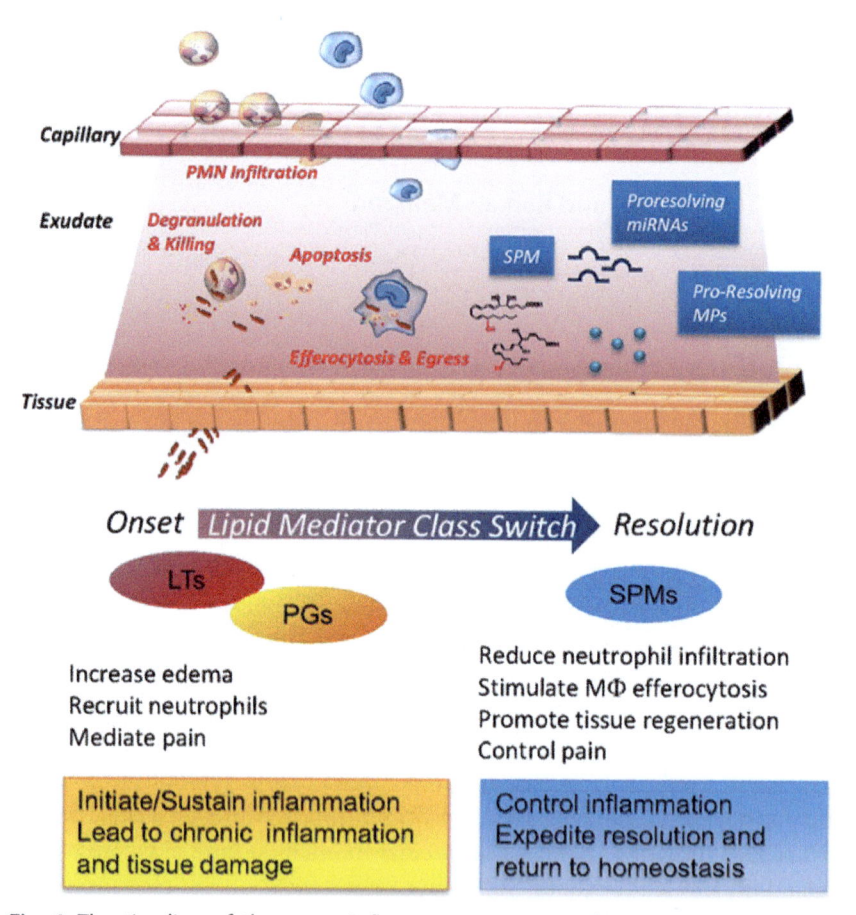

Fig. 1 The timeline of the acute inflammatory response from onset to resolution. *(Source: Serhan, Charles N, Antonio Recchiuti. Pro-resolving lipid mediators (SPMs) and their actions in regulating miRNA in novel resolution circuits in inflammation. Front Immunol 2012;3:298.)*

Cyclopentenone prostaglandins

Cyclopentenone Prostaglandins (CyPGs) are a small group of compounds that are a subset of the eicosanoid superfamily, which are metabolites of arachidonic acid, and are pivotal mediators of in a number of normal physiological and pathophysiological processes [4]. They are characterized by the common structural features of a five-membered carbocyclic ring containing an alfa-beta unsaturated keto group (see Fig. 2).

They are involved in a number of physiological activities (Fig. 3) including the ability to resolve chronic inflammation and suppress the growth as well as the survival of cells, especially those of cancerous or neurologic

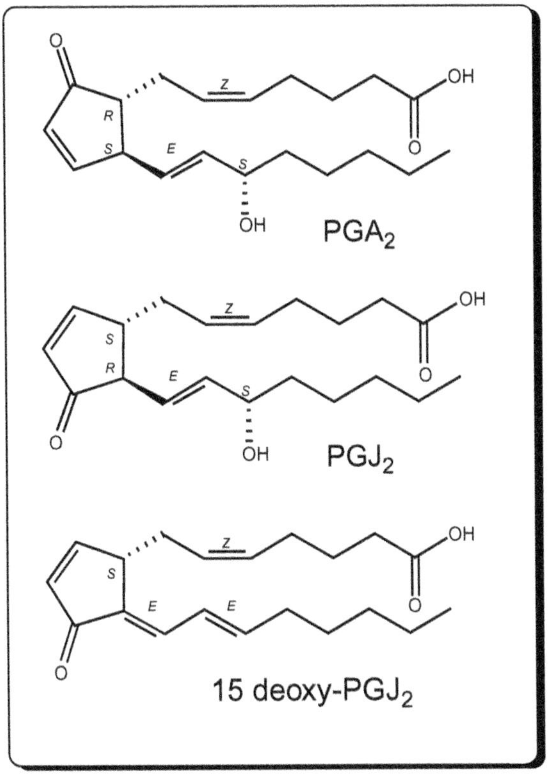

Fig. 2 CyPG structures showing the common structure of a prostane carbon skeleton and an alpha beta unsaturated ketone [4]. *(Source: Burstein, Sumner H. The chemistry, biology and pharmacology of the cyclopentenone prostaglandins. Prostaglandins Other Lipid Mediat 2020;148:106408.)*

origin [4]. Mechanisms of action include the activation of the prostaglandin D2 receptor as well as the ligand-dependent transcription factor PPAR-gamma [5].

Therapeutic applications

Despite over 20 years of applied research and multiple instances of proven in vitro and in vivo involvement in the initiation and cessation of inflammation (Fig. 4), there are no current clinical uses for CyPGs. Their ability to undergo a Michael addition reaction (nucleophilic addition of a carbanion or another nucleophile to an α,β-unsaturated carbonyl compound) without the necessity of an enzyme has been an impediment to consistent in vivo therapeutic results. Future clinical applications may require an agent that initiates the production of CyPGs in situ [4], thereby avoiding this modification and subsequent inactivation reaction.

Examples of physiological actions involving cyclopentenone prostaglandins.

Action	CyPG	System
Down-regulation of microglia	15d-PGJ$_2$	LPS-stimulated BV-2 cells & IL-1b-stimulated astrocytes
Increase astrocyte proliferation	PGE$_2$ PGD$_2$, 15d-PGJ$_2$ & PGA$_2$	C6 rat glioma cells and primary astrocytes
Induction of detoxification enzymes	15d-PGJ$_2$	RL34 RLN8, dRLN9,HeLa, HepG2, Hep3B and H4IIE cells
Neuroprotection against oxidative stress	PGD$_2$ & 15d-PGJ$_2$	Primary pericytes and endothelial cells
Induction of apoptosis	15d-PGJ$_2$	Dendritic cells
Down-regulation of an immune response	15d-PGJ$_2$	Human T lymphocytes
Activation of Akt/PKB	15d-PGJ$_2$ & PGA$_2$	Cancer cell line MCF-7
Regulation of growth-related and stress-induced genes	PGA$_1$ PGA$_2$, 15d-PGJ$_2$ & PGD$_2$	C6 rat glioma cells
Post-ischemic neuronal injury	15d-PGJ$_2$, PGD$_2$, PGJ2, & 15d-PGD$_2$	Cortical primary neuron-enriched cultures
Inhibition of axonal regeneration	15d-PGJ$_2$ & PGA$_1$	*Xenopus* dorsal root ganglia
Reduction of leukocyte migration	N-acyl amino acids 15d-PGJ$_2$	Mouse peritonitis assay
Inhibition of ubiquitin hydrolase	PGA$_1$, PGD$_2$, PGE$_2$, & PGJ$_2$	Microglia and astrocytes

Fig. 3 Physiological activities of CyPgs [4]. *(Source: Burstein, Sumner H. The chemistry, biology and pharmacology of the cyclopentenone prostaglandins. Prostaglandins Other Lipid Mediat 2020;148:106408.)*

Target	Agent	System	Results
Cancer chemoresistance	15d-PGJ$_2$, Δ^{12}-PGJ$_2$	Jurkat, A549, and primary rat mesangial cells (RMCs)	Induction of GSTP1-1 Cross-Linking
Sindbis virus replication	PGA$_1$	Vero cells	Inhibited the synthesis of the viral structural proteins
Early HTLV-1 infection	PGA$_1$ & 15d-PGJ$_2$	Infected blood-derived human mononuclear cells	No antiviral activity was found in this model
Infection with human T-cell leukemia virus	PGA$_1$ & 15d-PGJ$_2$	Human myeloid cell lines	Both CyPGs induced growth arrest prevalently at G1/S
Antiviral effects	PGA$_2$	Vesicular stomatitis virus RNA polymerase	Inhibition of vesicular stomatitis virus replication
HIV-1 replication	PGA$_1$ & 15d-PGJ$_2$	HIV-infected CEM-SS cells	Reduction in HIV-1 mRNA levels
Herpesvirus -induced HIV-1	PGA$_1$	Jurkat cells H9 and ACH-2 cells	Inhibits HSV-1-induced IKK and NF-kappaB activities
Regulation of BiP gene expression	Delta12-PGJ$_2$	HeLa cells	Stimulates the expression of the BiP gene
In vitro genotoxicity	PGA$_2$ & 15d-PGJ$_2$	V79 cells	Induced DNA damage
Resolution of inflammation	15d-PGJ$_2$	RAW 264.7 cells	Potentiation of apoptosis
Chronic inflammation	PGA$_1$ & 15d-PGJ$_2$	Jurkat and HeLa cells	Inhibition &modification of the IKK-beta subunit of IKK
NF-kappaB	15d-PGJ$_2$	Dendritic cells or macrophages	Modification of the IKKbeta subunit of IKK
Multiple sclerosis (MS	PGA$_2$	Mouse microglia and astrocytes	Inhibition of cytokine and chemokine production

Fig. 4 Pharmacological activities of CyPGs [4]. (Source: Burstein, Sumner H. The chemistry, biology and pharmacology of the cyclopentenone prostaglandins. Prostaglandins Other Lipid Mediat 2020;148:106408.)

Apoptotic cells and their clearance

PMN's apoptotic cells are rapidly removed by tissue-resident professional phagocytes and/or by neighboring nonprofessional phagocytes under homeostatic conditions. Clearance of apoptotic cells involves molecular steps that include the recruitment of phagocytes toward apoptotic cells through "find-me" signals and the recognition of "eat-me" signals on apoptotic cells that trigger engulfment. Apoptotic cell clearance under physiological conditions is generally antiinflammatory and immunologically silent. Defects in apoptotic cell removal are associated with the initiation and progression of a number of pathological conditions, including inflammation and autoimmunity [6].

Therapeutic applications

Several aspects of the apoptotic cell clearance cycle have therapeutic potential (Fig. 5) [6]:
- The molecules exposed on the apoptotic cells themselves appear to provide important differentiation signals.
- The phagocytic recognition step induces several antiinflammatory mediators that dampen the immune response.

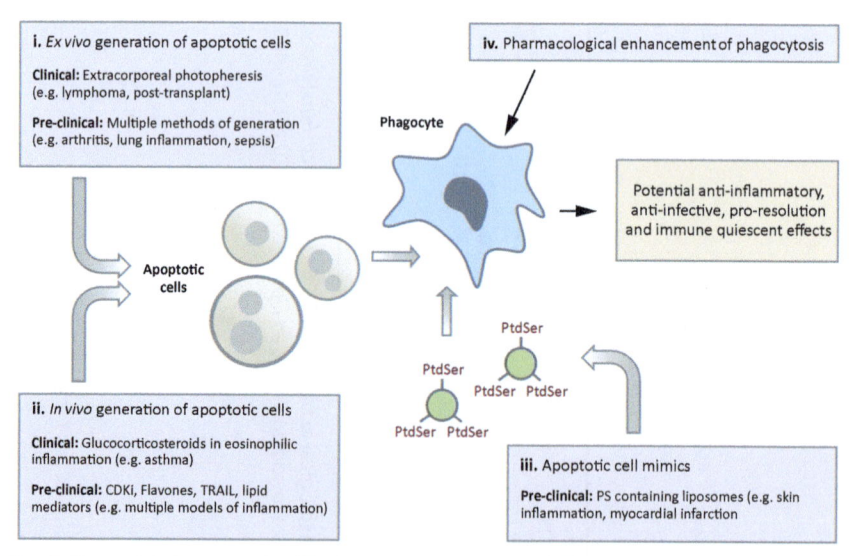

Fig. 5 Potential therapeutic effects utilizing apoptotic cells themselves, including current clinical applications and future applications (with corresponding disease states) under study [6]. *(Source: Poon, Ivan KH, Christopher D Lucas, Adriano G Rossi, Kodi S Ravichandran. Apoptotic cell clearance: basic biology and therapeutic potential. Nat Rev Immunol 2014;14(3): 166–180.)*

- The actual corpse internalization process appears to help limit certain infections.
- Depending on the type of apoptosis induction and the type of phagocyte, the engulfment process can also be made pro-immunogenic in specific conditions.

In the most recent reviews, apoptotic cell-based therapy demonstrates compelling evidence that it may dampen the inflammatory process of Rheumatoid Arthritis [7]. Continued research is necessary before novel therapeutic agents are available.

microRNA

microRNAs (miRNAs) are small noncoding ribonucleic acids (RNAs) that play critical roles in the regulation of host genome expression at the posttranscription level. Various functions can be attributed to them including: immune cell lineage commitment, differentiation, and maturation, and maintenance of immune homeostasis and immune function [8]. A single miRNA can exert diverse immune regulatory function which may be specific to developmental stages and the microenvironment of different types of immune cells [8]. miRNAs primarily regulate gene expression by promoting messenger RNA (mRNA) degradation or repressing mRNA translation [9].

MiRNA processing steps include:
- Transcription by RNA polymerase II to form a primary miRNA (pri-miRNA) transcript with 5'-end caps and 3'-end poly-A tails.
- It is then subsequently cleaved by the nuclease, Drosha, and its cofactor DiGeorge critical region 8 (DGCR8), thus generating a precursor miRNA (pre-miRNA).
- This pre-miRNA is transported from the nucleus to the cytoplasm by exportin-5 (Exp5) using RanGTP as a cofactor.
- It undergoes further processing in the cytoplasm by RNase III Dicer in a complex with trans-activation response RNA-binding protein (TRBP) to generate approximately 22-nucleotide duplex mature miRNA.
- Finally, the miRNA duplex unwinds and the functional strand of mature miRNA complexes with Argonaute (Ago2), forming an RNA-induced silencing complex (RISC). This RISC complex directs silencing via sequence-specific mRNAs target cleavage, translational repression, and mRNA deadenylation [10].

As is often the case with such influential bioactive molecules, disease states are related to dysregulated activity or expression. miRNA dysfunction can be implicated in multiple disease states, such as Systemic Lupus Erythematosus, Rheumatoid Arthritis, and Multiple Sclerosis [8], as well as various forms of cancer.

Therapeutic applications

Different miRNA species such as miRNA-122 and miRNA-155 are being studied for their therapeutic applications in cancer and various autoimmune diseases [9,11]. However, "despite the recent understanding of the biological functions and the role of miR-155 in inflammation and carcinogenesis, there are gaps in the identification and characterization of all miR-155 targets. Therefore, it is imperative to understand the physiological impact of miR-155 inhibition on these targets before anti-miR-155 therapy can be considered" [9]. Although directed specifically toward miRNA-155, these statements can be applied across the board for the clinical applications of miRNA inhibitors, as inhibition of miRNA may have unintended consequences.

Resolution-directed lipid mediators of inflammation

A lipid mediator is characterized by being stereoselective in its action and be produced in amounts that are commensurate with its potency and range of action [12].

As described previously in this chapter, during inflammation resolution, lipid mediators undergo a class switch where inflammation promoters are replaced by inflammation resolvers. These include lipoxins, protectins, maresins, and resolvins. Arachidonic Acid acts as the precursor of Lipoxins. The omega 3 fatty acids eicosapentaenoic acid (EPA)(e-series resolvins) and docosahexaenoic acid (DHA) (d-series resolvins, protectins, and maresins) (Fig. 6), via enzymatic reaction, are transformed into antiinflammatory, pro-resolving, and cytoprotective lipid mediators [2] (Fig. 7).

Eicosapentaenoic acid
(EPA, $C_{20}H_{30}O_2$)

Docosahexaenoic acid
(DHA, $C_{22}H_{32}O_2$)

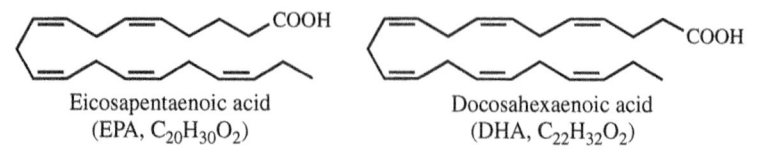

Fig. 6 Molecular structure of EPA and DHA [13]. *(Source: Yi, Tao, et al. Comparative analysis of EPA and DHA in fish oil nutritional capsules by GC-MS. Lipids Health Dis 2014;13(1):1–6.)*

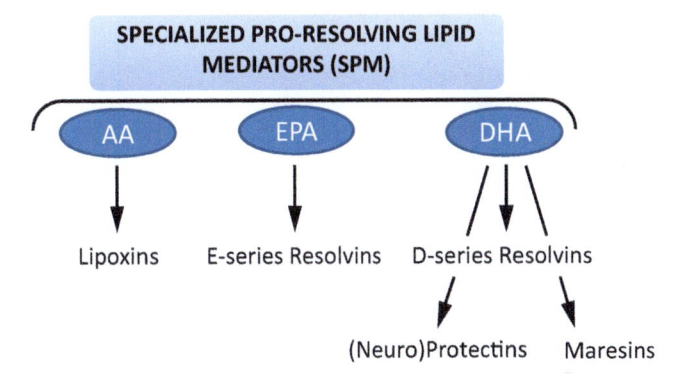

Fig. 7 Origins of lipid mediators from AA (arachidonic acid), EPA (eicosapentaenoic acid), DHA (docosahexaenoic acid) [2]. *(Source: Serhan, Charles N, Antonio Recchiuti. Pro-resolving lipid mediators (SPMs) and their actions in regulating miRNA in novel resolution circuits in inflammation. Front Immunol 2012;3:298.)*

Lipoxins

Lipoxins were the first lipid mediator recognized to possess pro-resolving actions [2]. They are lipoxygenase interaction products derived from the enzymatic conversion of arachidonic acid via transcellular biosynthesis during cell–cell interactions occurring during inflammation (Fig. 8) [14]. Its synthesis can also be initiated by aspirin. Among the nonsteroidal antiinflammatory drugs (NSAIDs), aspirin can accelerate and/or initiate inflammation resolution by triggering endogenous biosyntheses of "aspirin triggered" lipoxin (ATL) [2].

Lipoxins can act as "braking signals" of further PMN infiltration [15], as well as, stimuli for recruitment of monocytes [16] and efferocytosis [17].

Therapeutic applications

Evidence of aspirin-triggered biosynthesis of lipoxins was first published in 1995 [18]. As such, it appears that pharmaceutical application of lipoxin-mediated inflammation control has been going on for decades, even if we didn't know it.

Resolvins

Resolvins are designated e-series and d-series and have antiinflammatory and pro (inflammation)-resolving effects. E-series resolvins (e.g., RvE1) are generated from Eicosapentaenoic Acid (EPA) (Fig. 9). EPA, a component of fish oil, has long been promoted to have health benefits, but the molecular

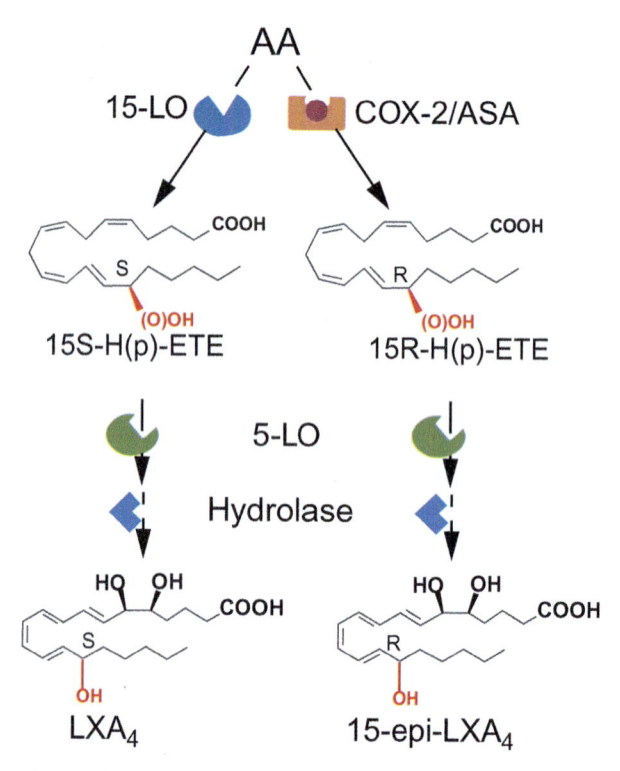

Fig. 8 Biosynthesis of lipoxins from arachidonic acid [2]. *(Source: Serhan, Charles N, Antonio Recchiuti. Pro-resolving lipid mediators (SPMs) and their actions in regulating miRNA in novel resolution circuits in inflammation. Front Immunol 2012;3:298.)*

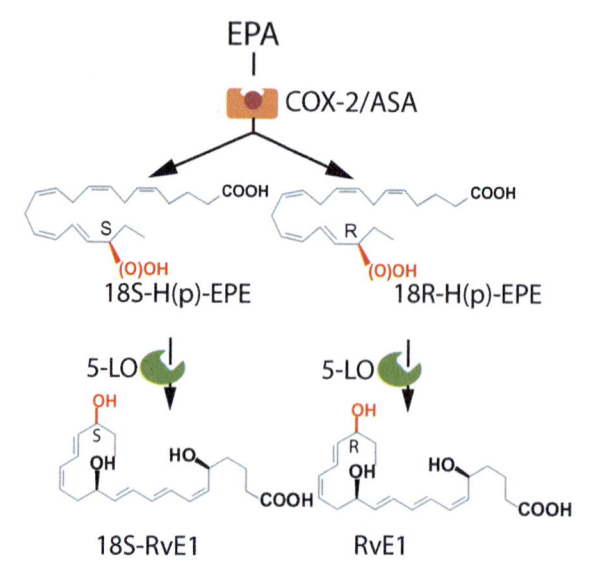

Fig. 9 Biosynthesis of e-series resolvins from EPA [2]. *(Source: Serhan, Charles N, Antonio Recchiuti. Pro-resolving lipid mediators (SPMs) and their actions in regulating miRNA in novel resolution circuits in inflammation. Front Immunol 2012;3:298.)*

basis of these was not known until its connection to e-series resolvins was discovered [19]. D-series resolvins (e.g., RvD1) are generated from the other significant component of fish oil, DHA or Docosahexaenoic Acid.

Functions of RvE1:
- Mitigation of PMN infiltration into inflammatory loci [20]
- Reduction of proinflammatory gene expression and protection against colitis [21]
- Promotion of macrophage ingestion of apoptotic PMNs [22]
- Protection against osteoclast-mediated bone destruction and prevention of periodontitis [23]
- Selective counterregulation of platelets and leukocytes [24]
- Reduction of inflammatory pain [25]

Functions of RvD1 and AT-RvD1 (Aspirin Triggered RvD1):
- Limit the infiltration of PMNs in the initial phase of inflammation [19]

The downstream antiinflammatory effects of EPA and DHA may account for the health benefits of fish oil and may be indicators for additional studies into the effectiveness of its supplementation.

Maresins

Maresins, Ma (macrophage) R (resolution) in (inflammation), are pro-resolving lipid mediators converted from DHA, which are biosynthesized in the macrophages present in inflammatory exudate [26].

Functions of Maresins:
- Stopping PMN infiltration to the site of inflammation
- Stimulation of macrophage phagocytosis. This stimulation of cellular activity can help shorten the inflammation resolution interval, thereby protecting tissues from damage and oxidative stress [27,28]

Therapeutic applications

Based on the current evidence, PUFAs, LXs, Rvs, and miRNAs play a significant role in various inflammatory conditions and that they themselves, or their more stable synthetic analogs, could be of significant benefit in the development of treatment strategies of several low-grade systemic inflammatory diseases.

Protectins

Protectins (PDs) are also derived from DHA. Their name derives from the role they play in the protection of neural and immune tissues. Based upon which tissue they are being observed, they may be referred to as neuroprotectins [2]. In vivo studies show that Protectin D1 inhibits leukocyte migration and PMN infiltration in murine (mouse) systems [29] and enhanced efferocytosis of apoptotic polymorphonuclear leukocytes by human Mα [29]. Protectins demonstrate the hallmark actions of pro-resolving lipid mediators by showing both antiinflammatory and pro-resolving in vitro and in vivo [2].

Therapeutic applications

There is no current clinical application of Protectins, per say. However, with its demonstrated pro-resolving action, it gives further credence to the supplementation of DHA (its antecedent molecule) as an antiinflammatory strategy.

References

[1] Kohli P, Levy BD. Resolvins and protectins: mediating solutions to inflammation. Br J Pharmacol 2009;158(4):960–71.
[2] Serhan CN, Recchiuti A. Pro-resolving lipid mediators (SPMs) and their actions in regulating miRNA in novel resolution circuits in inflammation. Front Immunol 2012;3:298.
[3] Majno G, Joris I. Cells, tissues, and disease: Principles of general pathology. Oxford University Press; 2004.
[4] Burstein SH. The chemistry, biology and pharmacology of the cyclopentenone prostaglandins. Prostaglandins Other Lipid Mediat 2020;148, 106408.
[5] Colville-Nash PR, Gilroy DW. COX-2 and the cyclopentenone prostaglandins-a new chapter in the book of inflammation? Prostaglandins Other Lipid Mediat 2000;62(1):33–43.
[6] Poon IKH, Lucas CD, Rossi AG, Ravichandran KS. Apoptotic cell clearance: basic biology and therapeutic potential. Nat Rev Immunol 2014;14(3):166–80.
[7] Toussirot E, et al. Mini-review: the administration of apoptotic cells for treating rheumatoid arthritis: current knowledge and clinical perspectives. Front Immunol 2021;12:493.
[8] Dai R, Ansar Ahmed S. MicroRNA, a new paradigm for understanding immunoregulation, inflammation, and autoimmune diseases. Transl Res 2011;157(4):163–79.
[9] Mahesh G, Biswas R. MicroRNA-155: a master regulator of inflammation. J Interferon Cytokine Res 2019;39(6):321–30.
[10] Winter J, et al. Many roads to maturity: microRNA biogenesis pathways and their regulation. Nat Cell Biol 2009;11(3):228–34.
[11] Pei ZJ, et al. miR-122-5p inhibits tumor cell proliferation and induces apoptosis by targeting MYC in gastric cancer cells. Pharmazie 2017;72(6):344–7.
[12] Serhan CN, Haeggström JZ, Leslie CC. Lipid mediator networks in cell signaling: update and impact of cytokines 1. FASEB J 1996;10(10):1147–58.
[13] Yi T, et al. Comparative analysis of EPA and DHA in fish oil nutritional capsules by GC-MS. Lipids Health Dis 2014;13(1):1–6.
[14] Samuelsson B, et al. Leukotrienes and lipoxins: structures, biosynthesis, and biological effects. Science 1987;237(4819):1171–6.
[15] Takano T, et al. Aspirin-triggered 15-epi-lipoxin A4 (LXA4) and LXA4 stable analogues are potent inhibitors of acute inflammation: evidence for anti-inflammatory receptors. J Exp Med 1997;185(9):1693–704.

[16] Maddox JF, et al. Lipoxin A4 stable analogs are potent mimetics that stimulate human monocytes and THP-1 cells via a G-protein-linked lipoxin A4 receptor. J Biol Chem 1997;272(11):6972–8.
[17] Godson C, et al. Cutting edge: lipoxins rapidly stimulate nonphlogistic phagocytosis of apoptotic neutrophils by monocyte-derived macrophages. J Immunol 2000;164(4):1663–7.
[18] Claria J, Serhan CN. Aspirin triggers previously undescribed bioactive eicosanoids by human endothelial cell-leukocyte interactions. Proc Natl Acad Sci 1995;92(21):9475–9.
[19] Serhan CN, Petasis NA. Resolvins and protectins in inflammation resolution. Chem Rev 2011;111(10):5922–43.
[20] Clish CB, et al. Local and systemic delivery of a stable aspirin-triggered lipoxin prevents neutrophil recruitment in vivo. Proc Natl Acad Sci 1999;96(14):8247–52.
[21] Arita M, et al. Resolvin E1, an endogenous lipid mediator derived from omega-3 eicosapentaenoic acid, protects against 2, 4, 6-trinitrobenzene sulfonic acid-induced colitis. Proc Natl Acad Sci 2005;102(21):7671–6.
[22] Schwab JM, et al. Resolvin E1 and protectin D1 activate inflammation-resolution programmes. Nature 2007;447(7146):869–74.
[23] Hasturk H, et al. RvE1 protects from local inflammation and osteoclastmediated bone destruction in periodontitis. FASEB J 2006;20(2):401–3.
[24] Dona M, et al. Resolvin E1, an EPA-derived mediator in whole blood, selectively counterregulates leukocytes and platelets. Blood 2008;112(3):848–55.
[25] Xu Z-Z, et al. Resolvins RvE1 and RvD1 attenuate inflammatory pain via central and peripheral actions. Nat Med 2010;16(5):592–7.
[26] Serhan CN, et al. Maresins: novel macrophage mediators with potent antiinflammatory and proresolving actions. J Exp Med 2009;206(1):15–23.
[27] Bannenberg GL, et al. Molecular circuits of resolution: formation and actions of resolvins and protectins. J Immunol 2005;174(7):4345–55.
[28] Schwab JM, et al. Resolvin E1 and protectin D1 activate inflammation-resolution programmes. Nature 2007;447(7146):869–74.
[29] Serhan CN, et al. Anti-inflammatory actions of neuroprotectin D1/protectin D1 and its natural stereoisomers: assignments of dihydroxy-containing docosatrienes. J Immunol 2006;176(3):1848–59.

CHAPTER 13

Physical activity in obesity and inflammation prevention and management

Ollin Venegas[a] and Raman Mehrzad[b]
[a]Department of Surgery, Rhode Island Hospital, Brown University, Providence, RI, United States
[b]Division of Plastic and Reconstructive Surgery, Rhode Island Hospital, The Warren Alpert School of Brown University, Providence, RI, United States

Introduction

Obesity is a significant public health concern that is associated with numerous health problems, including diabetes, cardiovascular disease, musculoskeletal disorders, and many forms of cancer [1,2]. Obesity develops when the quantity of calories consumed exceeds that of bodily energy expenditure, indicating that it is preventable through appropriate modifications to lifestyle [3–8]. Despite this knowledge, obesity is a major public health concern with prevalence rates dramatically rising in the United States and worldwide. In 2017–18, the age-adjusted prevalence of obesity in the United States was 42.4%, and the age-adjusted prevalence of severe obesity was 9.2% among adults aged 20 and over [9]. Overall prevalence of obesity was similar among men and women, but women had a higher prevalence of severe obesity [9]. Adults aged 40–59 had the highest prevalence of severe obesity. Thus, understanding the biological basis for the development of obesity-related disturbances is an important need. However, the disease process and its contribution to the aforementioned comorbidities are complex, with an innumerable amount of genetic and environmental factors influencing the effective outcome [10,11].

Body weight is a regulated body energy equation where energy balance is the sum of calories consumed minus the calories expended over a 24-h period [12]. Therefore, when energy intake is equal to energy expenditure, body weight remains stable in a homeostatic state. Studies have shown that an effective way to achieve a negative energy balance is through the combination of regular exercise and diet [13–16]. A negative energy balance can be achieved via two manners: decreasing energy intake through diet or increasing energy expenditure through physical activity [15]. As a result, appropriate and adequate weight management for an individual is dependent on a tailored dietary plan and exercise regimen. This chapter provides new scientific-based knowledge about the role of physical activity in the management and prevention of obesity-related inflammation.

Obesity-related inflammation

Inflammation is the process by which the body responds to injury or infection and represents the initial defense mechanism to restore tissue homeostasis and function. Chronic, low-grade adipose tissue inflammation has long been associated with obesity through the contribution of proinflammatory adipokines to circulating levels of inflammatory markers [17,18]. Obesity-associated inflammation is first triggered by excess nutrients and is primarily localized in specialized metabolic tissues such as white adipose tissue (WAT) [19]. WAT acts as a major source of energy and is primarily composed of adipocytes. Adipocytes are endocrine cells that secrete a large range of cytokines, hormones, and growth factors, also known as adipokines [20,21]. These specialized cytokines specialize in the storage of energy as triglycerides in lipid droplets in the cytoplasm of adipocytes. Excess nutrients lead to activation of metabolic signaling pathways such as the protein kinase R, c-Jun N-terminal kinase (JNK), and nuclear factor k B (NFkB) [19]. Activation of these pathways lead to an induction of low-level inflammatory cytokines resulting in the low-grade inflammation [18]. Also, excess nutrients and obesity lead to hyperplasia and hypertrophy of WAT as well as extensive tissue remodeling and an increase in free fatty acids. These changes result in adipokine production and feed into the low-grade inflammatory response [22].

Next, obesity leads to increased endoplasmic reticulum stress resulting in activation of the unfolded protein response (UPR). The three branches of the UPR implicated in cellular inflammatory response include: activating transcription factor 6 (ATF-6); inositol-requiring enzyme 1 (IRE-1); and PKR-like eukaryotic initiation factor 2 α kinase (PERK). Investigations reveal that ATF-6 leads to increased NFkB signaling [22]. Next, IRE-1, through its interaction with TNF receptor-associated factor 2 (TRAF2), can activate JNK and inhibitor of κ kinase (IKK), leading to increased expression of inflammatory cytokines [23,24]. Finally, PERK activation leads to decreased translation of IκBα (a negative regulator NFkB), allowing for more production of NFkB [25]. Together, these pathways all contribute to the initiation and perpetuation of obesity-associated inflammation.

Obesity-associated inflammation leads to changes in immune cell infiltration and polarization in WAT. Macrophages are the dominant innate immune cells that are recruited to the obese WAT (Fig. 1). Likewise, these macrophages are one of the major sources of inflammatory cytokines. The recruitment of macrophages into the white adipose tissue is mediated by

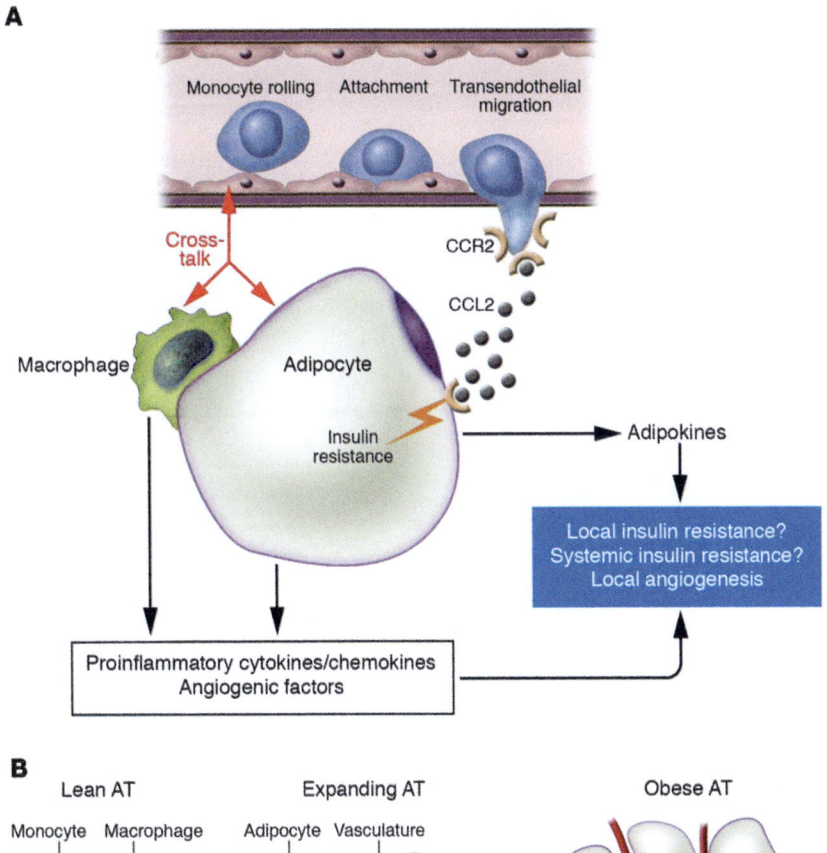

Fig. 1 Macrophage infiltration into white adipose tissue. (Source: Neels JG, Olefsky JM. Inflamed fat: what starts the fire? J Clin Invest. 2006 Jan;116(1):33–5. https://doi.org/10.1172/JCI27280. PMID: 16395402; PMCID: PMC1323268. Page 34.)

several mechanisms. First, adipose macrophages and adipocytes secrete a milieu of chemokines, including CCL2, CCL5, and RANTES/CCL5 [25]. These further promote the recruitment of macrophages into the WAT. Second, obesity-induced adipocyte hypertrophy leads to increased adipocyte cell death, which leads to the recruitment of macrophages [17]. Finally, adipocyte hypertrophy leads to increased levels of free fatty acids. These elevated levels act as TLR4 agonist and likely ligands for nod-like receptors to induce an inflammatory response and recruitment of macrophages to the WAT [22]. These mechanisms work in concert to induce a large influx of macrophages.

WAT can also shift the polarization of macrophages from an antiinflammatory M2-like phenotype in lean WAT, to a more proinflammatory M1-like phenotype seen in the WAT of obese patients (Fig. 2). Healthy adipose tissue expansion consists of an enlargement of the tissue through effective recruitment of adipogenic precursor cells, along with an appropriate remodeling of the extracellular matrix [22]. In contrast, pathological AT expansion consists of massive enlargement of existing adipocytes, limited angiogenesis, and ensuing hypoxia. Hypoxia-induced factor 1 α (HIF-1α), a

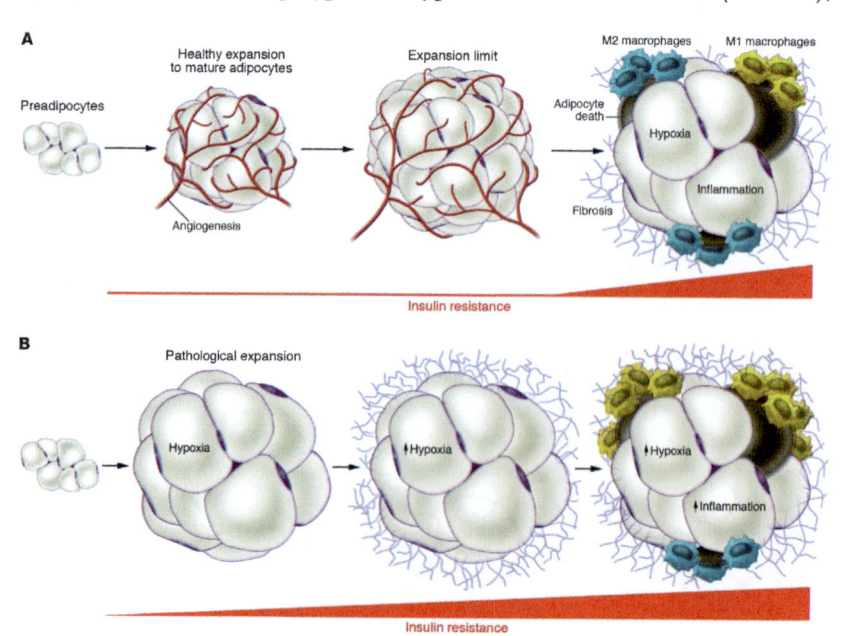

Fig. 2 Association of M1 macrophages and insulin resistance. (Source: Sun K, Kusminski CM, Scherer PE. Adipose tissue remodeling and obesity. J Clin Invest. 2011 Jun;121(6):2094–101. https://doi.org/10.1172/JCI45887. Epub 2011 Jun 1. PMID: 21633177; PMCID: PMC3104761. Page 2096.)

master regulator of oxygen homeostasis, is induced, which in turn can cause the induction of fibrosis [22]. As a result, M1-like macrophages prevail, leading to an inflammatory phenotype that is strongly associated with systemic insulin resistance [22].

Insulin resistance is partly due to the imbalance in leptin and adiponectin ratio [26]. Leptin is a product of the obese (*ob*) gene [27]. In humans, a major factor affecting leptin concentrations in plasma is adipose tissue mass [27]. Circulating levels of leptin exhibit a strong positive correlation with total body fat [27,28]. Moreover, higher concentrations of leptin in individuals with obesity are associated with increase fat mass and increased leptin release from larger adipocytes [28]. Finally, leptin expression can be induced under hypoxic conditions [29]. Chemical inducers of cellular hypoxia are able to activate the leptin promoter gene through the HIF-1 [27]. This evidence also supports other data that leptin regulates angiogenesis by itself and with vascular endothelial growth factor (VEGF) and fibroblast growth factor (FGF) 2 [29]. In summary, leptin is proinflammatory, proangiogenic, and proproliferative.

Physical activity and obesity-related inflammation

The impact of physical activity on inflammation has received significant attention in recent years. Physical activity is a major modifiable risk factor of obesity and therefore offers a potential therapeutic approach to modulate low-grade inflammation. The spectrum of physical activity is incredibly broad, ranging from the relatively new paradigm of physical inactivity/sedentary behavior physiology to adaptations associated with intermittent high-intensity exercise training (HIIT).

Often physical activity, physical exercise, and physical fitness are used as interchangeable concepts in reviews on this topic. However, it is important to point out the differences to highlight the potential differences in outcomes. For example, self-reported data of physical activity is easy and feasible to ask in a research questionnaire for a large sample population [30]. But this is a measurement subject to research biases. Exercise is planned, structured, and repetitive physical activity [30]. This is the objective data that is gathered in research studies. While physical fitness is the capacity to perform physical activity [30]. This makes reference to a full range of physiological and psychological qualities. Physical fitness also has been defined as "a set of attributes that people have or achieve that relates to the ability to perform physical activity." [30]

A major effect of an active lifestyle is to increase energy demands followed by a decrease of visceral fat mass. In this regard, exercise is known to mobilize fatty acids followed by a reduction in adipocyte size and increases blood flow and oxygen supply in adipose tissue [31]. In light of this, the potential for regular physical exercise as an antiinflammatory intervention is being studied for disorders of several body systems and tissues other than obesity. This includes but is not limited to circulatory (atherosclerosis, congestive heart failure), endocrine (metabolic syndrome), skeletal (arthritis, osteoporosis, and sarcopenia), pulmonary (obstructive lung diseases), and neurological (dementia and depression). Nevertheless, as will be pointed out below, the efficacy of exercise for reducing inflammation still requires further investigation.

Evidence from observational studies

Observational data from large population studies consistently demonstrate an association between physical activity and inflammation. Specifically, lower concentrations of inflammatory biomarkers are observed in individuals who perform more frequent, intense physical activity, leisure or non-leisure. This is true whether a single inflammatory biomarker is assessed or whether inflammation is depicted as a summary factor derived from multiple biomarkers.

Several large population cohorts provide strong evidence for an inverse, independent, dose-response relationship between systemic CRP concentration and level of physical activity. This includes the British Regional Heart Study [32], Third National Health and Nutrition Examination Survey (NHANES III) [33], Cardiovascular Health Study (CHS) [34], MacArthur Studies of Aging [35], Multi-Ethnic Study of Atherosclerosis (MESA) [36], InCHIANTI study [37], CoLaus Study [38], Heart and Soul Study [39], Indonesian Family Life Survey [40], and International Mobility in Aging Study(IMIAS) [41]. Table 1 summarizes the findings from 19 observational studies. In NHANES III, people who participated in jogging or dancing on 12 or more occasions per month showed the lowest odds for having elevated levels of CRP, odds ratio of 0.33 and 0.31, respectively [33]. In the Heart and Soul study, even light-intensity activity among patients with known coronary heart disease suggested a benefit for reducing or maintaining lower levels of inflammation in a medically complex population [39].

The inverse relationship between CRP and physical activity is seen across a wide age span, including the elderly [34,37,39,42–45] However, the association is seen more consistently in men than in women. For example,

Table 1 Observational studies showing association between inflammatory biomarkers and physical activity.

Author (year)	Sample size	Self-report physical activity measure	Association of greater PA measure to inflammatory biomarkers
Taaffe (2000)	880	Hours/year	↓ CRP and IL-6
Geffken (2001)	5888	Kcal/week	↓ CRP, factor VIII, WBC, and fibrinogen
Wannamethee (2002)	3810	physical activity index	↓ CRP, WBC, and fibrinogen
Reuben (2003)	13,748	Kcal/min/activity	↓ CRP and IL-6
Colbert (2004)	2798	mins/week	↓ TNF-α, CRP, and IL-6
Elousa (2005)	841	hours/week	↓ ESR, CRP, uric acid, and TNF-α
Hsu (2009)	1269	Kcal/week	↓ TNF-α, IL-6sR, and IL-2sR
Yu (2009)	3289	hours/week	↓ TNF-α, CRP, IL-6, adiponectin, and RBP4
Klenk (2012)	1253	mins/week	↓ WBC, hsTnT, Cr, and CysC
Bergström (2012)	391	hours/week	↓ CRP
Jennersjö (2012)	327	steps/day	↓ CRP and IL-6
Loprinzi (2013)	206	mins/day	↓ CRP
Moy (2014)	171	steps/day	↓ CRP and IL-6
Jarvie (2014)	656	mins/week	↓ CRP, IL-6, and fibrinogen
Nishida (2014)	1838	MET hour/day	↓ TNF-α, IL-6, and IL-15
Wu (2014)	1005	MET hour/week	↓ TNF-α, CRP, and IL-1β
Sujarwoto (2015)	2017	ADLs	↓ CRP
Vella (2016)	1970	MET min/week	↓ Leptin, IL-6, and resistin
Parsons (2017)	1274	mins/day	↓ CRP, tPA, vWF, D-dimer and IL-6

ADLs, activities of daily living; *CRP*, C-reactive protein; *Cr*, creatinine; *CysC*, cystatin C; *ESR*, erythrocyte sedimentation rate; *IL-6sR*, interleukin-6 soluble receptor; *IL2sR*, interleuking-2 soluble receptor; *MET*, metabolic equivalent; *RBP4*, retinol binding protein 4; *tPA*, tissue plasminogen activator; *TnT*, troponin T; *TNF-α*, tumor necrosis factor-alpha; *vWF*, Von Willebrand factor; *WBC*, white blood cells.

a stronger inverse relationship between CRP and physical activity was seen in men, compared with women, enrolled in the IMIAS [41]. When stratified by gender and ethnicity, the MESA study found that the strongest relationship between CRP and physical activity was seen in Hispanic men [36]. And for the InCHIANTI study, relationships between level of physical activity and inflammation were independent of body mass index (BMI) only in men [37]. This discrepancy may result from differences in body composition and/or regional fat distribution between women and men [46]. However, if this difference between sexes explained the discrepancy, it then becomes a potential confounding factor in the association between physical activity and inflammation.

While CRP is the most frequently studied biomarker of chronic inflammation, there are data regarding the association of other inflammatory markers with physical activity as well. In the Heart and Soul, there was a linear trend for IL-6, CRP, and insulin resistance biomarkers with increasing and high stable amounts of physical activity at 5-year follow-up [39]. In elderly men, both IL-6 and CRP concentrations were negatively related to the number of reported hours per year of moderate and strenuous exercise [43]. In addition, the lowest concentrations of both CRP and IL-6 were found in elderly persons with the highest levels of recreational physical activity [35]. Likewise, in a large study of leisure time exercise among Chinese women aged 40–70 years, levels of nonexercised physical activity were inversely associated with plasma concentrations of IL-6, IL-1β, and TNF-α [47]. Finally, among middle-aged Japanese people, step count and physical activity were inversely associated with TNF-α and IL-15 even after adjusting for BMI [48].

Results similar to those already mentioned have been reported from smaller studies as well. In the Cardiovascular Risk factors in Patients with Diabetes—a Prospective study in Primary care (CARDIPP), subjects who walked > 10,000 steps, compared with those with < 5000 steps, had lower levels of CRP and IL-6 [49]. Also, in the Leipzig University study for Adiposity Diseases, in participants with general obesity, levels of IL-4, IL-10, and IL-13 were significantly elevated in those with low physical activity [50].

Despite recent studies linking several inflammatory biomarkers to physical activity, it is not known whether one alone—or in specific combination with others—is a more robust indicator of the role of physical activity in the regulation of inflammation. The most recent study to compare multiple inflammatory factors was the Health, Aging, and Body Composition

(Health ABC) study [51]. This study utilized principal component analysis to identify inflammatory "components" and evaluated the associations between the identified components and measures of physical function. Results found two inflammatory components, TNF-α-related and CRP-related component, that had associations with physical performance [51]. However, the associations were inconsistent across different aspect of the physical function [51]. Future research is needed to clarify whether such an additive effect of inflammatory markers is reproducible in different disease states and populations.

A noteworthy limitation of the aforementioned studies is all assessed physical activity status via self-reporting surveys, without direct measurement of energy expenditure or activity. To our knowledge, there are no published studies on nondiseased individuals that examined the association between inflammation and physical activity energy expenditure measured via actigraphy or doubly labeled water. However, several studies report an inverse relationship exists between biomarkers of inflammation and direct measurement of cardiorespiratory fitness (VO_2max) assessed during an exercise test. In the Copenhagen Aging and Midlife Biobank, VO_2max was inversely associated with high sensitive CRP, IL-6, and IL-18, and directly associated with IL-10 [52]. There were no associations between VO_2max and IL-1β, TNF-α, or interferon gamma (IFN- γ) [52]. One statistically significant interaction between VO_2max and sex was in relation with IL-6. An increase in VO_2max of +1 mL/min/kg was associated with a decrease in IL-6 in both men and women of −1.44% and −2.80%, respectively [52].

Similar findings occurred in the HUNT3 Fitness study, where CRP was negatively associated with VO_{2peak} and positively associated with metabolic syndrome (with a stronger effect in men) and BMI (with a stronger effect in women) [53]. Owing to a significant interaction with sex, the influence of low fitness on CRP concentrations, when not considering BMI, was stronger in men [53]. The authors noted that the demonstration of a strong positive association between CRP and BMI showed that the negative relationship between CRP level and VO_{2peak} may be strongly confounded by BMI if it is not included in the analysis [53]. Importantly, it appears that differences in adiposity alone do not account for the strong inverse relationship seen between higher cardiorespiratory fitness and lower chronic inflammation. As discussed below, there are training adaptations observed in skeletal muscle and immune cells that can contribute to the lower levels of these inflammatory biomarkers, as observed in physically fit and active individuals.

The reasons for the observed inverse association between physical activity and inflammation are not entirely understood, but this relationship is likely related, in part, to the effects of physical activity on adiposity. Quantity of fat mass is irrefutably one of the strongest correlates of circulating inflammatory biomarkers [54]. Therefore, the amount needed to be accounted for when examining relationships between physical activity and inflammation. In most of the cohort studies, like in the HUNT3 Fitness Study, adjustment for adiposity (most often measured by BMI) attenuated the strength of the relationship between inflammatory biomarkers and physical activity. Also, in NHANESIII, the association between elevated CRP, fibrinogen, and physical activity was found to be independent of both BMI and waist-to-hip ratio [55]. However, in the InCHIANTI study, compared with sedentary women, women engaging in light and moderate-light physical activity had significantly IL-6 levels, and women practicing moderate-high activity had lower CRP [37]. But when the analysis adjusted for BMI, the association between physical activity and CRP, while the association with IL-6 was reduced [37]. Interestingly, in these models for the men in the study, the magnitude of the coefficients for physical activity was only slightly reduced and remained significant with lower levels of inflammatory biomarkers, including IL-6 and CRP [37].

BMI is not a direct measure of fat mass. As such, the strong associations observed between inflammation and physical activity/exercise may be confounded by variation in adiposity. To our knowledge, only the Health ABC Study has measured fat mass via dual-energy X-ray absorptiometry, as well as abdominal visceral fat via computed tomography [44]. Results found that adjustment for fat mass significantly reduced the association between IL-6 and physical activity and eliminated the association of CRP and TNFα with physical activity [44]. Consequently, a feasible explanation is that inflammation is decreased in physically active individuals primarily because of lower absolute amount of total and visceral body fat. The interaction of fat mass and physical activity and their effect on biomarkers is an important topic for future studies.

Overall, observational studies demonstrate the trend that the greater the volume of reported physical activity, the lower the risk of elevated levels of inflammatory biomarkers. In addition, the relationship between inflammation and physical activity is often independent of obesity when measured by BMI. However, as with all observational data, confirmation of whether inflammation and physical activity are causally related is not possible, nor to ascertain the directionality of the relationship. Several unanswered questions remain. First, are individuals with less inflammation more likely to maintain a greater level of physical fitness? Next, is a physically active lifestyle linked to lower inflammatory biomarkers linked through other health-related behavior, such as diet? And lastly, will an increase in physical activity/exercise result in a decrease in chronic inflammation? As summarized next, data from intervention studies may begin to answer these questions.

Evidence from interventional studies

Currently, data from intervention studies designed to examine the effects of exercise training on inflammation reflect less consistent findings than the data from observational studies (Table 2). Reasons for this are numerous, but are likely related to: (1) publication of findings from studies that are underpowered, (2) differences between studies in the caloric expenditure of the exercise leading to differences in the intervention's effect on body fat, (3) differences in the type (e.g., aerobic versus resistive), intensity, and duration of the exercise, (4) differences between studies in the baseline inflammatory status of study participants, and (5) lack of studies with an appropriate control group. This section summarizes the published exercise intervention studies (limited to those studies with exercise only treatments) and points to the need for additional fully powered and well-controlled studies to definitively assess the effects of exercise as a treatment for chronic inflammation.

Despite a large body of cross-sectional evidence showing that a higher volume of physical activity is associated with a lower systemic inflammation, a consensus does not exist between all intervention studies regarding an effect of increasing physical activity for reducing classical biomarkers of inflammation, especially CRP [55–64]. A recent meta-analysis that pooled 13 studies found that CRP and IL-6 were significantly decreased in response to chronic high-intensity endurance training [56]. Of the 13 studies, only four were included for the analysis of IL-6 and 10 for CRP [56]. Many studies were conducted with a smaller sample sizes than the observational studies. On the other hand, many of the studies that do show an effect of exercise training on CRP utilized an exercise intervention that resulted in slight to moderate decreases in body weight/fat [63,64]. However, in some studies, no significant differences were noted for CRP or IL-6 by the treatment arm, or changes in CRP were independent of the magnitude of weight/fat lost [64–67]. Nevertheless, because of the strong association between inflammation and adiposity, it is important to delineate the separate effects of exercise in the absence of weight or fat loss on inflammation.

Table 2 Randomized controlled trials examining the effect of exercise interventions on inflammatory biomarkers.

Author (year)	Sample size	Exercise intervention	Duration of intervention	Significance reported
Hammett (2004)	61	Aerobic exercise	6 months	↓ CRP
Rauramaa (2004)	140	Progressive aerobic exercises	6 years	↓ CRP
Campbell (2008)	202	Aerobic exercise	12 months	No effect to CRP levels
Beavers (2010)	368	Aerobic, strength, balance, and flexibility exercises	12 months	↓ IL-8
Donges (2010)	102	Aerobic and resistance exercises	10 weeks	↓ CRP
Arikawa (2011)	319	Aerobic exercise training	16 weeks	↓ CRP
Greene (2012)	18	Aerobic exercises	12 weeks	↓ CRP
Beavers (2013)	98	Walking and weight loss	18 months	↓ Leptin and IL-6
Keating (2013)	47	Walking and ergometers (cycle, row, and arm)	4 months	↓ CRP
Mediano (2013)	54	Home-based calisthenics	12 months	No effect to CRP levels
Khoo (2015)	80	Aerobic and resistance exercises	24 weeks	↓ Chemerin and CRP
Liu (2018)	1298	Walking; strength, flexibility, and balance training	24 months	↓ IL-8
Babatunde (2020)	337	Aerobic exercises	12 months	No reduction of CRP or IL-6

For the most part, intervention studies in participants with elevated inflammation due to chronic disease or obesity show a favorable exercise training effect (in the absence of weight loss) on specific inflammatory biomarkers. For instance, a meta-analysis of 23 studies found that exercise training is associated with reduced inflammatory activity (CRP and fibrinogen) in patients with coronary artery disease [68]. These results were re-enforced by a systemic review on atherosclerosis that the found high evidence that physical activity decreases CRP. Analysis also found moderate and low evidence for TNF-α and IL-6, respectively [68]. In a review of 20 randomized control trials on the antiinflammatory effects of exercise on metabolic syndrome patients, results demonstrated an overall significant decrease in serum levels of TNF- α, CRP, IL-8 and a significant increase in IL-10 [68]. For these variables, isolated aerobic exercise and combined aerobic and resistance exercise appeared to be optimal [68]. Exercise training did not change the level of IL-6 and IL-18 [68]. In one of the largest, yet nonrandomized, exercise studies conducted, the HERITAGE Family Study found that plasma CRP was significantly reduced with 20 weeks of exercise training program in the high baseline CRP group across all population groups [69]. Authors noted that individuals with a high baseline CRP represented one-fourth of the adult population in the United States, which highlights the importance of exercise in the prevention and management of cardiovascular and metabolic diseases [69].

Collectively, these studies support the hypothesis that regular aerobic exercise has the potential to lower concentrations of inflammatory biomarkers in individuals with conditions associated with elevated inflammation. However, the majority of interventional studies did not compare research subjects randomized to exercise versus a nonexercise control group. Furthermore, the wide variability and volatile nature of most biomarkers of inflammation within and among individuals necessitate the use of a control group and randomization of research subjects.

To date, there are relatively few adequately powered, randomized, controlled trials (RCTs) of an exercise intervention on inflammatory biomarkers. The included studies are limited to those with 20 or more subjects per primary treatment group, those that used supervised or center-based exercise interventions, and those where changes in body weight were not significantly related to changes in biomarkers of inflammation.

One of the larger nonrandomized clinically controlled trials demonstrated that a phase II cardiac rehabilitation and exercise training program reduced median CRP concentration by 41% in coronary heart disease (CHD) patients [67]. CRP did not change in CHD patients who did not undergo rehabilitation [67]. However, the effect of exercise training was more effective in patients with the highest CRP concentrations [67]. In addition, patients with intermittent claudication randomized to a 12-week exercise regimen reduced levels of CRP at the end, but with no changes observed in those randomized to the control group [70]. Interestingly, this change did not persist after 6 or 12 months [70]. In obese Asian men, the exercise group demonstrated greater reductions in fat mass, serum chemerin, CRP, and insulin resistance [71]. And in a 16-week study of women aged 18–30 years, the study demonstrated that the aerobic exercise program significantly decreased levels of CRP in young women, especially in those who were obese [72]. On the other hand, in obese African-American women, no difference was observed between the treatment and control group for CRP or IL-6 at 3 or 12 months [64]. Similarly, randomization in a 12-month aerobic exercise intervention did not affect CRP levels in men and women with normal CRP baseline values [73]. Finally, in a 6-month exercise training study of adults aged 60–85 years, serum CRP levels were not statistically altered, even when the reduction in CRP in the exercise group was twice that of the control arm [58]. Thus, some, but not all, randomized studies show a trend toward lowering of inflammation with exercise, especially in those with higher inflammation at baseline.

One stratum of the population where the relationship between physical activity and inflammatory markers is an active form of research is with elderly men and women. Chronic low-grade inflammation is associated with advanced age, thus the inflammatory pathway is a potential therapeutic target to reduce disease and disability in older adults. One such study was conducted as an ancillary study to the Cooperative Lifestyle Intervention Program, a randomized control trial of physical activity and weight loss on mobility in overweight or obese older adults with or at risk for cardiovascular disease [74]. The study was 18 months with a community infrastructure of cooperative extension centers in North Carolina on 288 participants community-dwelling men and women aged 60–79 years [74]. The physical intervention consisted of a combination of walking and interactive, group-mediated, behavioral focused session (total of 48 sessions) [74]. Several biomarkers of inflammation (adiponectin, leptin, IL-6, IL-8, and soluble TNF) were measured at three periods during the study (preintervention, 6 months, and 18 months) [74]. Overall, the physical activity plus weight loss reduced leptin and IL-6 levels more than physical activity alone and the successful aging health center intervention [74]. Findings for soluble TNF were not statistically significant, and no intervention effect was observed with adiponectin or IL-8 [74]. As a result, authors suggested that obesity is characterized by a state of chronic inflammation, directly related to the amount of stored body fat. And, more importantly, that the reduction in body fat mass is an effective means of reducing inflammatory burden

[74]. Thus, physical activity intervention reduces some, but certainly not all, biomarkers of systemic inflammation in elderly individuals, and this benefit is most pronounced in those often with more inflammation at baseline.

Although more attention has been paid to the effects of aerobic exercise on inflammation, resistance exercise training studies have been conducted, largely with negative results negative [75–85]. The first of such studies was conducted in 1996 and found that a 12-week regimen of progressive resistance strength training of men and women of all major muscle groups on a twice weekly basis did not affect IL-1β, TNF-α, IL-6, or IL-2 production [77]. However, this study only had a total of 30 research subjects complete the entire training regimen, with no more than eight subjects in each treatment or control group [77]. Thus, small sample sizes in this study may have contributed to this null effect. In addition, other more recent studies, with small sample sizes, have arrived at different conclusions. A 12-week study on the influence of resistance training on inflammatory biomarker in obese, postmenopausal women found that the training reduced markers of subclinical inflammation in the absence of changes in body composition [86]. Levels of CRP were reduced by 33%, leptin levels by 18%, and TNF-α by 29% [86]. Another 10-week study of moderate- to high-intensity resistance training on previously sedentary women (mean age, 72 years) observed a decrease in IL-6, IL-1β, TNF-α in circulation and lipopolysaccharide-stimulated whole blood [82]. Lastly, and in agreement with the notion that obesity plays an integral role in inflammatory biomarker expression, a 19-week study on progressive resistance training associated with dietetic advice, focusing on foods rich in antiinflammatory and antioxidant properties, in 40 elderly people found a reduction in inflammatory and metabolic variable [78].

In conclusion, data from RCTs indicate that aerobic exercise training interventions conducted in individuals with high inflammation are beneficial for reducing inflammatory biomarker levels. Moreover, individuals that had even a slight amount of weight reduction also found benefits. However, it appears that increasing physical activity alone has a small, often undetectable, effect on inflammation in normal, healthy individuals.

Weight loss and maintenance

As reviewed through the observational and interventional studies, the biological mechanisms by which physical activity/exercise prevents weight gain are multiple. Not only does activity increase total energy expenditure and basal metabolic rate, but also reduces fat mass and maintains lean muscle mass. However, the optimal amount of exercise needed to prevent weight gain in adults may vary by age, sex, and energy intake.

The consensus of evidence of recent reviews supports that the most effective plan for achieving initial weight loss should combine dietary changes focused on reduced calorie intake, increased physical activity, and behavior modification strategies [87–89]. Systematic reviews have reported that physical activity alone without dietary modification produces, at best, minimal to modest weight loss [87,90]. And this only occurs when the activity is moderately vigorous and of sufficient duration, approximately 60 min per session [87,90]. However, it should be noted that when dietary modifications alone were compared with physical activity alone, and when the same energy deficit was achieved, the weight loss was equivalent [91,92]. This means that weight loss can be achieved with exercise alone, but the exercise then must be sufficient—in intensity and duration—to influence metabolism and subsequent weight loss.

The current recommendation of 150 min per week of moderate-to-vigorous physical activity is required to influence body weight regulation and subsequent weight loss [93]. This equivocates to 30 min of exercise five times a week. Muscle-strengthening activities on 2 or more days a week is also recommended for adults [93]. Older adults should do multicomponent physical activity that includes balance training as well as aerobic and muscle-strengthening activities [93]. Adults with chronic conditions or disabilities, who are able, should follow the key guidelines for adults and do both aerobic and muscle-strengthening activities [93]. Recommendations emphasize that more movement and less sedentary habits benefit nearly everyone. Individuals performing the least physical activity benefit most by even modest increases in moderate-to-vigorous physical activity. Additional benefits occur with more physical activity.

In the MedWeight Registry study, results found a distinct difference between weight loss "maintainers" and weight loss "regainers." [94] The study looked at 756 participants, aged 18–65 years, who lost ≥ 10% initial weight, and either maintained their lost weight after 12 months or regained it [94]. For women who maintained their weight, averaged a total of 140 min of physical activity per week [94]. Although maintainers and regainers did similar activities, maintainers spent more time during these sessions by 12 min or more [94]. For every 10-min increment of weekly walking, or weekly total activity, the study observed 1% higher odds for weight loss maintenance, respectively [94]. Regarding men, maintainers were found to be largely more active than regainers, with greater differences observed in vigorous activities (intense aerobic exercises, lifting heavy weights, and strenuous gardening) [94]. Men maintainers participated in more vigorous activity sessions per week that lasted 27 min longer than the respective activity of regainers [94].

Conclusion

Obesity-related inflammation is an important contributor to the pathophysiology of several chronic health conditions. Given these widespread deleterious health effects of an augmented inflammatory state, identification of therapies that reduce inflammation is critical. Yet, to date, there is little definitive evidence for therapies that can effectively treat individuals with elevated markers of inflammation that are within the clinically normal range. Given that physical activity and obesity are often inversely related, it is not clear as to whether the antiinflammatory health benefits of a physically active lifestyle are due to exercise per se or result from favorable changes in body composition. However, consistent data from observational studies showing a link between self-reported levels of physical activity and inflammatory biomarkers, as well as some promising positive data from RCTS indicate that increasing aerobic physical activity could be effective for reducing chronic inflammation. This is especially the case in individuals with chronic diseases associated with a state of elevated inflammation. Nevertheless, exercise is uniquely positioned to reduce inflammation, and even small nonsignificant reductions in CRP levels may contribute to clinical benefits by reducing cardiovascular and metabolic risk. Additional trials targeting the magnitude of the effect of physical activity on inflammatory mediators and the amount of exercise necessary to produce clinically meaningful reductions in inflammation are needed.

References

[1] Jéquier E. Pathways to obesity. Int J Obes 2002;26(2):S12–7. https://doi.org/10.1038/sj.ijo.0802123.
[2] Ortega FB, Lavie CJ, Blair SN. Obesity and cardiovascular disease. Circ Res 2016;118(11):1752–70. https://doi.org/10.1161/CIRCRESAHA.115.306883.
[3] Hall KD, Heymsfield SB, Kemnitz JW, Klein S, Schoeller DA, Speakman JR. Energy balance and its components: implications for body weight regulation. Am J Clin Nutr 2012;95(4):989–94. https://doi.org/10.3945/ajcn.112.036350.
[4] Manore MM, Larson-Meyer DE, Lindsay AR, Hongu N, Houtkooper L. Dynamic energy balance: an integrated framework for discussing diet and physical activity in obesity prevention—is it more than eating less and exercising more? Nutrients 2017;9(8):905. https://doi.org/10.3390/nu9080905.

[5] Spiegelman BM, Flier JS. Obesity and the regulation of energy balance. Cell 2001;104(4):531–43. https://doi.org/10.1016/S0092-8674(01)00240-9.
[6] Astrup A, Raben A. Obesity: an inherited metabolic deficiency in the control of macronutrient balance? Eur J Clin Nutr 1992;46(9):611–20.
[7] Ravussin E, Lillioja S, Knowler WC, et al. Reduced rate of energy expenditure as a risk factor for body-weight gain. N Engl J Med 1988;318(8):467–72. https://doi.org/10.1056/nejm198802253180802.
[8] Flatt JP. Importance of nutrient balance in body weight regulation. Diabetes Metab Rev 1988;4(6):571–81. https://doi.org/10.1002/dmr.5610040603.
[9] Hales CM, Carroll MD, Fryar CDOC. Prevalence of obesity and severe obesity among adults: United States, 2017–2018. Hyattsville, MD., 2020, https://www.cdc.gov/nchs/data/databriefs/db360-h.pdf.
[10] Nicolaidis S. Environment and obesity. Metabolism 2019;100. https://doi.org/10.1016/j.metabol.2019.07.006, 153942.
[11] Albuquerque D, Nóbrega C, Manco L, Padez C. The contribution of genetics and environment to obesity. Br Med Bull 2017;123(1):159–73. https://doi.org/10.1093/bmb/ldx022.
[12] Hopkins M, Blundell JE. Energy balance, body composition, sedentariness and appetite regulation: pathways to obesity. Clin Sci 2016;130(18):1615–28. https://doi.org/10.1042/CS20160006.
[13] Anon. The effects of losing weight through diet or exercise programs on obesity. Ann Intern Med 2000;133(2):92. https://doi.org/10.7326/0003-4819-133-2-200007180-00022.
[14] Ross R, Dagnone D, Jones PJH, et al. Reduction in obesity and related comorbid conditions after diet-induced weight loss or exercise-induced weight loss in men: a randomized, controlled trial. Ann Intern Med 2000;133(2):92–103. https://doi.org/10.7326/0003-4819-133-2-200007180-00008.
[15] Hopkins M, Gibbons C, Caudwell P, et al. The adaptive metabolic response to exercise-induced weight loss influences both energy expenditure and energy intake. Eur J Clin Nutr 2014;68(5):581–6. https://doi.org/10.1038/ejcn.2013.277.
[16] Leibel RL, Rosenbaum M, Hirsch J. Changes in energy expenditure resulting from altered body weight. N Engl J Med 1995;332(10):621–8. https://doi.org/10.1056/nejm199503093321001.
[17] Neels JG, Olefsky JM. Inflamed fat: what starts the fire? J Clin Invest 2006;116(1):33–5. https://doi.org/10.1172/JCI27280.
[18] Mraz M, Haluzik M. The role of adipose tissue immune cells in obesity and low-grade inflammation. J Endocrinol 2014;222(3):113–27. https://doi.org/10.1530/JOE-14-0283.
[19] Gregor MF, Hotamisligil GS. Inflammatory mechanisms in obesity. Annu Rev Immunol 2011;29(1):415–45. https://doi.org/10.1146/annurev-immunol-031210-101322.
[20] Fasshauer M, Blüher M. Adipokines in health and disease. Trends Pharmacol Sci 2015;36(7):461–70. https://doi.org/10.1016/j.tips.2015.04.014.
[21] Sun S, Ji Y, Kersten S, Qi L. Mechanisms of inflammatory responses in obese adipose tissue. Annu Rev Nutr 2012;32:261–86. https://doi.org/10.1146/annurev-nutr-071811-150623.
[22] Sun K, Kusminski CM, Scherer PE. Adipose tissue remodeling and obesity. J Clin Invest 2011;121(6):2094–101. https://doi.org/10.1172/JCI45887.
[23] Hu P, Han Z, Couvillon AD, Kaufman RJ, Exton JH. Autocrine tumor necrosis factor alpha links endoplasmic reticulum stress to the membrane death receptor pathway through IRE1α-mediated NF-κB activation and down-regulation of TRAF2 expression. Mol Cell Biol 2006;26(8):3071–84. https://doi.org/10.1128/mcb.26.8.3071-3084.2006.

[24] Yamazaki H, Hiramatsu N, Hayakawa K, et al. Activation of the Akt-NF-κB pathway by subtilase cytotoxin through the ATF6 branch of the unfolded protein response. J Immunol 2009;183(2):1480–7. https://doi.org/10.4049/jimmunol.0900017.
[25] Deng J, Lu PD, Zhang Y, et al. Translational repression mediates activation of nuclear factor kappa B by phosphorylated translation initiation factor 2. Mol Cell Biol 2004;24(23):10161–8. https://doi.org/10.1128/mcb.24.23.10161-10168.2004.
[26] Zhang Y, Scarpace PJ. The role of leptin in leptin resistance and obesity. Physiol Behav 2006;88(3):249–56. https://doi.org/10.1016/j.physbeh.2006.05.038.
[27] Paracchini V, Pedotti P, Taioli E. Genetics of leptin and obesity: a HuGE review. Am J Epidemiol 2005;162(2):101–14. https://doi.org/10.1093/aje/kwi174.
[28] De Luis DA, Perez Castrillón JL, Dueñas A. Leptin and obesity. Minerva Med 2009;100(3):229–36. https://doi.org/10.2165/00023210-200014060-00001.
[29] Garofalo C, Surmacz E. Leptin and cancer. J Cell Physiol 2006;207(1):12–22. https://doi.org/10.1002/jcp.20472.
[30] Caspersen CJ, Powell KE, Christenson GM. Physical activity, exercise, and physical fitness: definitions and distinctions for health-related research. Public Health Rep 1985;100(2):126–31.
[31] Ringseis R, Eder K, Mooren FC, Krüger K. Metabolic signals and innate immune activation in obesity and exercise. Exerc Immunol Rev 2015;21:58–68.
[32] Wannamethee SG, Lowe GDO, Whincup PH, Rumley A, Walker M, Lennon L. Physical activity and hemostatic and inflammatory variables in elderly men. Circulation 2002;105(15):1785–90. https://doi.org/10.1161/hc1502.107117.
[33] King DE, Carek P, Mainous 3rd AG, Pearson WS. Inflammatory markers and exercise: differences related to exercise type. Med Sci Sports Exerc 2003;35(4):575–81. https://doi.org/10.1249/01.MSS.0000058440.28108.CC.
[34] Geffken DF, Cushman M, Burke GL, Polak JF, Sakkinen PA, Tracy RP. Association between physical activity and markers of inflammation in a healthy elderly population. Am J Epidemiol 2001;153(3):242–50. https://doi.org/10.1093/aje/153.3.242.
[35] Reuben DB, Judd-Hamilton L, Harris TB, Seeman TE. The associations between physical activity and inflammatory markers in high-functioning older persons: MacArthur studies of successful aging. J Am Geriatr Soc 2003;51(8):1125–30. https://doi.org/10.1046/j.1532-5415.2003.51380.x.
[36] Vella CA, Allison MA, Cushman M, et al. Physical activity and adiposity-related inflammation: the MESA. Med Sci Sports Exerc 2017;49(5):915–21. https://doi.org/10.1249/MSS.0000000000001179.
[37] Elosua R, Bartali B, Ordovas JM, Corsi AM, Lauretani F, Ferrucci L. Association between physical activity, physical performance, and inflammatory biomarkers in an elderly population: the InCHIANTI study. J Gerontol A Biol Sci Med Sci 2005;60(6):760–7. https://doi.org/10.1093/gerona/60.6.760.
[38] Marques-Vidal P, Bochud M, Bastardot F, et al. Association between inflammatory and obesity markers in a Swiss population-based sample (CoLaus study). Obes Facts 2012;5(5):734–44. https://doi.org/10.1159/000345045.
[39] Jarvie JL, Whooley MA, Regan MC, Sin NL, Cohen BE. Effect of physical activity level on biomarkers of inflammation and insulin resistance over 5 years in outpatients with coronary heart disease (from the Heart and Soul Study). Am J Cardiol 2014;114(8):1192–7. https://doi.org/10.1016/j.amjcard.2014.07.036.
[40] Sujarwoto S, Tampubolon G. Inflammatory markers and physical performance in middle-aged and older people in Indonesia. Age Ageing 2015;44(4):610–5. https://doi.org/10.1093/ageing/afv052.
[41] Sousa ACPA, Zunzunegui M-V, Li A, Phillips SP, Guralnik JM, Guerra RO. Association between C-reactive protein and physical performance in older populations: results from the International Mobility in Aging Study (IMIAS). Age Ageing 2016;45(2):274–80. https://doi.org/10.1093/ageing/afv202.

[42] Yu Z, Ye X, Wang J, et al. Associations of physical activity with inflammatory factors, adipocytokines, and metabolic syndrome in middle-aged and older chinese people. Circulation 2009;119(23):2969–77. https://doi.org/10.1161/CIRCULATIONAHA.108.833574.

[43] Taaffe DR, Harris TB, Ferrucci L, Rowe J, Seeman TE. Cross-sectional and prospective relationships of interleukin-6 and C-reactive protein with physical performance in elderly persons: MacArthur studies of successful aging. J Gerontol A Biol Sci Med Sci 2000;55(12):M709–15. https://doi.org/10.1093/gerona/55.12.m709.

[44] Colbert LH, Visser M, Simonsick EM, et al. Physical activity, exercise, and inflammatory markers in older adults: findings from the health, aging and body composition study. J Am Geriatr Soc 2004;52(7):1098–104. https://doi.org/10.1111/j.1532-5415.2004.52307.x.

[45] Wärnberg J, Cunningham K, Romeo J, Marcos A. Physical activity, exercise and low-grade systemic inflammation. Proc Nutr Soc 2010;69(3):400–6. https://doi.org/10.1017/S0029665110001928.

[46] Karastergiou K, Smith SR, Greenberg AS, Fried SK. Sex differences in human adipose tissues—the biology of pear shape. Biol Sex Differ 2012;3(1):13. https://doi.org/10.1186/2042-6410-3-13.

[47] Wu SH, Shu XO, Chow W-H, et al. Nonexercise physical activity and inflammatory and oxidative stress markers in women. J Women's Health (Larchmt) 2014;23(2):159–67. https://doi.org/10.1089/jwh.2013.4456.

[48] Nishida Y, Higaki Y, Taguchi N, et al. Objectively measured physical activity and inflammatory cytokine levels in middle-aged Japanese people. Prev Med (Baltim) 2014;64:81–7. https://doi.org/10.1016/j.ypmed.2014.04.004.

[49] Jennersjö P, Ludvigsson J, Länne T, Nystrom FH, Ernerudh J, Östgren CJ. Pedometer-determined physical activity is linked to low systemic inflammation and low arterial stiffness in Type 2 diabetes. Diabet Med 2012;29(9):1119–25. https://doi.org/10.1111/j.1464-5491.2012.03621.x.

[50] Schmidt FM, Weschenfelder J, Sander C, et al. Inflammatory cytokines in general and central obesity and modulating effects of physical activity. PLoS ONE 2015;10(3). https://doi.org/10.1371/journal.pone.0121971, e0121971.

[51] Hsu F-C, Kritchevsky SB, Liu Y, et al. Association between inflammatory components and physical function in the health, aging, and body composition study: a principal component analysis approach. J Gerontol A Biol Sci Med Sci 2009;64(5):581–9. https://doi.org/10.1093/gerona/glp005.

[52] Wedell-Neergaard A-S, Krogh-Madsen R, Petersen GL, et al. Cardiorespiratory fitness and the metabolic syndrome: roles of inflammation and abdominal obesity. PLoS One 2018;13(3). https://doi.org/10.1371/journal.pone.0194991, e0194991.

[53] Madssen E, Skaug E-A, Wisløff U, Ellingsen Ø, Videm V. Inflammation is strongly associated with cardiorespiratory fitness, sex, BMI, and the metabolic syndrome in a self-reported healthy population: HUNT3 fitness study. Mayo Clin Proc 2019;94(5):803–10. https://doi.org/10.1016/j.mayocp.2018.08.040.

[54] Nicklas BJ, You T, Pahor M. Behavioural treatments for chronic systemic inflammation: effects of dietary weight loss and exercise training. Can Med Assoc J = J l'Association medicale Can 2005;172(9):1199–209. https://doi.org/10.1503/cmaj.1040769.

[55] Abramson JL, Vaccarino V. Relationship between physical activity and inflammation among apparently healthy middle-aged and older US adults. Arch Intern Med 2002;162(11):1286–92. https://doi.org/10.1001/archinte.162.11.1286.

[56] Tesema G, George M, Hadgu A, Haregot E, Mondal S, Mathivana D. Does chronic high-intensity endurance training have an effect on cardiovascular markers of active populations and athletes? Systematic review and meta-analysis. BMJ Open 2019;9(10). https://doi.org/10.1136/bmjopen-2019-032832, e032832.

[57] Donges CE, Duffield R, Drinkwater EJ. Effects of resistance or aerobic exercise training on interleukin-6, C-reactive protein, and body composition. Med Sci Sports Exerc 2010;42(2):304–13. https://doi.org/10.1249/MSS.0b013e3181b117ca.

[58] Hammett CJK, Oxenham HC, Baldi JC, et al. Effect of six months' exercise training on C-reactive protein levels in healthy elderly subjects. J Am Coll Cardiol 2004;44(12):2411–3. https://doi.org/10.1016/j.jacc.2004.09.030.

[59] Kelley GA, Kelley KS. Effects of aerobic exercise on C-reactive protein, body composition, and maximum oxygen consumption in adults: a meta-analysis of randomized controlled trials. Metabolism 2006;55(11):1500–7. https://doi.org/10.1016/j.metabol.2006.06.021.

[60] Church TS, Barlow CE, Earnest CP, Kampert JB, Priest EL, Blair SN. Associations between cardiorespiratory fitness and C-reactive protein in men. Arterioscler Thromb Vasc Biol 2002;22(11):1869–76. https://doi.org/10.1161/01.atv.0000036611.77940.f8.

[61] Rauramaa R, Halonen P, Väisänen SB, et al. Effects of aerobic physical exercise on inflammation and atherosclerosis in men: the DNASCO Study: a six-year randomized, controlled trial. Ann Intern Med 2004;140(12):1007–14. https://doi.org/10.7326/0003-4819-140-12-200406150-00010.

[62] Mikkelsen UR, Couppé C, Karlsen A, et al. Life-long endurance exercise in humans: circulating levels of inflammatory markers and leg muscle size. Mech Ageing Dev 2013;134(11-12):531–40. https://doi.org/10.1016/j.mad.2013.11.004.

[63] Greene NP, Martin SE, Crouse SF. Acute exercise and training alter blood lipid and lipoprotein profiles differently in overweight and obese men and women. Obesity (Silver Spring) 2012;20(8):1618–27. https://doi.org/10.1038/oby.2012.65.

[64] Babatunde OAP, Arp Adams SP, Truman S, et al. The impact of a randomized dietary and physical activity intervention on chronic inflammation among obese African-American women. Women Health 2020;60(7):792–805. https://doi.org/10.1080/03630242.2020.1746950.

[65] Oberbach A, Tönjes A, Klöting N, et al. Effect of a 4 week physical training program on plasma concentrations of inflammatory markers in patients with abnormal glucose tolerance. Eur J Endocrinol 2006;154(4):577–85. https://doi.org/10.1530/eje.1.02127.

[66] Okita K, Nishijima H, Murakami T, et al. Can exercise training with weight loss lower serum C-reactive protein levels? Arterioscler Thromb Vasc Biol 2004;24(10):1868–73. https://doi.org/10.1161/01.ATV.0000140199.14930.32.

[67] Milani RV, Lavie CJ, Mehra MR. Reduction in C-reactive protein through cardiac rehabilitation and exercise training. J Am Coll Cardiol 2004;43(6):1056–61. https://doi.org/10.1016/j.jacc.2003.10.041.

[68] Swardfager W, Herrmann N, Cornish S, et al. Exercise intervention and inflammatory markers in coronary artery disease: a meta-analysis. Am Heart J 2012;163(4):663–6. https://doi.org/10.1016/j.ahj.2011.12.017.

[69] Lakka TA, Lakka H-M, Rankinen T, et al. Effect of exercise training on plasma levels of C-reactive protein in healthy adults: the HERITAGE family study. Eur Heart J 2005;26(19):2018–25. https://doi.org/10.1093/eurheartj/ehi394.

[70] Tisi PV, Hulse M, Chulakadabba A, Gosling P, Shearman CP. Exercise training for intermittent claudication: does it adversely affect biochemical markers of the exercise-induced inflammatory response? Eur J Vasc Endovasc Surg 1997;14(5):344–50. https://doi.org/10.1016/s1078-5884(97)80283-3.

[71] Khoo J, Dhamodaran S, Chen D-D, Yap S-Y, Chen RY-T, Tian RH-H. Exercise-induced weight loss is more effective than dieting for improving adipokine profile, insulin resistance, and inflammation in obese men. Int J Sport Nutr Exerc Metab 2015;25(6):566–75. https://doi.org/10.1123/ijsnem.2015-0025.

[72] Arikawa AY, Thomas W, Schmitz KH, Kurzer MS. Sixteen weeks of exercise reduces C-reactive protein levels in young women. Med Sci Sports Exerc 2011;43(6):1002–9. https://doi.org/10.1249/MSS.0b013e3182059eda.

[73] Campbell KL, Campbell PT, Ulrich CM, et al. No reduction in C-reactive protein following a 12-month randomized controlled trial of exercise in men and women. Cancer Epidemiol Biomarkers Prev 2008;17(7):1714–8. https://doi.org/10.1158/1055-9965.EPI-08-0088.

[74] Beavers KM, Ambrosius WT, Nicklas BJ, Rejeski WJ. Independent and combined effects of physical activity and weight loss on inflammatory biomarkers in overweight and obese older adults. J Am Geriatr Soc 2013;61(7):1089–94. https://doi.org/10.1111/jgs.12321.

[75] Ihalainen JK, Schumann M, Eklund D, et al. Combined aerobic and resistance training decreases inflammation markers in healthy men. Scand J Med Sci Sports 2018;28(1):40–7. https://doi.org/10.1111/sms.12906.

[76] Kolahdouzi S, Baghadam M, Kani-Golzar FA, et al. Progressive circuit resistance training improves inflammatory biomarkers and insulin resistance in obese men. Physiol Behav 2019;205:15–21. https://doi.org/10.1016/j.physbeh.2018.11.033.

[77] Rall LC, Roubenoff R, Cannon JG, Abad LW, Dinarello CA, Meydani SN. Effects of progressive resistance training on immune response in aging and chronic inflammation. Med Sci Sports Exerc 1996;28(11):1356–65. https://doi.org/10.1097/00005768-199611000-00003.

[78] Lopes LMP, de Oliveira EC, Becker LK, et al. Resistance training associated with dietetic advice reduces inflammatory biomarkers in the elderly. Biomed Res Int 2020;2020:7351716. https://doi.org/10.1155/2020/7351716.

[79] Ihalainen JK, Inglis A, Mäkinen T, et al. Strength training improves metabolic health markers in older individual regardless of training frequency. Front Physiol 2019;10:32. https://doi.org/10.3389/fphys.2019.00032.

[80] Sardeli AV, Tomeleri CM, Cyrino ES, Fernhall B, Cavaglieri CR, Chacon-Mikahil MPT. Effect of resistance training on inflammatory markers of older adults: a meta-analysis. Exp Gerontol 2018;111:188–96. https://doi.org/10.1016/j.exger.2018.07.021.

[81] Phillips MD, Flynn MG, McFarlin BK, Stewart LK, Timmerman KL, Ji H. Resistive exercise blunts LPS-stimulated TNF-alpha and Il-1 beta. Int J Sports Med 2008;29(2):102–9. https://doi.org/10.1055/s-2007-965115.

[82] Phillips MD, Flynn MG, McFarlin BK, Stewart LK, Timmerman KL. Resistance training at eight-repetition maximum reduces the inflammatory milieu in elderly women. Med Sci Sports Exerc 2010;42(2):314–25. https://doi.org/10.1249/MSS.0b013e3181b11ab7.

[83] Phillips MD, Patrizi RM, Cheek DJ, Wooten JS, Barbee JJ, Mitchell JB. Resistance training reduces subclinical inflammation in obese, postmenopausal women. Med Sci Sports Exerc 2012;44(11):2099–110. https://doi.org/10.1249/MSS.0b013e3182644984.

[84] Hagstrom AD, Marshall PWM, Lonsdale C, et al. The effect of resistance training on markers of immune function and inflammation in previously sedentary women recovering from breast cancer: a randomized controlled trial. Breast Cancer Res Treat 2016;155(3):471–82. https://doi.org/10.1007/s10549-016-3688-0.

[85] Rech A, Botton CE, Lopez P, Quincozes-Santos A, Umpierre D, Pinto RS. Effects of short-term resistance training on endothelial function and inflammation markers in elderly patients with type 2 diabetes: a randomized controlled trial. Exp Gerontol 2019;118:19–25. https://doi.org/10.1016/j.exger.2019.01.003.

[86] Franklin NC, Robinson AT, Bian J-T, et al. Circuit resistance training attenuates acute exertion-induced reductions in arterial function but not inflammation in obese women. Metab Syndr Relat Disord 2015;13(5):227–34. https://doi.org/10.1089/met.2014.0135.

[87] Swift DL, McGee JE, Earnest CP, Carlisle E, Nygard M, Johannsen NM. The effects of exercise and physical activity on weight loss and maintenance. Prog Cardiovasc Dis 2018;61(2):206–13. https://doi.org/10.1016/j.pcad.2018.07.014.

[88] Jakicic JM, Rogers RJ, Davis KK, Collins KA. Role of physical activity and exercise in treating patients with overweight and obesity. Clin Chem 2018;64(1):99–107. https://doi.org/10.1373/clinchem.2017.272443.

[89] Garvey WT, Mechanick JI, Brett EM, et al. American Association of Clinical Endocrinologists and American College of Endocrinology comprehensive clinical practice guidelines for medical care of patients with obesity. Executive summary complete guidelines available at https://www.aace.com/publication, Endocr Pract 2016;22(7):842–84. https://doi.org/10.4158/EP161356.ESGL.

[90] Cox CE. Role of physical activity for weight loss and weight maintenance. Diabetes Spectr 2017;30(3):157–60. https://doi.org/10.2337/ds17-0013.

[91] Pourhassan M, Glüer C-C, Pick P, Tigges W, Müller MJ. Impact of weight loss-associated changes in detailed body composition as assessed by whole-body MRI on plasma insulin levels and homeostatis model assessment index. Eur J Clin Nutr 2017;71(2):212–8. https://doi.org/10.1038/ejcn.2016.189.

[92] Ross R, Janssen I, Dawson J, et al. Exercise-induced reduction in obesity and insulin resistance in women: a randomized controlled trial. Obes Res 2004;12(5):789–98. https://doi.org/10.1038/oby.2004.95.

[93] Piercy KL, Troiano RP, Ballard RM, et al. The physical activity guidelines for Americans. JAMA 2018;320(19):2020–8. https://doi.org/10.1001/jama.2018.14854.

[94] Poulimeneas D, Maraki MI, Karfopoulou E, et al. Sex-specific physical activity patterns differentiate weight loss maintainers from regainers: the medweight study. J Phys Act Health 2020;17(2):225–9. https://doi.org/10.1123/jpah.2019-0407.

CHAPTER 14

Diet and inflammation in obesity: Prevention and management

Kathryn Ottaviano and Jessica A. Zaman
Department of Surgery, Albany Medical Center, Albany, NY, United States

The obesity epidemic

Obesity is defined as a body mass index (BMI) that is higher than what is considered healthy, 30.0 kg/m^2 or greater (Table 1). While this numeric threshold may seem arbitrary, it is based on well-established data that demonstrates an increased risk of obesity-related comorbidities such as hypertension, diabetes, and heart disease in comparison to those who are not obese [1]. According to the most recent National Health and Nutrition Examination Survey reporting on data from 2017 to 2018, the prevalence of obesity in the United States is 42.4% [2]. Globally, the World Health Organization reports that 39% of adults over the age of 18 are overweight and 13% are obese [3]. What is even more problematic is the increasing prevalence of obesity over time. It is projected that at the current rate of increase, nearly 50% of Americans will be obese by 2030 [4]. While obesity is associated with significant psychosocial distress, obesity-related comorbidities and long-term health-related quality of life are major concerns and place considerable burden on healthcare systems. Obesity-related medical costs exceed 140 billion dollars a year [5,6], and this does not account for overall economic impact in terms of lost productivity due to obesity-related health problems.

Pathophysiology of obesity

Obesity results from an energy imbalance due to an excessive intake of calories when compared with energy expenditure. The pathophysiology of obesity is a complex phenomenon that is multifactorial, based on patient genetic and environmental factors. The physiology of obesity hinges on an increase in size and number of adipose cells (largely size in the adult patient) [7]. These adipose cells release cytokines, also known as adipokines, such as

Table 1 Obesity classification according to body mass index (BMI, kg/m^2) based on the National Institutes of Health guidelines.

Body mass index (kg/m^2)	Obesity classification
< 18.5	Underweight
18.5–24.9	Normal weight
25.0–29.9	Overweight
30.0–34.9	Class I obesity
35.0–39.9	Class II obesity
≥ 40.0	Class II obesity

leptin, adiponectin, and resistin. Proinflammatory adipokines include leptin and resistin, which upregulate IL-6 and TNF-a and reduce antiinflammatory adiponectin [8,9]. This contributes to the chronic low-grade inflammatory state in obesity. Adiponectin is a hormone downregulated in obese individuals, which has both antiinflammatory and insulin-sensitizing effects [9]. Resistin is an adipokine found to generate insulin resistance in mice fed a high-fat diet [8]. Leptin is an adipokine that exerts negative feedback to the hypothalamic axis, regulating energy intake and expenditure. Leptin has higher levels in individuals with higher amounts of adipose tissue. Leptin receptors are located throughout the body and can affect multiple organ systems ranging from secretion of hormones by the reproductive system to bone demineralization in the musculoskeletal system. Obesity is a state of leptin resistance and is driven by genetic mutations in leptin receptors, altered transport of leptin across the blood–brain barrier, and regulation of leptin expression [10].

Leptin and inflammation

This process of leptin resistance has direct implications on inflammation as leptin is also a proinflammatory cytokine. At the molecular level, leptin is a 16 kDa peptide that resembles other long-chain cytokines including IL-6, IL-11, IL-12, IFNy, and GCSF [11]. This structural similarity is further translated into parallel functionality. Leptin plays a critical role in both innate and adaptive immunity and acts as an acute-phase reactant by upregulating other proinflammatory cytokines such as IL-6 and TNF alpha [12]. The elevated proinflammatory cytokines along with insulin resistance affect body composition—they increase breakdown of muscle and increase energy use in an inflammatory response [9]. Leptin also plays an integral role for inflammation in chronic diseases such as atherosclerosis, diabetes

II, COPD, Bechet's disease, and cancer [13]. While increased leptin levels contribute to low-grade chronic inflammation in obese patients, decreased leptin in malnourished patients or during phases of fasting can lead to increased susceptibility to infection [14–16].

Obesity and markers of inflammation—Are they adequate?

It is well established that the inflammation induced by obesity is considered a chronic, low-grade inflammation. There is no consensus, however, on which biomarker represents low-grade inflammation. Cells such as total leukocytes, cytokines such as TNF-a, IL-6, IL-1, IL-8, adipokines such as adiponectin, and acute-phase reactants such as CRP and fibrinogen are all measured as surrogates [17,18]. Most studies look at high-sensitivity C-reactive protein (hsCRP), TNF-a, and IL-6. For example, in a meta-analysis of 51 studies, obesity was found to be associated with elevated hsCRP levels. BMI to hsCRP levels had an $r=0.36$ (CI 0.22–0.44), and waist circumference to hsCRP levels had an $r=0.4$ (CI 0.31–0.48). There was some variability in the correlation between men and women and different ethnicities, for example, women have a stronger correlation as do North Americans compared with Asians [19]. However, these biomarkers are elevated with any insult whether it's an acute reaction to an injury or chronic inflammation, they are not specific to obesity-induced inflammation or metabolic low-grade inflammation [20]. Factors that influence inflammatory markers include age, body habitus, diet, physical activity, stress, and genetics [17]. A change in diet or weight can have effects on multiple physiological processes, and no single biomarker has been identified that can consistently and sufficiently predict disease [20].

As an example, a cross-sectional study of 5440 people found that 8.1% of metabolically abnormal individuals were of normal weight, conversely 31.7% of obese individuals were metabolically normal with no elevations in the inflammatory marker CRP. This study used hypertension, triglycerides, fasting glucose, CRP, insulin resistance, and HDL levels as surrogates for metabolic health, defining a metabolically healthy individual as having 0 or 1 of these abnormalities [21]. Another study looked at 24 morbidly obese individuals classified as insulin-resistant or insulin-sensitive and, using biopsies of visceral adipose tissue, found that hypertrophy of visceral adipose tissue is more likely to confer increased inflammation; findings that macrophage infiltration and proinflammatory gene expression are more likely to lead to insulin resistance [22]. This study showed that insulin resistance is mediated by inflammation, and obese individuals may not necessarily have increased risk of cardiometabolic abnormalities. It is not as simple as obesity leads to inflammation, as these processes are multifactorial rather than linear, which should be kept in mind throughout the course of this chapter.

Diet and obesity

The energy imbalance associated with obesity is applicable at the individual as well as at the broader, societal level. Industrialized, urbanized societies have an abundance of inexpensive, processed, and nutrient-poor food with an increased reliance on mechanical transport and decreased mobility that has cultivated an obesogenic environment [23]. Phenotypic plasticity is a phenomenon in which environment can impact gene transcription resulting in expression of a different phenotype. We know that diet plays a role in phenotypic plasticity in both animals and humans [24]. Although there is no single obesogenic diet, the primary "offenders" leading to obesity and leptin resistance are high sugar and fat content [25]. The relationship is complex, and while there is abundant evidence, the data is controversial.

Sugar and obesity

In the early 2000s, high-fructose corn syrup was thought to be a primary culprit in the cause of obesity with the proposed mechanism being a decrease in insulin and leptin secretion despite excessive intake of calories leading to weight gain [26,27]. Dietary trends based on USDA per capita nutrient consumption in the United States in the 20th century demonstrated an initial, steady decrease in carbohydrate consumption that was linked to a decline in whole grain consumption [28]. Beginning in the early 1960s, however, carbohydrate consumption increased without a corresponding increase in fiber indicating an increase in the consumption of refined carbohydrates. At the same time, the prevalence of diabetes and obesity increased. This epidemiologic relationship has since been tested in multiple animal models that have demonstrated that a high-fructose, high-fat, or combination high-fat/high-fructose diet can lead to leptin resistance and weight gain [28, 29]. In the context of inflammation most interestingly, IL-6 and TNF-a levels were evaluated by one group and were found to be normal [30]. Ultimately, however, the link between obesity and high-fructose corn syrup was likely oversimplified as the epidemiologic trends were not maintained, and humans are not consuming high-fructose corn syrup in high, isolated amounts as they were in many animal studies [31,32].

There is a more consistent link between sugar-sweetened beverages to risk of obesity [33]. A prospective study of a large group of men and women demonstrated that consumption of one or more sugar-sweetened beverage per day increased the combined genetic effects on BMI and obesity by two times, when compared with individuals consuming less than one per month [34]. Similarly, a systematic review and meta-analysis found that every additional daily serving of a sugar-sweetened beverage increases BMI by 0.06 kg/m^2 in children and 0.22 kg/m^2 in adults [35]. The direct correlation between sugar-sweetened beverages and predisposition to obesity has held true in other nations as well [36].

Some have attempted to generalize the trends between obesity and high dietary sugar to high carbohydrate intake, although the same conclusions cannot be consistently made due to the complex nature of carbohydrates [37]. In a simplistic view, 1 g of consumed carbohydrates (similar to protein) leads to 4 kcal of energy, while one 1 of fat leads to 9 kcal of energy. However, not all carbohydrates are created equally. Simple carbohydrates are mono- or disaccharides with a high glycemic index, while complex carbohydrates such as starches and fibers have a lower glycemic index. Refined sugars are highly processed and mimic the glycemic profile of simple carbohydrates. Current dietary recommendations are for 50%–55% of total daily calories to consist of carbohydrates and that less than 10% of total daily calorie intake should come from added sugar [38]. Many low-carbohydrate diets go a step further and target a goal between 25 and 150 g per day [39]. The success of many low-carbohydrate diets in recent years has led many to wonder if high-carbohydrate diets alter metabolism to increase risk of obesity.

The carbohydrate insulin model of obesity posits that a high-carbohydrate diet (including large amounts of refined starches and sugar) leads to disproportionate weight gain when compared with low-carbohydrate diets [40]. In this theory, high-glycemic-index foods lead to excess insulin secretion, which due to its anabolic nature leads to lipogenesis and less circulating energy. The lack of availability of metabolic products increases hunger and less activity to conserve energy, which leads to weight gain. While this is an interesting theory that would help explain the obesity epidemic, it has been met with considerable resistance [41]. A recent mouse model was created to test the theory partially validated two of five tenants of the carbohydrate insulin model, the elevation of postprandial insulin levels, and decrease in fasting glucose, but ultimately the model was not found to be valid in mice [42]. Further study is needed to help further investigate these mechanisms.

Sugar and inflammation

Some have also postulated that elevated sugar intake directly mediates inflammatory processes in addition to its indirect effect through obesity potentiation. For example, it is well known in diabetic patients that hyperglycemia leads to oxidative stress and inflammatory biomarkers [43]. Increase in mitochondrial superoxide production leads to micro- and macrovascular endothelial damage through a myriad of biochemical pathways [44]. These pathways ultimately lead to chronic cardiovascular, liver, kidney, and neuroendocrine disease. Dietary sugar intake in the form of fructose, sucrose, high-fructose corn syrup, and glucose is well demonstrated in multiple studies to elevate inflammatory biomarkers such as CRP, IL-6, IL-11, TNF a, and adiponectin [45]. When sugar is consumed in the form of complex carbohydrates, however, many of these adverse effects are mitigated due to the production of short-chain fatty acids, which exert an antiinflammatory effect [46] (Fig. 1).

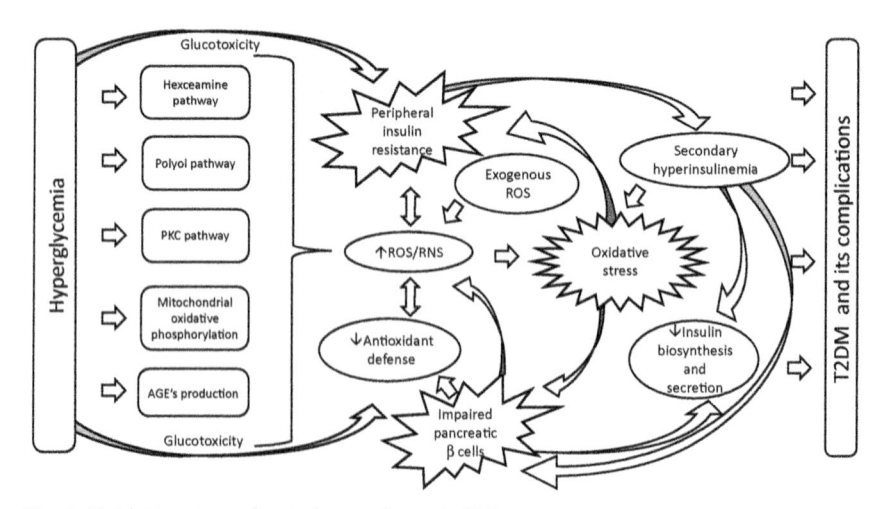

Fig. 1 Oxidative stress due to hyperglycemia [47].

High fat

Excessive consumption of high-fat diets has also potentiated the obesity epidemic and is clearly linked with inflammation and immune system activation [48,49]. Hypertrophic adipocytes of obese individuals are responsible for high levels of inflammatory markers mediated by macrophages within these adipocytes secreting IL-6 and TNF-a [50]. When fat is consumed in excess, it is stored in adipose tissue but can also accumulate in ectopic tissue such as the liver and muscle when the initial reservoir is filled. This is known as visceral fat and is considered more inflammatory as it increases cytokine production [17,18]. This ultimately leads to an increase in circulating fatty acyl-CoA, diacylglycerols, and ceramides that act as important intermediaries in the development of hepatic steatosis, glucose intolerances, and type II diabetes [51].

Essential fatty acids

Essential fatty acids play a direct role on inflammation through their inherent metabolic pathways. Nomenclature is dictated by the location of the double bond near the methyl terminus of the acyl chain of the fatty acid. Linolenic acid is the simplest omega 6 poly unsaturated fatty acid (n-6 PUFA), and linolenic acid is the simplest omega 3 polyunsaturated fatty acid (n-3PUFA). These are considered essential fatty acids because they cannot be produced by the human body. N-6 PUFA increases eicosanoid production and modulates the NF B and PPAR pathways that cause a proinflammatory response [52].

In contrast, n-3 PUFA is considered antiinflammatory. Humans lack the enzyme to convert linoleic acid to linolenic acid, so n-3 PUFA must be derived from diet, such as oily fish, seeds, and nuts [52]. The antiinflammatory mechanisms of n-3 PUFA include: the production of fewer inflammatory cytokines (TNF-a, IL-6, or IL-1b), decreased adhesion with leukocytes and endothelial cells, and decreased chemotactic responses to leukocytes. Several studies have demonstrated the benefits of marine omega 3 fatty acids, which are high in the n-3 PUFAs eicosapentaenoic acid (EPA) and docosahexaenoic acid (DHA). For example, marine n-3 PUFAs can influence skeletal muscle metabolism in athletes and can mitigate oxidative stress during periods of training [53]. Similarly, there is an extensive body of literature about the health benefits of marine n-3 PUFA in patients with heart disease [54] and rheumatoid arthritis [55]. Some suggest that there is also utility in considering marine oil for inflammatory bowel disease and asthma, but the evidence is more controversial [56].

Saturated and unsaturated fat

Saturated fatty acids lack a double bond between carbon atoms, while unsaturated fatty acids have at least one double bond present (Fig. 2). Saturated fat tends to be solid and is generally found in butter, meats, and dairy. Unsaturated fats are often liquid at room temperature and found in vegetable and olive oils. Excessive consumption of saturated fatty acids, especially in obese and overweight individuals, leads to an increase in inflammatory markers COX-2, IL-6, IL-1β, TNF-a, as well as activation of NFκB and the toll-like receptor 4 (TLR4) pathways, which activate the innate immune system [48,49,58].

Unsaturated fats can come as a trans or cis isomer, depending on the hydrogenation process and orientation of carbon atoms across the double bond (a straight orientation for a trans bond and bent orientation for a cis bond) [57]. Although some small quantities of trans fats are found in meat and dairy, most dietary consumption is from processed foods. Trans fats raise epidemiologic health concerns as they increase low-density lipoprotein

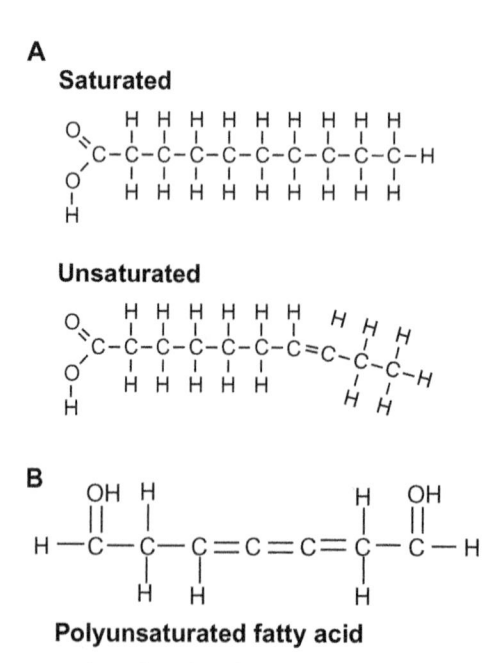

Fig. 2 Fatty acid structure based on classification [57].

(LDL) and decrease high-density lipoprotein (HDL) leading to increased risk of cardiovascular disease.

Trans fats

The impact of trans fatty acids on chronic disease has been studied extensively. Multiple studies have demonstrated that trans fatty acid intake is associated with insulin resistance [59,60]. Increased risk of atherosclerosis and cardiovascular disease is also well established [61] and is related to the impact of trans fatty acids on lipid profile including elevated LDL, decreased HDL, and an elevated total cholesterol to HDL ratio [62]. Likewise, fatty liver disease has been directly linked to plasma trans fatty acid levels and may be due to de novo lipogenesis and inhibition of fatty acid beta-oxidation [63].

The direct correlation between trans-fatty acid and inflammation, however, is less clear and data are often conflicting. An example of a trans-fat is partially hydrogenated vegetable oil, which has been shown to increase inflammatory markers TNF-a, IL-6, and CRP [64]. Elevation of TNF-a in association with increased trans fatty acid intake was demonstrated using a large population of otherwise healthy nurses and was found to be independent of body mass index, smoking, physical activity, aspirin and nonsteroidal antiinflammatory drug use, alcohol consumption, and intakes of saturated fat, protein, n-6 and n-3 fatty acids, fiber, and total energy [65]. The increase in CRP has also been studied in a randomized controlled fashion in multiple studies [66,67]. However, other studies suggest that trans-fats may not necessarily be associated with inflammation. For example, one study found that it was actually the n-6 PUFA to n-3 PUFA ratio that leads to elevated inflammatory markers and that unsaturated n-6 PUFA was found to be antiinflammatory, hypocoagulant, and inversely correlated with IL-6, CRP, arachidonic acid, and fibrinogen [68]. Similarly, when 49 postmenopausal women studied after 4 months of a diet with trans-fat (using partially hydrogenated vegetable oils) compared with a control group, there was a significant difference in serum TNF-a, but no differences in mRNA expression of IL-6, IL-8, TNF-a, or adiponectin in subcutaneous abdominal adipose tissue. Nor was there any significant difference in systemic markers of endothelial dysfunctions E-selectin or sVCAM-1 or sICAM-1 [66]. These discrepancies in data are likely due to the complex nature of the biochemical pathways that are potentiated by different environmental factors (Fig. 3) [69].

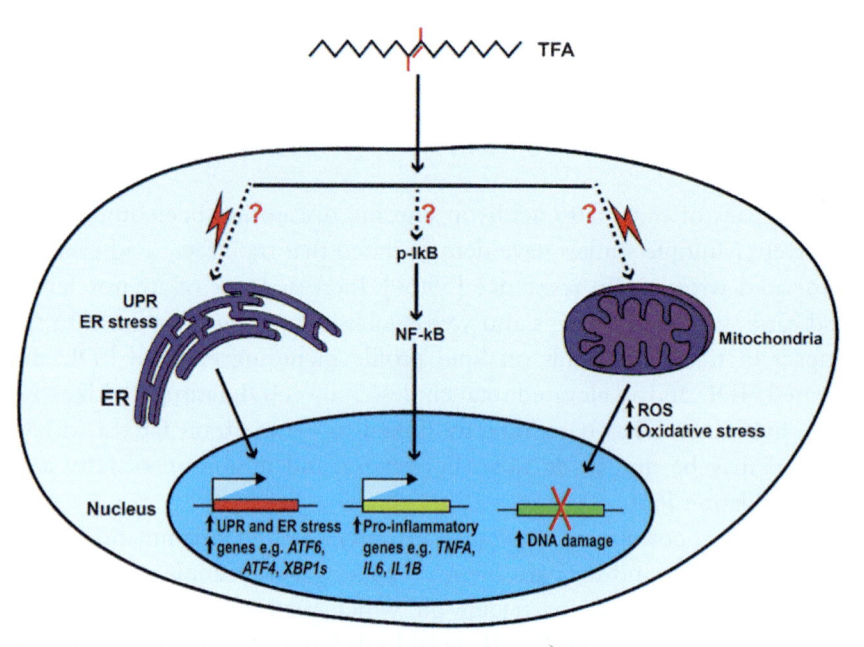

Fig. 3 Proposed molecular mechanisms of trans fatty acids. ATF4, activating transcription factor 4; ATF6, activating transcription factor 6; ER, endoplasmic reticulum; p-IκB, phosphorylated IκB; ROS, reactive oxygen species; TFA, trans fatty acid; UPR, unfolded protein response; XBP1s, X-box binding protein 1, spliced form;?, represents unclarified mechanism [69].

What is an antiinflammatory diet

While there is no single definition of an antiinflammatory diet, there is consensus regarding the balance of specific macronutrients for such diets. These diets are high in omega-3 fatty acids and low in omega-6 fatty acids and trans-fats. They generally include higher proportions of olive oil, whole grains, vegetables and fruits, and minimal amounts of starch and red meat. For protein, antiinflammatory diets call for low-fat options, such as nuts, poultry, and fish [4,70]. High-glycemic foods and those containing a high proportion of omega-6 fatty acids—such as oils derived from corn, peanut, or soybean—are thought to induce an inflammatory immune response and are to be avoided [71]. Several relatively well-known, plant-based diets have emerged, including the Mediterranean diet, the Okinawa diet, and the Zone diet by Dr. Barry Sears, who coined the term "antiinflammatory diet." [64]

For Sears, chronic "silent" inflammation leads to hypothalamus–pituitary axis dysfunction and adipose tissue signaling cascades that cause weight gain.

Sears hypothesizes that omega-6 fatty acids paired with high-glycemic foods induce arachidonic acid production. Specifically, insulin activates the enzymes that break down linoleic acid to arachidonic acid, which is a polyunsaturated fatty acid (PUFA) that has the downstream effect of inducing inflammation via prostaglandins and NFκB activation. Similarly, saturated fats bind to TLR4 and activate NFκB, a transcription factor that induces cytokine production. Further, "overnutrition"—that is, excessive caloric consumption—also induces inflammation [71]. Sears's Zone diet calls for 1500 cal a day, which should come 40% from carbohydrates, 30% from protein, and 30% from fat. It differs from the Mediterranean diet in that it is more restrictive of carbohydrates and specifies that, for fruits and vegetables, the colorful varieties, which contain more polyphenols, should be consumed.

Several studies have indicated that antiinflammation diets are closely correlated with a decrease in bodily inflammation and in all-cause mortality (i.e., deaths from any cause). For instance, a meta-analysis looking at 25 studies involving 2689 predominantly obese patients consuming a plant-based diet compared with control patients consuming a "Western" diet showed that the mean difference in inflammatory biomarker concentrations in the plant-based group was -0.55 mg/L ($-0.78, -0.32$) [72]. These diets were mostly Mediterranean (17) though some used the Nordic (4), Dash (2), and Paleolithic (1) diets. The serum levels of the inflammatory markers IL-6, CRP, and sICAM were most often studied and found to have the most pronounced decrease in the experimental group. In contrast, the serum levels of TNF-alpha, adiponectin, leptin, and resistin did not significantly differ among the experimental and control groups. This study is important because it indicates that across populations of obese or metabolically abnormal individuals, chronic inflammation can be addressed with diet alone [72].

Relatedly, a large prospective cohort study [73] (the PREDIMED and SUN studies in Spain) looked at 18,566 individuals over a median of 5 years to assess dietary inflammatory index and all-cause mortality. Using food frequency questionnaires, diets were analyzed with dietary inflammatory index (DII) scores that assessed whether each food increased, decreased, or had no effect on inflammatory markers in the serum (IL-1B, IL-4, IL-6, IL-10, TNF-a, hsCRP). Meat, dairy, and baked goods increased DII scores. Consumption of vegetables, fruit, fish, legumes, olive oil, and nuts decreased DII scores. Diets with elevated inflammatory potential, as deduced by DII scores, were linked to all-cause mortality. A "proinflammatory" diet was found to have a relative risk of 1.23 (CI 1.16–1.32) for all-cause mortality across all cohorts [73].

Similar results were detected by a large population-based Swedish prospective cohort that spanned 16 years. It found that study participants who consumed an antiinflammatory diet experienced a decrease in all-cause mortality, cardiovascular disease, and cancer mortality (in men only) as compared with those consuming a proinflammatory diet [74].

Additional research could help further refine the foods consumed as part of the antiinflammatory diets. For instance, there are few human randomized control trials that evaluate the antiinflammatory effects of flavonoids (a type of polyphenol), in particular the anthocyanin group, which include blueberries and strawberries that have been associated with a decrease in cognitive decline [17]. At the same time, large cohort studies have found that total flavonoid intake is inversely correlated with CRP levels in serum [17,75,76].

Antiinflammatory diet and weight loss

Notably, there is no consensus that the macronutrient balance for antiinflammatory diets best achieves weight loss. Many studies have evaluated different macronutrient balances yet they do not agree on which combination of fats, carbohydrates, and protein most effectively leads to weight loss [77]. A meta-analysis of 121 randomized trials looking at 21,942 participants consuming 14 diets of different macronutrient balances, including low-fat diet, low-carbohydrate diet, and Mediterranean diets, found that there was no difference in weight loss or decrease in blood pressure (BP) at 12 months [78]. Yet modest reductions in weight loss and BP were seen at 6 months, thus suggesting that lack of adherence to the diet, rather than the diet itself, may have played a significant role in the results [78].

Regardless, this lack of consensus as to weight-loss potential does not necessarily suggest a lack of consensus for other health benefits of antiinflammatory diets. Studies with exclusive findings as to weight loss found that the diets that were most frequently found to improve cardiovascular risks and mortality were antiinflammatory, such as the Mediterranean diet, Zone, and the high-fiber DASH diet [78–80].

Antiinflammatory benefits of popular diets

The Mediterranean Diet is high in vegetables, fruits, whole grains, beans, nuts and seeds, and olive oil. The Lyon Diet Heart Study was one of the first randomized trials regarding cardiovascular disease that demonstrated a clear benefit in preventing a second heart attack in patients who consumed the Mediterranean diet after initial myocardial infarction [81]. Numerous other studies have demonstrated a preventative impact on cardiovascular disease and other chronic diseases such as cancer, obesity, and cognitive decline [82]. Although the exact pathways are not known, the five most likely mechanisms include a lipid lowering effect, protection against oxidative stress, modifications of hormones and growth factors causing cancer, inhibition of nutrient sensing pathways by specific amino acid restriction, and gut microbiota-mediated production of metabolites influencing metabolic health [83].

Intermittent fasting diets consist of either complete fasting on certain days, consuming only water or a 70% restriction in calorie intake every other day, or long periods during the day of fasting, with between 6 and 8 h of food intake each day. Overall health and longevity are some of the purported benefits of the diet, which have been demonstrated in animal models. Human studies have shown reduction in weight, body fat, cholesterol, and triglycerides [84]. Randomized controlled trials have not found a difference in weight loss between intermittent fasting and continuous calorie restriction, however [84]. A randomized controlled trial of 76 obese women undergoing every other day fasting found no difference in serum TNF-alpha, IL-6 and IL-10. Weight loss was greater in intermittent fasting with 70% calorie restriction group compared with continuous calorie restriction and intermittent fasting without calorie restriction; however, the serum inflammatory markers were unchanged [85]. After fasting, however, macrophage infiltration into adipose tissue was increased compared with continuous calorie restriction, which the authors attributed to adipose tissue lipolysis.

The standard ketogenic diet consists of very low carbohydrates (approximately 10%), moderate protein (20%), and high fat (70%). The ketogenic diet has been used since the 1920s for patients with refractory epilepsy [86]. The theoretical basis of this treatment involves a shift from glucose to fatty acid metabolism, which leads to ketone bodies as a primary source of energy for the brain. The therapeutic effects of a ketogenic diet may apply to other disease processes as well, such for chronic pain, as some believe the ketogenic metabolic pathway leads to fewer free radicals and a decrease in oxidative stress. Several animal studies have shown potential benefits in processing thermal and neuropathic pain for rodents fed a ketogenic diet [87]. However, data about these benefits in humans is sparse and must be weighed against adverse effects such as a substantial rise in LDL cholesterol levels [88].

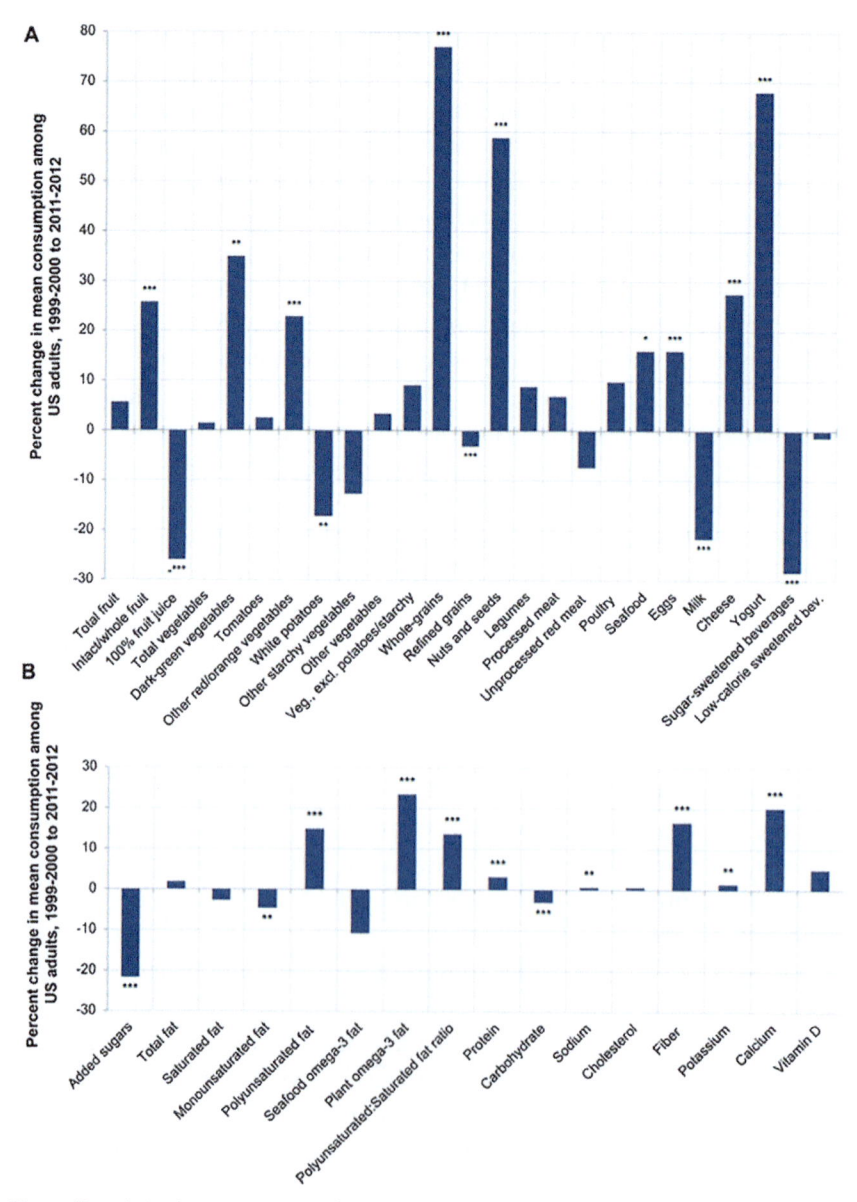

Fig. 4 Trends in the proportion of US adults meeting dietary recommendations based on NHANES data from 1999 to 2012 [89].

Diets low in oligosaccharides, disaccharides, monosaccharides, and polyols (low FODMAPS) are increasingly utilized in the treatment of inflammatory bowel disease (IBD) and irritable bowel syndrome (IBS) and have implications on inflammation. The primary principle is to avoid fermentable carbohydrates to reduce gas, bloating, and abdominal discomfort. Multiple randomized controlled trials have been performed and demonstrate that the diet effectively leads to symptom relief in patients [89]. However, the impact on inflammatory markers is variable with some studies showing no change in inflammatory markers in the short term [90], but others demonstrating a change in inflammatory marker profile after long-term adherence to a low FODMAP diet [91].

The long-term outlook

While much of the data and trends discussed have been present over time, changes in dietary patterns are slow but positive. Trends in AHA dietary recommendations showed that over a decade, survey respondents increased intake of whole grains, nuts and seeds, and fish and decreased sugar-sweetened beverages marginally (Fig. 4). However, there was no increase in total fruits and vegetables, processed meat, saturated fat, or sodium [92]. Greater education among patients and providers, particularly with regard to inflammation and chronic disease, is needed.

References

[1] Clinical Guidelines on the Identification. Evaluation, and treatment of overweight and obesity in adults—the evidence report. National Institutes of Health. Obes Res 1998;6(Suppl. 2):51S–209S.
[2] Hales CM, Carroll MD, Fryar CD, Ogden CL. Prevalence of obesity and severe obesity among adults: United States, 2017–2018. NCHS Data Brief 2020;360:1–8.
[3] Ricker MA, Haas WC. Anti-inflammatory diet in clinical practice: a review. Nutr Clin Pract 2017;32(3):318–25.
[4] Ward ZJ, Bleich SN, Cradock AL, et al. Projected U.S. State-Level prevalence of adult obesity and severe obesity. N Engl J Med 2019;381(25):2440–50.
[5] Biener A, Cawley J, Meyerhoefer C. The impact of obesity on medical care costs and labor market outcomes in the US. Clin Chem 2018;64(1):108–17.
[6] Finkelstein EA, Trogdon JG, Cohen JW, Dietz W. Annual medical spending attributable to obesity: payer-and service-specific estimates. Health Aff (Millwood) 2009;28(5):w822–31.
[7] Brunicardi FC, et al. Schwartz's Principles of Surgery. 11th. New York: McGraw-Hill Education; 2019.
[8] Qatanani M, Szwergold NR, Greaves DR, Ahima RS, Lazar MA. Macrophage-derived human resistin exacerbates adipose tissue inflammation and insulin resistance in mice. J Clin Invest 2009;119(3):531–9.
[9] Nimptsch K, Konigorski S, Pischon T. Diagnosis of obesity and use of obesity biomarkers in science and clinical medicine. vol. 92. W.B. Saunders; 2019. p. 61–70.
[10] Gruzdeva O, Borodkina D, Uchasova E, Dyleva Y, Barbarash O. Leptin resistance: underlying mechanisms and diagnosis. Diabetes Metab Syndr Obes 2019;12:191–8.

[11] Hegyi K, Fulop K, Kovacs K, Toth S, Falus A. Leptin-induced signal transduction pathways. Cell Biol Int 2004;28(3):159–69.
[12] La Cava A, Matarese G. The weight of leptin in immunity. Nat Rev Immunol 2004;4(5):371–9.
[13] La Cava A. Leptin in inflammation and autoimmunity. Cytokine 2017;98:51–8.
[14] Iikuni N, Lam QL, Lu L, Matarese G, La Cava A. Leptin and inflammation. Curr Immunol Rev 2008;4(2):70–9.
[15] Matarese G, La Cava A, Sanna V, et al. Balancing susceptibility to infection and autoimmunity: a role for leptin? Trends Immunol 2002;23(4):182–7.
[16] Gregor MF, Hotamisligil GS. Inflammatory mechanisms in obesity. Annu Rev Immunol 2011;29:415–45.
[17] Minihane AM, Vinoy S, Russell WR, et al. Low-grade inflammation, diet composition and health: current research evidence and its translation. Br J Nutr 2015;114(7):999–1012.
[18] Calder PC, Ahluwalia N, Albers R, et al. A consideration of biomarkers to be used for evaluation of inflammation in human nutritional studies. Br J Nutr 2013;109(Suppl. S1).
[19] Choi J, Joseph L, Pilote L. Obesity and C-reactive protein in various populations: a systematic review and meta-analysis. Obes Rev 2013;14(3):232–44.
[20] De Vries J, Antoine JM, Burzykowski T, et al. Markers for nutrition studies: review of criteria for the evaluation of markers. vol. 52. Springer; 2013. p. 1685–99.
[21] Wildman RP, Muntner P, Reynolds K, et al. The obese without cardiometabolic risk factor clustering and the normal weight with cardiometabolic risk factor clustering: prevalence and correlates of 2 phenotypes among the US population (NHANES 1999-2004). Arch Intern Med 2008;168(15):1617–24.
[22] Barbarroja N, López-Pedrera R, Mayas MD, et al. The obese healthy paradox: is inflammation the answer? Biochem J 2010;430(1):141–9.
[23] Hruby A, Hu FB. The epidemiology of obesity: a big picture. Pharmacoeconomics 2015;33(7):673–89.
[24] Bradley P. Refined carbohydrates, phenotypic plasticity and the obesity epidemic. Med Hypotheses 2019;131, 109317.
[25] Vasselli JR, Scarpace PJ, Harris RB, Banks WA. Dietary components in the development of leptin resistance. Adv Nutr 2013;4(2):164–75.
[26] Bray GA, Nielsen SJ, Popkin BM. Consumption of high-fructose corn syrup in beverages may play a role in the epidemic of obesity. Am J Clin Nutr 2004;79(4):537–43.
[27] Teff KL, Elliott SS, Tschop M, et al. Dietary fructose reduces circulating insulin and leptin, attenuates postprandial suppression of ghrelin, and increases triglycerides in women. J Clin Endocrinol Metab 2004;89(6):2963–72.
[28] Gross LS, Li L, Ford ES, Liu S. Increased consumption of refined carbohydrates and the epidemic of type 2 diabetes in the United States: an ecologic assessment. Am J Clin Nutr 2004;79(5):774–9.
[29] Scarpace PJ, Zhang Y. Leptin resistance: a prediposing factor for diet-induced obesity. Am J Physiol Regul Integr Comp Physiol 2009;296(3):R493–500.
[30] Shapiro A, Tumer N, Gao Y, Cheng KY, Scarpace PJ. Prevention and reversal of diet-induced leptin resistance with a sugar-free diet despite high fat content. Br J Nutr 2011;106(3):390–7.
[31] Rippe JM. The health implications of sucrose, high-fructose corn syrup, and fructose: what do we really know? J Diabetes Sci Technol 2010;4(4):1008–11.
[32] White JS. Straight talk about high-fructose corn syrup: what it is and what it ain't. Am J Clin Nutr 2008;88(6):1716S–21S.
[33] Heianza Y, Qi L. Gene-diet interaction and precision nutrition in obesity. Int J Mol Sci 2017;18(4).
[34] Qi Q, Chu AY, Kang JH, et al. Sugar-sweetened beverages and genetic risk of obesity. N Engl J Med 2012;367(15):1387–96.

[35] Malik VS, Pan A, Willett WC, Hu FB. Sugar-sweetened beverages and weight gain in children and adults: a systematic review and meta-analysis. Am J Clin Nutr 2013;98(4):1084–102.
[36] Brunkwall L, Chen Y, Hindy G, et al. Sugar-sweetened beverage consumption and genetic predisposition to obesity in 2 Swedish cohorts. Am J Clin Nutr 2016;104(3):809–15.
[37] Sartorius K, Sartorius B, Madiba TE, Stefan C. Does high-carbohydrate intake lead to increased risk of obesity? A systematic review and meta-analysis. BMJ Open 2018;8(2), e018449.
[38] Youdim A. Overview of nutrition. Merck Manuals; 2019.
[39] Oh R, Gilani B, Uppaluri KR. Low carbohydrate diet [Updated 2021 July 12]. In: StatPearls [Internet]. Treasure Island, FL: StatPearls Publishing; 2022. Available from: https://www.ncbi.nlm.nih.gov/books/NBK537084/.
[40] Ludwig DS, Hu FB, Tappy L, Brand-Miller J. Dietary carbohydrates: role of quality and quantity in chronic disease. BMJ 2018;361, k2340.
[41] Hall KD, Guyenet SJ, Leibel RL. The carbohydrate-insulin model of obesity is difficult to reconcile with current evidence. JAMA Intern Med 2018;178(8):1103–5.
[42] Hu S, Wang L, Togo J, et al. The carbohydrate-insulin model does not explain the impact of varying dietary macronutrients on the body weight and adiposity of mice. Mol Metab 2020;32:27–43.
[43] Luc K, Schramm-Luc A, Guzik TJ, Mikolajczyk TP. Oxidative stress and inflammatory markers in prediabetes and diabetes. J Physiol Pharmacol 2019;70(6).
[44] Giacco F, Brownlee M. Oxidative stress and diabetic complications. Circ Res 2010;107(9):1058–70.
[45] Della Corte KW, Perrar I, Penczynski KJ, Schwingshackl L, Herder C, Buyken AE. Effect of dietary sugar intake on biomarkers of subclinical inflammation: a systematic review and meta-analysis of intervention studies. Nutrients 2018;10(5).
[46] Freeman CR, Zehra A, Ramirez V, Wiers CE, Volkow ND, Wang GJ. Impact of sugar on the body, brain, and behavior. Front Biosci (Landmark Ed) 2018;23:2255–66.
[47] Wozniak LA. In: Marzena Wojcik MK, Zieleniak A, Marcjanek KM, Preuss DB HG, editors. Dietary sugar, salt and fat in human health. Academic Press; 2020. p. 305–23.
[48] Lee H, Lee IS, Choue R. Obesity, inflammation and diet. Pediatr Gastroenterol Hepatol Nutr 2013;16(3):143–52.
[49] Joffe YT, Collins M, Goedecke JH. The relationship between dietary fatty acids and inflammatory genes on the obese phenotype and serum lipids. Nutrients 2013;5(5):1672–705.
[50] Joffe YT, Collins M, Goedecke JH. The relationship between dietary fatty acids and inflammatory genes on the obese phenotype and serum lipids. vol. 5. MDPI AG; 2013. p. 1672–705.
[51] Feillet-Coudray C, Fouret G, Vigor C, et al. Long-term measures of dyslipidemia, inflammation, and oxidative stress in rats fed a high-fat/high-fructose diet. Lipids 2019;54(1):81–97.
[52] Calder PC. Omega-3 polyunsaturated fatty acids and inflammatory processes: nutrition or pharmacology? Br J Clin Pharmacol 2013;75(3):645–62.
[53] Gammone MA, Riccioni G, Parrinello G, D'Orazio N. Omega-3 polyunsaturated fatty acids: benefits and endpoints in sport. Nutrients 2018;11(1).
[54] Innes JK, Calder PC. Marine omega-3 (N-3) fatty acids for cardiovascular health: an update for 2020. Int J Mol Sci 2020;21(4).
[55] Senftleber NK, Nielsen SM, Andersen JR, et al. Marine oil supplements for arthritis pain: a systematic review and Meta-analysis of randomized trials. Nutrients 2017;9(1).
[56] Calder PC. Marine omega-3 fatty acids and inflammatory processes: effects, mechanisms and clinical relevance. Biochim Biophys Acta 2015;1851(4):469–84.
[57] Marchand V. Trans fats: what physicians should know. Paediatr Child Health 2010;15(6):373–5.

[58] Zhou H, Urso CJ, Jadeja V. Saturated fatty acids in obesity-associated inflammation. J Inflamm Res 2020;13:1–14.
[59] Angelieri CT, Barros CR, Siqueira-Catania A, Ferreira SR. Trans fatty acid intake is associated with insulin sensitivity but independently of inflammation. Braz J Med Biol Res 2012;45(7):625–31.
[60] Thompson AK, Minihane AM, Williams CM. Trans fatty acids, insulin resistance and diabetes. Eur J Clin Nutr 2011;65(5):553–64.
[61] Mozaffarian D, Aro A, Willett WC. Health effects of trans-fatty acids: experimental and observational evidence. Eur J Clin Nutr 2009;63(Suppl 2):S5–21.
[62] Mensink RP, Katan MB. Effect of dietary trans fatty acids on high-density and low-density lipoprotein cholesterol levels in healthy subjects. N Engl J Med 1990;323(7):439–45.
[63] Mazidi M, Katsiki N, Mikhailidis DP, Banach M. Link between plasma trans-fatty acid and fatty liver is moderated by adiposity. Int J Cardiol 2018;272:316–22.
[64] Ricker MA, Haas WC. Anti-inflammatory diet in clinical practice: a review. Nutr Clin Pract 2017;32(3):318–25.
[65] Mozaffarian D, Pischon T, Hankinson SE, et al. Dietary intake of trans fatty acids and systemic inflammation in women. Am J Clin Nutr 2004;79(4):606–12.
[66] Bendsen NT, Stender S, Szecsi PB, et al. Effect of industrially produced trans fat on markers of systemic inflammation: evidence from a randomized trial in women. J Lipid Res 2011;52(10):1821–8.
[67] Baer DJ, Judd JT, Clevidence BA, Tracy RP. Dietary fatty acids affect plasma markers of inflammation in healthy men fed controlled diets: a randomized crossover study. Am J Clin Nutr 2004;79(6):969–73.
[68] Kalogeropoulos N, Panagiotakos DB, Pitsavos C, et al. Unsaturated fatty acids are inversely associated and n-6/n-3 ratios are positively related to inflammation and coagulation markers in plasma of apparently healthy adults. Clin Chim Acta 2010;411(7–8):584–91.
[69] Oteng AB, Kersten S. Mechanisms of action of trans fatty acids. Adv Nutr 2020;11(3):697–708.
[70] Galland L. Diet and inflammation. Nutr Clin Pract 2010;25(6):634–40.
[71] Sears B, Ricordi C. Anti-inflammatory nutrition as a pharmacological approach to treat obesity. J Obes 2011;2011.
[72] Eichelmann F, Schwingshackl L, Fedirko V, Aleksandrova K. Effect of plant-based diets on obesity-related inflammatory profiles: a systematic review and meta-analysis of intervention trials. Obes Rev 2016;17(11):1067–79.
[73] Garcia-Arellano A, Martínez-González MA, Ramallal R, Salas-Salvado J, Hebert JR. Dietary inflammatory index and all-cause mortality in large cohorts: the SUN and PREDIMED studies—ClinicalKey. Clin Nutr 2019;38(3):1221–31.
[74] Kaluza J, Hakansson N, Harris HR, Orsini N, Michaelsson K, Wolk A. Influence of anti-inflammatory diet and smoking on mortality and survival in men and women: two prospective cohort studies. J Intern Med 2019;285(1):75–91.
[75] Chun OK, Chung SJ, Claycombe KJ, Song WO. Serum C-reactive protein concentrations are inversely associated with dietary flavonoid intake in U.S. adults. J Nutr 2008;138(4):753–60.
[76] Landberg R, Sun Q, Rimm EB, et al. Selected dietary flavonoids are associated with markers of inflammation and endothelial dysfunction in U.S. women. J Nutr 2011;141(4):618–25.
[77] Hwalla N, Jaafar Z. Dietary management of obesity: a review of the evidence. Diagnostics 2020;11(1):24.
[78] Ge L, Sadeghirad B, Ball GDC, et al. Comparison of dietary macronutrient patterns of 14 popular named dietary programmes for weight and cardiovascular risk factor reduction in adults: Systematic review and network meta-analysis of randomised trials. vol. 369. BMJ Publishing Group; 2020.

[79] Soltani S, Arablou T, Jayedi A, Salehi-Abargouei A. Adherence to the dietary approaches to stop hypertension (DASH) diet in relation to all-cause and cause-specific mortality: a systematic review and dose-response meta-analysis of prospective cohort studies. vol. 19. BioMed Central Ltd; 2020.
[80] Carlos S, De La Fuente-Arrillaga C, Bes-Rastrollo M, et al. Mediterranean diet and health outcomes in the SUN cohort. Nutrients 2018;10(4).
[81] de Lorgeril M, Salen P, Martin JL, Monjaud I, Delaye J, Mamelle N. Mediterranean diet, traditional risk factors, and the rate of cardiovascular complications after myocardial infarction: final report of the Lyon diet heart study. Circulation 1999;99(6):779–85.
[82] Widmer RJ, Flammer AJ, Lerman LO, Lerman A. The Mediterranean diet, its components, and cardiovascular disease. Am J Med 2015;128(3):229–38.
[83] Tosti V, Bertozzi B, Fontana L. Health benefits of the Mediterranean diet: metabolic and molecular mechanisms. J Gerontol A Biol Sci Med Sci 2018;73(3):318–26.
[84] Mattson MP, Longo VD, Harvie M. Impact of intermittent fasting on health and disease processes. Ageing Res Rev 2017;39:46–58.
[85] Liu B, Hutchison AT, Thompson CH, Lange K, Heilbronn LK. Markers of adipose tissue inflammation are transiently elevated during intermittent fasting in women who are overweight or obese. Obes Res Clin Pract 2019;13(4):408–15.
[86] Ulamek-Koziol M, Czuczwar SJ, Januszewski S, Pluta R. Ketogenic diet and epilepsy. Nutrients 2019;11:10.
[87] Masino SA, Ruskin DN. Ketogenic diets and pain. J Child Neurol 2013;28(8):993–1001.
[88] O'Neill B, Raggi P. The ketogenic diet: pros and cons. Atherosclerosis 2020;292:119–26.
[89] Gibson PR. The evidence base for efficacy of the low FODMAP diet in irritable bowel syndrome: is it ready for prime time as a first-line therapy? J Gastroenterol Hepatol 2017;32(Suppl. 1):32–5.
[90] Cox SR, Lindsay JO, Fromentin S, et al. Effects of low FODMAP diet on symptoms, fecal microbiome, and markers of inflammation in patients with quiescent inflammatory bowel disease in a randomized trial. Gastroenterology 2020;158(1):176–188 e177.
[91] Orlando A, Tutino V, Notarnicola M, et al. Improved symptom profiles and minimal inflammation in IBS-D patients undergoing a long-term low-FODMAP diet: a lipidomic perspective. Nutrients 2020;12(6).
[92] Rehm CD, Penalvo JL, Afshin A, Mozaffarian D. Dietary intake among US Adults, 1999–2012. JAMA 2016;315(23):2542–53.

CHAPTER 15

Management of obesity and related inflammatory disorders

Nisrine I. Kawa[a] and Souheil W. Adra[b]
[a]Department of Internal Medicine, Waterbury Hospital, Yale School of Medicine, Waterbury, CT, United States
[b]Department of Surgery, Beth Israel Deaconess Medical Center, Harvard Medical School, Boston, MA, United States

Introduction

Obesity has been associated with a myriad of inflammatory disorders and demonstrates characteristically elevated levels of circulating inflammatory markers. This is possibly due to increased production of proinflammatory cytokines from several tissues and cells, including adipose tissue, vascular endothelial cells, and peripheral blood mononuclear cells. Adipose tissue inflammation is a central mechanism for local-grade inflammation in many systemic conditions, including cardiovascular disease [1,2], insulin resistance, fatty liver disease, reproductive dysfunction, neurological diseases, rheumatoid arthritis, changes to the gut microbiome and periodontal flora, and cancers [3]. Weight loss has successfully reversed many of these abnormalities, as described in prior chapters.

In this chapter, we will start by reviewing the traditional treatments for obesity and inflammation, illustrating their shortcomings, and consider why new strategies beyond calorie counting and exercise are essential. We will then explore more novel approaches for tackling obesity-related inflammation, including minimally invasive procedures, pharmacological therapies, microbiome manipulation, and bariatric surgery.

Behavioral weight management strategies and inflammation
Impact of diet

Many of the strategies for weight loss have been ineffective to provide long-term results. The effectiveness of calorie counting has been evaluated in many studies. In the dietary intervention randomized control trial (DIRECT) published in 2008 in the New England Journal of Medicine, 322 overweight and obese adults were studied. Males made up 85% of

enrolled participants, and they were randomized to one of three diets for 2 years. Each of the three groups followed structures versions of commonly adopted diets as follows:
- The low-fat diet in conformity with the American Health Association guidelines:
    o Composed of 30% fat, 1500 cal for women, and 1800 cal for men,
    o Includes grains, vegetables, fruits, and beans.
- The Mediterranean diet:
    o Composed of 35% fat, 1500 cal for women, and 1800 cal for men,
    o Includes olive oil, nuts, vegetables, and fish.
- The low-carbohydrate diet:
    o Composed of 20 g per day of carbohydrates for 2 months, then 120 g per day carbohydrates,
    o No calorie limit for fat and protein from vegetable sources

The three groups were assessed at the end of the 2-year intervention [4], then once again 4 years after the completion of trial [5] (Table 1).

Overall, the study had a completion rate of 85%, more specifically 90% in the low-fat diet, 85% of the Mediterranean diet, and 78% of the low-carbohydrate diet. The low-carbohydrate diet was associated with the most significant reductions in total cholesterol/HDL ratio and C-Reactive Protein (CRP), while the Mediterranean diet was associated with the greatest reduction in fasting blood glucose among diabetics. Interestingly, at 6 years, 67% of the subjects continued the original diets, while 11% switched, and 22% were not following any regulated diet. Still, the total weight loss was greatest for

Table 1 The DIRECT study compared three groups of diets: low-fat, Mediterranean, and low-carb.

Weight loss	Low-fat (kg)	Mediterranean (kg)	Low-carb (kg)
All subjects, 2 years	2.9	4.4	4.7
Completers, 2 years ($n=272$)	3.3	4.6	5.5
Completers, 6 years ($n=259$)	0.6	3.1	1.7

The outcomes for weight loss of all subjects vs. those who completed the study at 2 years and 6 years are shown.
Adapted from Golan R, Schwarzfuchs D, Shai I. Four-year follow-up after two-year dietary interventions. N Engl J Med 2012;367:1373–4. https://doi.org/10.1056/NEJMc1204792 and Shai I, Schwarzfuchs D, Henkin Y, Shahar DR, Witkow S, Greenberg I, Golan R, Fraser D, Bolotin A, Vardi H, Tangi-Rozental O, Zuk-Ramot R, Sarusi B, Brickner D, Schwartz Z, Sheiner E, Marko R, Katorza E, Thiery J, Fiedler GM, Blüher M, Stumvoll M, Stampfer MJ. Weight loss with a low-carbohydrate, Mediterranean, or low-fat diet. N Engl J Med 2008;359:229–41. https://doi.org/10.1056/NEJMoa0708681.

the Mediterranean diet (3.1 kg deficit), followed by the low-carbohydrate diet (1.7 kg deficit), and the low-fat diet (0.6 kg deficit). This revealed that despite weight regain in the Mediterranean and low-carbohydrates diet groups, subjects had beneficial changes that persisted. Indeed, on 4-year follow-up, their triglycerides and LDL levels showed persistent improvement.

Many dietary interventions have been studied in that context. A systematic review of metaanalyses and randomized control trials (RCTs) evaluated the impact of the Mediterranean diet on adults with or at risk for type 2 diabetes mellitus (prediabetes). Measured outcomes assessed metabolic control and cardiovascular risk factors. Five metaanalyses revealed a favorable effect of the Mediterranean diet on weight, lipids as compared with other diets. Two long-term RCTs showed a 49% increased probability of remission from the metabolic syndrome [6].

The benefit of dietary interventions is enhanced when meal replacement programs are used. They not only improve dietary structure and provide calorie and portion control, but also limit intake of calorie-dense foods. The "Look AHEAD" trial showed that such plans led to significant improvements in weight loss outcomes, reducing the risk of diabetes in the intervention group by 60% [7]. Nevertheless, the effectiveness of meal replacement diets is limited by their cost, as well as the capacity for long-term adherence, which undermines their usefulness.

Looking beyond large-scale dietary modifications, additional studies assessed outcomes of more minor changes. For instance, a Danish RCT evaluated the impact of consuming whole grain carbohydrates on inflammation, obesity, and insulin resistance. Their findings noted significant reduction in both weight and inflammatory markers interleukin-6 (IL-6) and CRP, surprisingly without any change in fecal microbiome or insulin sensitivity [8].

Researchers at the University of South Carolina created a Dietary Inflammation Index (DII) using an extensive review of literature focusing on impact of dietary parameters on inflammatory markers. They evaluated levels of IL-1β, IL-4, IL-6, IL-10, tumor necrosis factor-alpha (TNF-α), and CRP. This provided them with a metric to classify a diet along a spectrum of inflammation promoting vs. preventing [9]. The highest scoring diet on the inflammation scale was the fast-food diet, and the lowest was the Mediterranean and macrobiotic. This index has been validated and used extensively in the literature since. Inflammatory diets have been correlated with a wide range of outcomes in relation to this measure, including cardiovascular disease, asthma, depression, and cancers, among others. The general recommendations for an antiinflammatory diet center on avoidance of foods that induce inflammation and increased consumption of those with antiinflammatory effects. Inflammation-associated foods include refined carbohydrates (such as white bread, pastries, and sugary beverages), red meat—especially when processed—, and saturated fats.

Using this tool, a recent study associated a more prominent prevalence of *Ruminococcus torques*, *Eubacterium nodatum*, *Acidaminococcus intestini*, and *Clostridium leptum* in the most proinflammatory diets and a more notable presence of *Akkermansia muciniphila* in the most antiinflammatory diet group [10].

The impact of "timing of food intake" is another avenue that has been explored. Intermittent fasting and periodic fasting have been evaluated extensively in animal models and more recently in some human studies. Associated metabolic benefits mimic effects of exercise, with favorable metabolic outcomes, weight loss, and delayed aging in animal models [11]. That being said, a more recent metaanalysis of RCTs and systematic review showed that the intermittent fasting was associated with a drop in CRP but without a drop in TNF-α or IL-6 [12].

It is important to remember that metabolic adaptation plagues dietary approaches for weight loss. A study evaluating participants in the "Biggest Loser" competition serves as a perfect illustration to that effect. There was a significant initial drop in participants' residual basal metabolic rate (RMR). Upon follow-up 6 years after their participation, significant weight regain was noted; however, the RMR remained reduced. RMR was about 500 kcal/day below expected for the change in their body composition and their increased age. This essentially presented participants with the daunting task of maintaining a deficit of 500 kcal/day over at least 6 years after completion of their weight loss [13].

The impact of exercise

Exercise training, aerobic, and resistance training have been associated with decreased levels of inflammatory mediators. CRP in particular was one of the earlier markers to be inversely associated with physical activity [14]. Physiologic levels of epinephrine released during exercise have inhibitory effects on monocyte TNF production in vitro. Therefore, exercise may mediate some antiinflammatory effects through epinephrine inhibition of TNF [15]. Subsequently, many markers of inflammation were examined in the setting of obesity. Evidence suggested a role for adipocyte hypoxia in the pathophysiology of adiposopathy [16,17].

In the setting of obesity, exercise has a profound effect on reduction of inflammation, beyond its impact on weight, and beyond its impact on normal weight individuals. In those individuals with obesity who are undergoing prolonged physical activity interventions, exercise further reduced inflammation, as the baseline levels of inflammatory mediators are elevated. Many studies have shown that this is not weight loss related. Instead, several mechanisms have been proposed, including muscle generated antiinflammatory myokines, of which IL-6, with an impact on inflammation and hypoxia. This is thought to enhance endothelial cell function while decreasing proinflammatory cytokine production. Downstream effects may include improved oxygenation of adipose tissue, enhanced angiogenesis, and reversal of adiposopathy [16].

The intensity of exercise does matter. A study of 62 adolescents with obesity (mean BMI 34.8) randomized participants to either low-intensity training (LIT) or high-intensity training (HIT) for 24 weeks. Cytokines levels were measured, and while groups had improved inflammatory profiles, those undergoing HIT showed more prominent improvement compared with the LIT counterpart [18].

Despite the wide range of effects with diet and exercise, compliance with lifestyle changes and exercise has always challenged patients with obesity. With the medical weight loss programs that include medical follow-up, support, and exercise regimens, the majority of patients still regain the weight they had lost [19]. The physiological basis of this was not a lack of willpower as was demonstrated in many studies. Rather, a multifactorial etiology has been reported, including physiologic adaptation, hormonal changes, and the sustained drop in the resting metabolic rate compromising the long-term maintenance of weight loss [13].

The role of the microbiome in treatment of obesity and inflammation

Gut microbes far outnumber our own cells, with more than 7×10^{13} microbes for every human cell [20]. These microbes include a large variety of bacteria, unicellular eukaryotes, archaeas, and viruses. More than 50 phyla of bacteria exist in the gut, dominated by Bacteroidetes and Fermicutes [21].

Until recently, the relationship of the enteric microbiome to health and inflammation in the setting of obesity was merely anecdotal and corollary at best [22,23]. Further data from weight loss patients, and most notably bariatric surgery patients, revealed very strong associations. In the past decade, this field has witnessed a boom, propelling it to become one of the most interesting areas of translational research and medicine. A quick search on Pubmed shows an exponential growth in publications starting in the mid 2000s. Of these studies, most were based on murine models of obesity, with growing expansion into human clinical trials.

A fine balance exists between potentially proinflammatory and antiinflammatory cells at the level of the gut. The former are T helper (Th) cells that produce interferon gamma (IFN-γ), Th17 cells that secrete IL-17 and IL-22. While the latter are the regulatory T cells (Treg) that are FoxP3 + T cells. Changes of the gut microbiome have been shown to have a significant impact on this balance in animal and human models. Indeed, many bacteria have been shown to directly stimulate Treg cell maturation and increase production of IL-10. The inoculation of the mouse colon with a mix of subtypes of naturally occurring Clostridium promoted Treg cell accumulation in the wall and protected from the occurrence of colitis [24].

A proposed mechanism considers a plant-rich diet coupled with an environment of food scarcity. In such settings, the ability of the gut to extract more nutrients from plant complex carbohydrates depends on a several enzymes produced by the microbiome. This diversity is usually associated with an increase in the variety of Bacteroidetes. In contrast, abundant diets rich in fat and simple carbohydrates, and depleted of plant-derived complex carbohydrates, resulted in a dramatic and specific change in the microbiome, namely an increase in the *Firmicutes* [25]. This has been further compounded by the use of emulsifiers [26] and artificial sweeteners in the diet [27], the abuse of antibiotics in agriculture, and the liberal administration of antibiotics in children [28,29].

The microbiome can regulate the host metabolism and energy balance, by influencing the satiety/reward centers in the brain utilizing direct vagal stimulation or neuro-immuno-endocrine pathways. The latter modulate gene expression and downstream antiinflammatory effects, including upregulation of FOXP3 gene, downregulation of retinoic-acid-receptor-related orphan nuclear receptor gamma-t (ROR-gt), controlling the T-reg (regulatory T cells) [24], or increasing the production of IL-10 [30]. Many substrates have been implicated including short-chain fatty acids (SCFAs) as we will discuss [31,32].

Probiotics

The marked heterogeneity among the different probiotic preparations contributes to the difficulty in evaluating their impact. While a variety of bacteria and/or yeast combinations are available on the market, they do not all share similar properties. Unfortunately, the beneficial effects of a particular strain of bacteria may not extend to other members of its genus or species. Furthermore, the manufacturing guidelines are not strict, whereby shelf life and microbial count may vary among different batches of the same product. Many available studies have not controlled for the impact of comorbidities in the subjects. This leads to additional ambiguity given that such factors are well known to alter the composition of the microbiome.

Therefore, it is not surprising that a significant portion of the literature shows negative findings with respect to weight loss. Even more, some studies showed an increase in weight with the addition of probiotics [33–35]. This underlines the importance of a microbial strain-specific supplement evaluation.

Studies were able to show specific changes in the microbiome correlating with weight loss and decreased inflammatory markers. A metaanalysis of studies of leans vs. high-fat diet (HFD)-induced obese rodents evaluated the raw sequenced data of the gut microbiomes. Findings suggested an increased prevalence of bacterial families known for fermenting polysaccharides into SCFA (*Dorea*, *Oscillospira*, and *Ruminococcus*), this also coincided with a decrease in *Turicibacter* and an increase in *Lactococcus*, which are consistent with elevated inflammation in obesity [36].

An increased Firmicutes-to-Bacteroidetes ratio serves as a marker of obesity and by extension of the obesogenic impact of a diet. An increase in this ratio is noted with Western diets as well as with the use of preservatives and emulsifiers [32].

In an RCT performed by Tagliamonte et al., patients with diagnoses of overweight and obesity were changed from a usual Western diet to an equicaloric Mediterranean diet. They were noted to have an increase in endocannabinoids and fecal *A. muciniphila*. They also exhibited simultaneous improvements in their insulin sensitivity as measured by the homeostatic model assessment of insulin resistance index (HOMA-IRA) and serum high-sensitive CRP (hs-CRP) [37].

An MIT group of researchers conducted a long series of experiments that evaluated diet supplementation of experimental mice. They administered a specific strain of *Lactobacillus reuterii*, with remarkable effects. Indeed, those mice displayed a variety of health benefits ranging from preventing age-associated weight gain, reversal of the obesogenic effect of fast-food diet, and enhanced wound healing. Even more impressive was the ability to transfer these effects to probiotic naïve mice, solely through the transfer of CD4+ cells. The positive effects of this microbiome manipulation were mediated by CD25+ immune cells. Treg also utilized a pathway driven by IL-10 to downregulate proinflammatory processes where IL-6 and IL-17 are essential [38,39].

Through microbiome manipulation, antibiotics have been demonstrated to significantly impact obesity, its progression, and even development of metabolic disorders [40,41]. Moreover, we are now gaining further insight into the pathway through which high-fat diets alter gut microbiota. Evidently, the process requires a functional Toll-Like Receptor (TLR), specifically TLR-4, which allows weight balance and glucose metabolism to be altered, resulting in the systemic inflammation seen in diet-induced obesity.

Clearly these results cannot be extrapolated to humans at this time, but the premise is very seductive. We will delve deeper into the relationship between the microbiome and bariatric surgery in a subsequent section, as newer data suggests that the positive impacts of bariatric surgery are in no small part affected by the changes in the microbiome.

Prebiotics

Prebiotics have gained attention and are considered a crucial chapter of the microbiome story. Indeed, they make up the environment that will to a great deal provide probiotics with the substrate and milieu to support their growth. One can imagine that this could explain some of the heterogeneous results of probiotic supplementation.

A study evaluated the impact of oligofructose-enriched inulin (OI) in a single-center placebo-controlled randomized controlled trial. Children aged 7–12 years with overweight or obesity were followed over 16 weeks. The subjects receiving OI experienced significant decreases in weight as well as body fat in comparison to the placebo control group. They also experienced significant decreases of IL-6 (increased in placebo group) and significantly decreased LDL cholesterol levels. The intestinal microbiome contained increased proportions of Bifidobacterium species and decreases in *Bacteroides vulgatus* [42].

Another study revealed that prebiotics may help modulate the composition of the microbiome and, in turn, regulate inflammatory markers. A metaanalysis by Borges et al. looked at the markers of obesity. They contacted the authors for unpublished findings and independently extracted data. Ultimately, they evaluated the relationship between inflammatory markers and obesity such as leptin, ghrelin, CRP, ACTH, among others. They were able to demonstrate that supplementation of inulin type fructans resulted in a drop in blood concentrations of ghrelin and CRP in overweight or obese individuals [43].

Further data was reported in a triple-blind randomized trial by Dehghan et al. in which 52 type-2 diabetic females with BMI > 25 and BMI < 35 were given 10 g of OI for 8 weeks. Findings were significant for a decrease in fasting plasma glucose, glycosylated controlled hemoglobin (HbA1c), IL-6, TNF-α, and plasma lipopolysaccharide [44].

The mechanisms of action of prebiotics on individual's gut physiology are detailed in a review by Ferrarese et al. The prebiotics appear to cause a delay in gastric emptying that could modulate satiety and decrease the amount of bile acids and dietary cholesterol absorbed [45]. The increased colonic fermentation results in an increase in the production of SCFA. Many downstream benefits of SCFA include an increased ratio of propionate to acetate, which decreases liver lipogenesis. The SCFA also decreases the gut permeability to lipopolysaccharide from Gram-negative enteric bacteria. This reduces systemic markers of inflammation in human models. Another impact of the SCFA is the production of incretins such as GLP-1 and PYY, which impacts satiety centers along with many gut effects [31]. As a result, prebiotics have shown potentially beneficial outcomes for intervention to address inflammation and obesity.

Synbiotics

The presence of both a probiotic and prebiotic can have a positive synergistic effect. This was demonstrated in a double-blinded randomized trial comparing the impact of combined supplementation of probiotic yogurt vs. control milk along with or without probiotic capsules in subjects with obesity. The probiotic yogurt resulted in a significantly increased HOMA-IR. The impact of a similar combination of bacteria only impacted the HOMA-IR in the presence of prebiotic milk in the yogurt [46]. This indicates that a probiotic supplement may not be effective unless in the presence of the proper prebiotic milieu.

Fecal transformation is likely to provide an important therapeutic target for future prevention and management of obesity and inflammation. The potential for supplements to restore the microbiome content is an exciting frontier in medicine. Interesting research has demonstrated that some consumers of junk food appear resistant to weight gain. Evaluation of their stool showed signature fecal microbiome, which may confer this desirable effect. One can imagine dietary supplements designed to restore the microbiome to healthier strains (such as *Lactobacillus gasseri* strains), administered with prebiotics such as galactomannan and/or inulin fibers, with potential enhanced impacts on weight management and treatment of inflammation [31].

Role of weight loss medications

Pharmacotherapy for weight management has existed for several decades. Nevertheless, for various reasons, such medications had not garnered much favor. Evaluation of prescription trends over the years demonstrates that only a small percentage of eligible patients received drugs to support weight loss. In one retrospective review of 987 million visits of patients with obesity, a mere 2% were noted to have received antiobesity medication [47]. Barriers to prescription included safety concerns, stringent substance control regulation, and lack of insurance coverage, among others. More recently, however, as the understanding of obesity, inflammation, and hormonal signaling has progressed, the development of novel agents has shifted the paradigm of medical management. As of mid-2021, the FDA lists five weight loss drugs approved for long-term use with an additional four listed as suitable for short-term appetite suppression [48]. While earlier drug formulations relied on monotherapies with a single downstream target, newer products make use of combination therapies, reducing the potential for counter-regulatory pathways. The detailed signaling mechanisms of hunger, satiety, and adipogenesis are beyond the scope of this chapter; however, we will consider pharmacological agents that make use of them to support weight loss. More specifically, we will consider the ways in which these medications affect inflammatory processes.

There is some overlap between the pharmacologic management of obesity and that of diabetes. Glucagon-like peptide-1 receptor agonists (GLP1-RAs) in particular were associated with weight reduction, allowing Liraglutide (*Saxenda, Victoza*) to gain FDA approval as a weight loss agent. This drug works by delaying gastric emptying and suppressing appetite [49]. In addition, GLP1 therapies are thought to produces multisystem antiinflammatory effects, causing downregulation in the production of cytokines (TNF-α, IFN-γ, IL-1β, IL-2, IL-6, and IL-17), adhesion molecules (VCAM, ICAM and E-Selectin), and chemokines (CXCL10 and MCP1) [50]. Affected organs include the brain, vascular system, liver, pancreas, lungs, kidneys, testes, and skin. Studies pertaining specifically to the cardioprotective effects of Liraglutide illustrated the drug's significant antioxidative properties. In a human umbilical vein model, Liraglutide inhibited signaling from PKC-α, NF-κB, and NADPH oxidase, resulting in reduced inflammation in the endothelium [51]. The drug is also thought to downregulate the endoplasmic reticulum stress pathway. In the presence of hypoxia, ischemia, or oxidative stress, these organelles accumulate unfolded proteins, leading to cell death and disease development. In a murine model, treatment with Liraglutide was associated with reduced expression of apoptosis-associated caspases and improved histological and functional outcomes [52].

In June 2021, Semaglutide (*Ozempic, Wegovy*), a weekly administered GLP1-RA, was added to the list of approved drugs. In a retrospective analysis of long-term treatment with Semaglutide, authors reported a significant dose-dependent and weight-loss-based reduction in ALT and hs-CRP [53]. Nevertheless, results from human studies have been conflicting [54], and the exact relationship between GLP1-RA treatment and redox homeostasis remains uncertain. When weight adjustment was conducted, some studies assessing reduction in inflammatory markers did not find any significant changes, potentially indicating that the antiinflammatory effect was related to weight loss rather than a direct effect of GLP1-RA therapy [55].

Tirzepatide is a promising drug under evaluation [56]. In addition to its GLP1-RA activity, it also functions as a GIP agonist. Histological studies from murine models demonstrated superiority of the dual-acting drug compared with Liraglutide in reducing inflammation-associated astrogliosis and microgliosis [57]. Overall, the reported data on GLP1-RA appears to correlate with reduction in multisystem inflammatory processes, but further evaluation of the causal pathway is needed. Assessment of other diabetes therapies is also worthwhile.

Although Metformin is not formally recognized as a weight loss therapy, it is often prescribed off label for this purpose with a mere 3%–5% weight loss. Several studies have highlighted the drug's antiinflammatory effect beyond simple glucose control [58,59].

In contrast to the glucose-regulatory effect of the aforementioned drugs, inhibition of lipid absorption is another notable weight loss mechanism adopted by the FDA-approved agent Orlistat (*Xenical*). A lower-dose over-the-counter form of the lipase inhibitor also exists (Alli). From an inflammation standpoint, it has previously been shown that high-fat diets are associated with acute and chronic states of systemic inflammation. High fat intake is highly associated with states of Endoplasmic Reticular stress, neurotoxicity in the appetite regulating centers of the brain, and other deleterious states [60]. With that in mind, one may question whether a reduced absorption of dietary fat may in turn lead to a decreased inflammatory state.

In studies assessing the impact of lipase inhibitor treatment on circulating inflammatory markers, consistent treatment with Orlistat was found to increase levels of adiponectin. This oligomer has antiinflammatory properties, and its secretion is inversely proportional to adiposity [61]. Although the placebo groups that were randomized to lifestyle modifications alone showed mild increase in adiponectin, this was significantly less than what was noted in the treatment group [62].

Once again, one may question whether the antiinflammatory effect is due to weight loss rather than a direct effect of the medications. When comparing average weight loss in both groups, the placebo/lifestyle modification group did not show significant change in weight (91.7 ± 8.7 kg at baseline to 89.1 ± 7.8 kg at 12 months), unlike the Orlistat cohort (94.5 ± 9.6 kg at baseline to 85.0 ± 5.9 kg at 12 months). Nevertheless, these findings further emphasize the difficulty in achieving antiinflammatory benefits of weight loss in the absence of pharmacological support.

Changes in other markers of inflammation were evaluated, once again comparing treatment group (Orlistat + hypocaloric diet) with control group (hypocaloric diet alone). In this study, even after controlling for differences in groups' weight loss, the treatment cohort had a more significant decrease in levels of TNF-α, CPR, and isoprostane [63]. Positive downstream effects may also be noted at the organ system level. In a study assessing short course of Orlistat treatment versus diet alone control, levels of periostin, an inflammatory protein highly associated with progression of NAFLD, were significantly reduced in the treatment group [64]. Although the treatment course was too brief to induce significant changes in weight, ultrasound imaging of the liver demonstrated improvement in degree of fatty changes in the Orlistat group. This further elucidates the weight-loss-independent antiinflammatory effect. Murine models of inflammation in the testes [65] and vascular system [66] showed similar protective effects of treatment.

Of all the currently approved weight loss agents, Phentermine was able to stand the test of time, having gained FDA approval as early as 1959. At the time, this noradrenergic agent was prescribed as a short course monotherapy. More recently, the combined formulation with the antiepileptic Topiramate was approved for long-term use (*Qsymia, Vivus*). Several large-scale blinded placebo control trials were able to prove the significant impact this medication had on weight reduction [67,68]. Despite impressive availability of information about the effectiveness of phentermine/topiramate for weight reduction, there is a paucity of data relating to potential effects on inflammation. Even when evaluating each of the components separately, little is known about the mechanisms of action of these drugs. Some reports have noted that topiramate aided in the reduction of oxidative stress and glutathione levels in hyperglycemic states [69].

While other weight-regulation drugs modulate the homeostatic aspect of food intake, the final category of approved drugs tackles the hedonistic and motivational aspects. The Naltrexone-Bupropion combination (*Contrave*) exerts downstream effects on the μ-opioid, NE, and DA receptors, reducing food seeking behavior. Used separately for drug and smoking dependence, respectively, the joint formulation stimulates POMC neurons in hypothalamus, releasing α-MSH and reducing appetite, while simultaneously inhibiting negative feedback inhibition.

Studies pertaining to the effects on inflammation evaluate the two drugs independently. In murine models, Bupropion successfully reduced TNF and increased antiinflammatory IL-10, protecting against otherwise lethal doses of injected lipopolysaccharide [70]. Similar results were noted in mice models of NASH treated with Bupropion, but the treatment failed to induce any changed on vascular relaxation response [71].

On the other hand, naltrexone was able to produce significant reduction in neuroinflammation. By attenuating the NF-κB pathway, Naltrexone resulted in inhibition of the mitochondrial apoptotic pathway, reducing ischemia-induced brain injury [72]. The drug was also found to reduce microglial activation [73], potentially acting via TLR4 antagonism. Despite existing evidence of their antiinflammatory effects, studies pertaining specifically to the combined therapy's effect on weight loss and related information are still lacking.

Patients living with obesity generally require a reduction of > 15% body weight to achieve optimal health outcomes with greater weight loss associated with better results. As of yet, the overall efficacy of medications in achieving this goal has yet to be achieved. Further pharmacological therapies must be developed to this end. Nevertheless, weight loss of even 5%–10% body weight can significantly improve health outcomes, especially for those who did not have successful outcomes from lifestyle modification and who are not candidates for more invasive options. As noted throughout this section, such pharmacologic interventions may provide benefits beyond the weight reduction, supporting generalized reduction in inflammation (Table 2).

Table 2 Overview of pharmacological agents for weight loss.

Category	Mechanism of action	Drug	Dosing and administration	Indication	Expected outcome from trials	Potential side effects
GLP1	POMC neuron stimulation	Liraglutide (Saxenda, Victoza)	Daily subcutaneous administration Starting dose: 1 week of 0.6 mg/d. dose increases by 0.6 per week till 3.0 mg/d	Long term use	Approximately 10% by 1 year	Theoretical risk for Medullary thyroid carcinoma pancreatitis
		Semaglutide (Ozempic, Wegovy)	Weekly subcutaneous administration Gradually increased over 16–20 weeks to 2.4 mg/week	Long term use	Average of 12.4% weight loss	
		Tirzepatide[a] Additional GIP activity	Still under investigation	*Anticipated FDA approval Late 2021*	—	Still unknown
Noradrenergic	Unclear	Phentermine (Adipex)	8–37.5 mg Use least dose possible	Short term use, only for 12 weeks	Approximately 5% weight loss	Constipation, dry mouth, and trouble sleeping

	Drug	Dose	Duration	Efficacy	Side effects/notes
Lipase inhibitor	Orlistat (Alli, Xenical)	Prescription: 120 mg TID with meals OTC – 60 mg TID	Long term use	5% weight loss when used alone vs greater when combined with behavioral intervention	Reduced absorption of fat-soluble vitamins
Decreased absorption	Phentermine/topiramate ER (Qsymia, Vivus)	7.5/46 recommended Discontinue or increase dose if <3% wt loss after 12 weeks	Long term use	In cases of extreme obesity, up to 20% body weight loss is possible at high dose	
Dopamine, NE reuptake inhibitor/opioid receptor antagonist	Bupropion SR/Naltrexone SR (Contrave)	32 mg/360 mg BID Recommend discontinuing if <5% weight loss after 16 weeks	Long term use	Synergistic effect Up to 15% weight loss	Not to be used with opioid pain medication Possible increase in suicidal thoughts
Unclear/increases satiety					
Increase satiety					
[b]5 HT2C receptor agonist	Lorcaserin (Belviq)	10 mg BID Recommend discontinuing if <5% weight loss after 12 weeks	Long term use *Recently withdrawn*	8%	***Increased cancer risk***

This table includes drugs that are in progress[a] as well as drugs that were recently withdrawn[b] for completion.

Bariatric interventions endoscopic/surgical and inflammation

Impact of endoscopic interventions

In 2015, the FDA approved the first intragastric balloon (IGB) for use in the United States. These had been available in many countries and trialed since the 1990s outside the United States. The current treatment course is a placement of the IGB for 6 months during which the patients follow strict dietary protocols. Following this period, the IGB is removed. After the IGB is removed, the patient is maintained on a strict diet to enhance the weight loss outcomes and minimize weight regain.

This presented an attractive nonoperative technique for weight loss as an alternative to a surgical intervention. A recent study from Brazil published in 2019 evaluated the impact of IGB placement on weight loss and adipokines and cytokines. In that study, it was noted that the levels of leptin, hs-CRP, glucose, insulin, HOMA-IR, and triglycerides all decreased appropriately. Adiponectin/leptin ratio was otherwise increased [74].

Unfortunately, the above study was only for a period of 6 months, and no long-term studies are currently available for the IGB. The course of treatment with the IGB is short, 6 months. Other studies have evaluated the impact of IGB on serum levels of hs-CRP showing a significant decrease [75,76]. We look forward to longer-term studies. One can imagine that these may reflect longer-term benefits that may persist in some cases when the weight loss does not.

The AspireAssist is a procedure that relies on the endoscopic placement of a modified gastrostomy tube for the postprandial aspiration of about 30% of the ingested calories from the stomach [77,78]. There is no data regarding its impact on inflammatory markers, that being said, evidence of improvement of weight, HbA1C, triglycerides, LFTs, and blood pressure are reported [79].

Another technique is the endoscopic sleeve gastroplasty, where the stomach is plicated endoluminally, thereby reducing its lumen along the greater curvature of the stomach. Again, the literature has focused solely on weight loss rather than its impact on inflammatory markers. The mean is 15.9% of total body weight loss at 5 years [80]. This underlines the need for more research to fully understand the impact of these techniques.

Impact of bariatric surgery

In the severely obese, bariatric surgery has been demonstrated as the only intervention providing long-term sustained weight loss and improvement of comorbidities. This is associated with an improvement in life expectancy and medical comorbidities as shown in many studies, the longest running of which is the Swedish Obese Subjects trial [19]. The term "metabolic surgery" was coined to reflect the marked impact of bariatric surgery on metabolic endpoints and medical comorbidities including diabetes. The NIH consensus statement for GI surgery in 1991 determined that bariatric surgery was indicated for BMI of 35 or greater with comorbidities and BMI greater than 40 without comorbidities [81]. More recent data has challenged the NIH criteria, ultimately calling for their revision and expansion. In the 2nd Diabetes Surgery Summit, a multidisciplinary panel including endocrinologist, surgeons, and internists called for the consideration of metabolic surgery as an option for the treatment of adults with type 2 diabetes and BMI $30.0–34.9\,kg/m^2$ ($27.5–32.4\,kg/m^2$ in Asians) if hyperglycemia is poorly controlled despite appropriate medical therapy by either oral or injectable medications (including insulin) [82]. The American Diabetes Association upheld their recommendations in their subsequent revisions of the document. Alas, very few health insurances have adopted these recommendations yet, despite the mounting body of evidence.

Many bariatric surgical procedures are available: adjustable gastric banding (or lap banding), sleeve gastrectomy (SG), Roux-en-Y gastric bypass (RYGB), and biliopancreatic diversion with duodenal switch (BPD/DS). Newer procedures are being explored with some early adoption: the one anastomosis gastric bypass (OAGB), and the Single Anastomosis Duodeno-Ileal bypass (SADI). Currently, the SG and the RYGB are the most performed procedures in the United States and worldwide, accounting for about 85% of all procedures. These are also the most widely studied procedures, allowing better understanding of their mechanism of action, both affecting weight loss and independently affected physiologic alterations.

The mechanism of action of bariatric procedures was postulated to be a combination of restrictive and malabsorptive mechanisms. It is clear now that the impact is far more complex, involving interactions of the gut-brain axis, including immune, microbiome, and gut hormonal pathways.

Following bariatric surgery, signature bacteria are noted to change. There is enhanced development of Proteobacteria and Virrucomicrobia. These organisms lead to fermentation in the gut, increasing SCFAs, which improve the intestinal barrier function, reduce solubility of free bile acids, and prevent the growth of pH-sensitive pathogens [83]. As such, this provides protection against obesity and carcinogenesis.

While inflammation appears to improve most studied procedures—RYGB, SG, lap band, and OAGB [84], we will consider them in further detail in the following section.

Roux-en-y gastric bypass (RYGB)

Roux-en-Y Gastric bypass (RYGB) is considered the "gold standard" for bariatric surgery, as it has been performed for the longest period of time. A small gastric pouch is separated from the rest of the stomach and is connected to a limb of early jejunum, the Roux limb. The food moves through the gastric pouch into the jejunum, thereby bypassing the distal stomach and duodenum. The RYGB provides a loss of about 70% of excess weight. The RYGB was the first weight loss surgery procedure to be extensively studied. In addition, animal models have allowed evaluation of outcomes in a lab setting.

The impact of the RYGB on weight is accompanied by improved insulin sensitivity, leptin, oxidative stress, as well as adipose tissue inflammation [85,86]. This procedure reduces levels of multiple inflammatory mediators and the expression of TLR-4 and TLR-2 on mononuclear cells [87]. In addition, there was a reduced activation of mononuclear cells as evidenced by a fall in the expression of the CD14 surface marker. Evidence of reduced inflammation may precede significant weight loss, occurring as early as 1-month postop, when CRP levels begin declining [88]. In fact, surgery was found to reduce the expression of TLRs within the small intestines of diabetic women with obesity, independently of weight loss [89].

The impact of the RYGB on the enteric flora has been well documented. These changes are so marked, that it is now thought to be a major mechanism for the weight loss [90]. The anatomical rearrangement that takes place following RYGB results in alteration of local pH, bile acid metabolism, and nutrient flow, leading to selective development of microbial flora. Following RYGB, the reduced caloric intake allows expansion of Bacteroides growth [91]. While specific findings vary, studies have shown expansion of Gammaproteobacteria (Escherichia) and Verrucomicrobia (Akkermansia) and a decreased abundance of Firmicutes following surgical interventions [32] [90]. Downstream effects are thought to be modulated by changes in the SCFA previously described.

In addition, the antiinflammatory effect associated with RYGB can potentially benefit chronic conditions beyond metabolic syndrome. In a recent review, the relation between the gut microbiome in obesity and asthma was evaluated. After bariatric surgery, *A. muciniphila* is known to increase, potentially helping against inflammation and hyperactive airway disease. The impact of the microbiome modulation is through an increase in SCFA potentially aiding in modulating asthma severity in patients with obesity [92].

The microbial changes associated with RYGB are so pronounced that they may confer beneficial effects even when transferred outside the host. In a murine model, fecal transplantation from donor mice that underwent RYGB to untreated mice resulted in weight loss in the recipients [90]. Nevertheless, some studies claim that the alterations in gut microbiome post RYGB are transient and revert back to baseline findings a year after the intervention [93]. Additional long-term studies will be needed to validate and verify these findings.

Obesity is associated with elevated adipocyte secretion of adipokines with some proinflammatory potential [94]. This includes leptin, visfatin, vaspin, omentin, adipsin, retinol-binding protein 4, adiponectin, apelin, resistin, and perilipin. In addition to the markers of systemic inflammation discussed throughout this chapter, the effect of the RYGB on adipokine secretion has also been documented. Although studies are still inconclusive, we are beginning to see trends in postintervention levels of these substances [95]. Further evaluations are needed to better understand the specific relationship between bariatric surgery-mediated alteration in local adipocyte inflammation and broader systemic effects. As of yet, some findings even point to possible post-RYGB reduction in hypothalamic inflammation with induction of similar downstream effect [96].

Sleeve gastrectomy

The sleeve gastrectomy is currently the most performed procedure worldwide and in the United States. The stomach is divided along its length based on the lesser curvature, removing about 70%–80% of its volume. The sleeve affords about 60% loss of excess weight. The mechanism for the sleeve gastrectomy has not been completely elucidated; however, there is an impact for a decrease in ghrelin levels post gastrectomy. In terms of its antiinflammatory effect, most evaluations were done in comparison to the RYGB. Studies demonstrated similar patterns of reduced IL-17, IL-23, and IFN-γ in both procedures [97], but the RYGB had a broader effect, reducing other cytokines and increasing IL-33 [98]. These differences may be in part due to the variation in underlying mechanisms associated with the gut hormones, microbiota, and resulting weight loss [99].

Less common surgical procedures

In terms of their effect on inflammation, the remaining bariatric procedures are less widely studied. In this section, we will consider some of these additional procedures as well as comparative studies. The lap band procedure was very common in the 1990–early 2000s; however, currently it has largely been supplanted. The excess weight loss afforded is in the range of ~50% of the excess weight.

As reviewed in the section on probiotics, gut microbial has been associated with obesity. A recent study showed that 75% of obese study patients showed a decrease in microbial gene richness, a surrogate measure of variability of bacteria. After bariatric surgery, microbial variability was noted to increase, however, more so with the adjustable lap band than with the RYGB [100]. Nevertheless, RYGB continues to afford better metabolic outcomes than its counterpart. When comparing these procedures in terms of markers of systemic inflammation, there seems to be discrepancies in the reduction in TNF-α [101]. Following the lap band procedure, there appears to be no change in TNF-α. In contrast, levels have varied in patients who underwent RYGB.

Other procedures such as the biliopancreatic diversion with duodenal switch (BPD/DS) are far less studied. In the United States, it is uncommonly performed due to the high risk of malabsorption, accounting for ~0.3% of all procedures. A study comparing the effect of BPD to RYGB noted more pronounced reduction in ALT, GGT, and BMI in the former group [102]. They extrapolate that this difference may be related to even further reduction in inflammation, yet there is insufficient evidence to support that claim.

Similarly, there is a paucity of information related to OAGB and SADI with available inflammation-related data pertaining to animal models. In a study comparing these procedures to the RYGB and sleeve gastrectomy, OAGB, SADI, and RYGB had similar changes in microbiome [103]. The implications of these findings require further follow-up in the future as significance is corollary at best.

Overall, the consistent findings related to microbiome manipulation with bariatric surgery have led researchers to question whether preoperative interventions may optimize long-term results. Further evaluations are still needed to determine whether this is feasible.

A standardized evaluation of inflammation in patients with obesity

Evidence-based recommendations for the evaluation of overweight and obese adults have been released by the NHLBI (National Heart, Lung, and

Blood Institute), in cooperation with the National Institute of Diabetes and Digestive and Kidney Diseases in 1998 [104]. A comprehensive history and physical exam should be obtained on all patients. This should focus on obesity-related comorbid conditions and inflammatory disorders. Clinical evaluation should include the determination of the BMI, which grades the patient's obesity. Then, an assessment of the presence of abdominal obesity based on waist circumference should be performed as central obesity is associated with metabolic syndrome and inflammation. During the history taking, emphasis should be placed on assessing the presence of underlying diseases and conditions (diabetes mellitus, hypertension, coronary artery disease, etc.) as well as the presence of risk factors of cardiovascular disease (smoking, impaired fasting glucose, high LDL, etc.). Also an evaluation for the presence of physical inactivity should be performed [105].

Laboratory data should be obtained and should include a complete blood count (CBC) with a differential count, which will allow the evaluation of the WBC, monocyte, and neutrophil counts. Further specific values include ESR and hs-CRP, which are easily obtained as a serum test. CRP is a sensitive inflammatory marker, which can be elevated with a range of mild inflammatory processes throughout the body, and therefore lacks specificity. IL-6 level could also be obtained to assess inflammation as a simple lab test.

Glucose level, insulin, and GLP-1 levels can be helpful to assess insulin resistance. HOMA-IR is a score obtained by the multiplication of (Fasting insulin) × (Fasting glucose)/405. Units for glucose are mg/dl. The usual normal range for HOMA-IR is from 0.7 to 2, but this range varies between different populations. ACTH also helps in the assessment of insulin resistance. Leptin is occasionally ordered to rule out congenital etiologies for obesity and evaluate the degree of adiposopathy.

Other tests that were mentioned through our review are mostly research tools that are not widely available for clinical use. These include TNF-alpha, soluble intercellular adhesion molecule-1 (ICAM-1), soluble vascular cell adhesion molecule-1 (V-CAM-1), ghrelin levels, and other interleukins [18].

A stepwise approach for managing inflammation and weight in the obese patients

We have reviewed possible therapies to impact inflammation in the setting of obesity. This reinforces the usual approach used in general weight management. There is very little data regarding a positive impact of behavioral counseling on inflammation in the setting of obesity [106]. However, due to its established impact on weight loss maintenance, it should probably be included as a standard approach to all patients with weight issues.

Dietary interventions should be advised in all patients with increased proinflammatory states, irrespective of weight. We reviewed many strategies for dieting, including a Mediterranean diet or macrobiotic diet, which are associated with the lowest scores for proinflammation. This can be attributed in part to the high amounts of prebiotics and fiber in these diets. Also an avoidance of proinflammatory additives such as emulsifiers and artificial sweeteners is advisable, in part due to their nefarious impact on the microbiome. Intermittent fasting further enhances the impact of the caloric restriction, with decreases in inflammatory markers.

High-intensity exercise with a target of 250 min of endurance training and 2–3 times of weight training per week should help enhance the antiinflammatory markers. This impact occurs even before any weight change is noted. More intense training is also associated with further antiinflammatory outcomes.

Probiotics and prebiotics have very encouraging outcomes on weight and inflammation with some mixed data at the time of writing, probably due to many factors including the lack of standardization of probiotic strains, purity, and the dosage of the probiotics. Microbiome restoration with the administration of specific prebiotics/probiotic strain combinations, the transplantation of feces, and the use of antibiotics to treat pervasive proinflammatory strains are all exciting avenues of future management. Further human research will undoubtedly uncover avenues for prevention and management of obesity and inflammation.

Many medications for weight management have proven beneficial on inflammation; however, some of the newer medications have not been specifically evaluated vis-a-vis their impact on inflammation. This underlines the need for further research. These medications are prescribed by physicians specializing in weight management and who are ideally a part of a multidisciplinary team for weight management including a dietitian, an exercise physiologist, and a metabolic/bariatric surgeon.

The intragastric balloon and other noninvasive endoscopic interventions could be considered in the obese, without comorbidities (as they do not qualify for weight loss surgery). The impact is notable on inflammatory markers, albeit more modestly than that of bariatric surgical procedures. The lack of insurance coverage for these procedures limits their utility at this time.

Since surgical interventions are the most effective in treating weight and weight-related comorbidities in the severely obese patients, counseling patients to obtain bariatric metabolic procedures as early as patients qualify will prevent further deterioration of metabolic reserve and progression of comorbidities. Bariatric surgery is also the most impactful with respect to inflammation, the most studied of which is the RYGB. The sleeve gastrectomy is also proving very effective in reversing inflammation, albeit less than the RYGB. Further expansion of the criteria of these procedures to patients with lower BMI has been well supported by the literature, however, not yet by insurers. Persistent education of the public and advocacy to widen access to patients is essential.

References

[1] Xiao X, Liu Y-Z, Cheng Z-B, Sun J-X, Shao Y-D, Qu S-L, Huang L, Zhang C. Adipokines in vascular calcification. Clin Chim Acta 2021;516:15–26. https://doi.org/10.1016/j.cca.2021.01.009.

[2] Robinson T, Martin RM, Yarmolinsky J. Mendelian randomisation analysis of circulating adipokines and C-reactive protein on breast cancer risk. Int J Cancer 2020;147:1597–603. https://doi.org/10.1002/ijc.32947.

[3] Mannelli M, Gamberi T, Magherini F, Fiaschi T. The adipokines in cancer cachexia. Int J Mol Sci 2020;21:4860. https://doi.org/10.3390/ijms21144860.

[4] Shai I, Schwarzfuchs D, Henkin Y, Shahar DR, Witkow S, Greenberg I, Golan R, Fraser D, Bolotin A, Vardi H, Tangi-Rozental O, Zuk-Ramot R, Sarusi B, Brickner D, Schwartz Z, Sheiner E, Marko R, Katorza E, Thiery J, Fiedler GM, Blüher M, Stumvoll M, Stampfer MJ. Weight loss with a low-carbohydrate, Mediterranean, or low-fat diet. N Engl J Med 2008;359:229–41. https://doi.org/10.1056/NEJMoa0708681.

[5] Golan R, Schwarzfuchs D, Shai I. Four-year follow-up after two-year dietary interventions. N Engl J Med 2012;367:1373–4. https://doi.org/10.1056/NEJMc1204792.

[6] Esposito K, Maiorino MI, Bellastella G, Chiodini P, Panagiotakos D, Giugliano D. A journey into a Mediterranean diet and type 2 diabetes: a systematic review with meta-analyses. BMJ Open 2015;5:e008222. https://doi.org/10.1136/bmjopen-2015-008222.

[7] Espeland M, Pi-Sunyer X, Blackburn G, Brancati FL, Bray GA, Bright R, Clark JM, Curtis JM, Espeland MA, Foreyt JP, Graves K, Haffner SM, Harrison B, Hill JO, Horton ES, Jakicic J, Jeffery RW, Johnson KC, Kahn S, Kelley DE, Kitabchi AE, Knowler WC, Lewis CE, Maschak-Carey BJ, Montgomery B, Nathan DM, Patricio J, Peters A, Redmon JB, Reeves RS, Ryan DH, Safford M, Van Dorsten B, Wadden TA, Wagenknecht L, Wesche-Thobaben J, Wing RR, Yanovski SZ. Reduction in weight and cardiovascular disease risk factors in individuals with type 2 diabetes—one-year results of the Look AHEAD trial. Diabetes Care 2007;30:1374–83. https://doi.org/10.2337/dc07-0048.

[8] Roager HM, Vogt JK, Kristensen M, Hansen LBS, Ibrügger S, Mærkedahl RB, Bahl MI, Lind MV, Nielsen RL, Frøkiær H, Gøbel RJ, Landberg R, Ross AB, Brix S, Holck J, Meyer AS, Sparholt MH, Christensen AF, Carvalho V, Hartmann B, Holst JJ, Rumessen JJ, Linneberg A, Sicheritz-Pontén T, Dalgaard MD, Blennow A, Frandsen HL, Villas-Bôas S, Kristiansen K, Vestergaard H, Hansen T, Ekstrøm CT, Ritz C, Nielsen HB, Pedersen OB, Gupta R, Lauritzen L, Licht TR. Whole grain-rich diet reduces body weight and systemic low-grade inflammation without inducing major changes of the gut microbiome: a randomised cross-over trial. Gut 2019;68:83–93. https://doi.org/10.1136/gutjnl-2017-314786.

[9] Shivappa N, Steck SE, Hurley TG, Hussey JR, Hébert JR. Designing and developing a literature-derived, population-based dietary inflammatory index. Public Health Nutr 2014;17:1689–96. https://doi.org/10.1017/S1368980013002115.
[10] Zheng J, Hoffman KL, Chen J-S, Shivappa N, Sood A, Browman GJ, Dirba DD, Hanash S, Wei P, Hebert JR, Petrosino JF, Schembre SM, Daniel CR. Dietary inflammatory potential in relation to the gut microbiome: results from a cross-sectional study. Br J Nutr 2020;124:931–42. https://doi.org/10.1017/S0007114520001853.
[11] Longo VD, Mattson MP. Fasting: molecular mechanisms and clinical applications. Cell Metab 2014;19:181–92. https://doi.org/10.1016/j.cmet.2013.12.008.
[12] Wang X, Yang Q, Liao Q, Li M, Zhang P, Santos HO, Kord-Varkaneh H, Abshirini M. Effects of intermittent fasting diets on plasma concentrations of inflammatory biomarkers: a systematic review and meta-analysis of randomized controlled trials. Nutrition 2020;79–80. https://doi.org/10.1016/j.nut.2020.110974, 110974.
[13] Fothergill E, Guo J, Howard L, Kerns JC, Knuth ND, Brychta R, Chen KY, Skarulis MC, Walter M, Walter PJ, Hall KD. Persistent metabolic adaptation 6 years after "The Biggest Loser" competition. Obesity (Silver Spring, Md) 2016;24:1612–9. https://doi.org/10.1002/oby.21538.
[14] Ford ES. Does exercise reduce inflammation? physical activity and C-reactive protein among U.S adults. Epidemiology (Cambridge, Mass) 2002;13:561–8. https://doi.org/10.1097/00001648-200209000-00012.
[15] Dimitrov S, Hulteng E, Hong S. Inflammation and exercise: inhibition of monocytic intracellular TNF production by acute exercise via β2-adrenergic activation. Brain Behav Immun 2016;61:60–8. https://doi.org/10.1016/j.bbi.2016.12.017.
[16] You T, Arsenis NC, Disanzo BL, LaMonte MJ. Effects of exercise training on chronic inflammation in obesity: current evidence and potential mechanisms. Sports Med (Auckland) 2013;43:243–56. https://doi.org/10.1007/s40279-013-0023-3.
[17] Bays HE. Adiposopathy: is "sick fat" a cardiovascular disease? J Am Coll Cardiol 2011;57:2461–73. https://doi.org/10.1016/j.jacc.2011.02.038.
[18] Tenorio TRS, Balagopal PB, Andersen LB, Ritti-Dias RM, Hill JO, Lofrano-Prado MC, Prado WL. Effect of low-versus high-intensity exercise training on biomarkers of inflammation and endothelial dysfunction in adolescents with obesity: a 6-month randomized exercise intervention study. Pediatr Exerc Sci 2018;30:98–107. https://doi.org/10.1123/pes.2017-0067.
[19] Sjöström L, Narbro K, Sjöström CD, Karason K, Larsson B, Wedel H, Lystig T, Sullivan M, Bouchard C, Carlsson B, Bengtsson C, Dahlgren S, Gummesson A, Jacobson P, Karlsson J, Lindroos A-K, Lönroth H, Näslund I, Olbers T, Stenlöf K, Torgerson J, Ågren G, Carlsson LMS. Effects of bariatric surgery on mortality in Swedish obese subjects. N Engl J Med 2007;357:741–52. https://doi.org/10.1056/NEJMoa066254.
[20] Walsh CJ, Guinane CM, O'Toole PW, Cotter PD. Beneficial modulation of the gut microbiota. FEBS Lett 2014;588:4120–30. https://doi.org/10.1016/j.febslet.2014.03.035.
[21] Sekirov I, Russell SL, Antunes LCM, Finlay BB. Gut microbiota in health and disease. Physiol Rev 2010;90:859–904. https://doi.org/10.1152/physrev.00045.2009.
[22] Duncan SH, Lobley GE, Holtrop G, Ince J, Johnstone AM, Louis P, Flint HJ. Human colonic microbiota associated with diet, obesity and weight loss. Int J Obes (Lond) 2008;32:1720–4. https://doi.org/10.1038/ijo.2008.155.
[23] Nadal I, Santacruz A, Marcos A, Warnberg J, Garagorri JM, Garagorri M, Moreno LA, Martin-Matillas M, Campoy C, Martí A, Moleres A, Delgado M, Veiga OL, García-Fuentes M, Redondo CG, Sanz Y. Shifts in clostridia, bacteroides and immunoglobulin-coating fecal bacteria associated with weight loss in obese adolescents. Int J Obes (Lond) 2009;33:758–67. https://doi.org/10.1038/ijo.2008.260.
[24] Atarashi K, Tanoue T, Shima T, Imaoka A, Kuwahara T, Momose Y, Cheng G, Yamasaki S, Saito T, Ohba Y, Taniguchi T, Takeda K, Hori S, Ivanov II, Umesaki Y, Itoh K, Honda

K. Induction of colonic regulatory T cells by indigenous clostridium species. Science 2011;331:337–41. https://doi.org/10.1126/science.1198469.
[25] Ley RE, Bäckhed F, Turnbaugh P, Lozupone CA, Knight RD, Gordon JI. Obesity alters gut microbial ecology. Proc Natl Acad Sci U S A 2005;102:11070–5. https://doi.org/10.1073/pnas.0504978102.
[26] Chassaing B, Koren O, Goodrich JK, Poole AC, Srinivasan S, Ley RE, Gewirtz AT. Dietary emulsifiers impact the mouse gut microbiota promoting colitis and metabolic syndrome. Nature 2015;519:92–6. https://doi.org/10.1038/nature14232.
[27] Suez J, Korem T, Zeevi D, Zilberman-Schapira G, Thaiss CA, Maza O, Israeli D, Zmora N, Gilad S, Weinberger A, Kuperman Y, Harmelin A, Kolodkin-Gal I, Shapiro H, Halpern Z, Segal E, Elinav E. Artificial sweeteners induce glucose intolerance by altering the gut microbiota. Nature 2014;514:181–6. https://doi.org/10.1038/nature13793.
[28] Cox LM, Blaser MJ. Antibiotics in early life and obesity. Nat Rev Endocrinol 2015;11:182–90. https://doi.org/10.1038/nrendo.2014.210.
[29] De Filippo C, Cavalieri D, Di Paola M, Ramazzotti M, Poullet JB, Massart S, Collini S, Pieraccini G, Lionetti P. Impact of diet in shaping gut microbiota revealed by a comparative study in children from Europe and rural Africa. Proc Natl Acad Sci U S A 2010;107:14691–6. https://doi.org/10.1073/pnas.1005963107.
[30] Round JL, Lee SM, Li J, Tran G, Jabri B, Chatila TA, Mazmanian SK. The toll-like receptor 2 pathway establishes colonization by a commensal of the human microbiota. Science 2011;332:974–7. https://doi.org/10.1126/science.1206095.
[31] Ferrarese R, Ceresola ER, Preti A, Canducci F. Probiotics, prebiotics and synbiotics for weight loss and metabolic syndrome in the microbiome era. Eur Rev Med Pharmacol Sci 2018;22:7588–605. https://doi.org/10.26355/eurrev_201811_16301.
[32] Torres-Fuentes C, Schellekens H, Dinan TG, Cryan JF. The microbiota-gut-brain axis in obesity. Lancet Gastroenterol Hepatol 2017;2:747–56. https://doi.org/10.1016/S2468-1253(17)30147-4.
[33] Chouraqui JP, Grathwohl D, Labaune JM, Hascoet JM, de Montgolfier I, Leclaire M, Giarre M, Steenhout P. Assessment of the safety, tolerance, and protective effect against diarrhea of infant formulas containing mixtures of probiotics or probiotics and prebiotics in a randomized controlled trial. Am J Clin Nutr 2008;87:1365–73. https://doi.org/10.1093/ajcn/87.5.1365.
[34] Maldonado J, Lara-Villoslada F, Sierra S, Sempere L, Gómez M, Rodriguez JM, Boza J, Xaus J, Olivares M. Safety and tolerance of the human milk probiotic strain *Lactobacillus salivarius* CECT5713 in 6-month-old children. Nutrition 2010;26:1082–7. https://doi.org/10.1016/j.nut.2009.08.023.
[35] Robinson EL, Thompson WL. Effect on weight gain of the addition of *Lactobacillus acidophilus* to the formula of newborn infants. J Pediatr 1952;41:395–8. https://doi.org/10.1016/s0022-3476(52)80121-0.
[36] Jiao N, Baker SS, Nugent CA, Tsompana M, Cai L, Wang Y, Buck MJ, Genco RJ, Baker RD, Zhu R, Zhu L. Gut microbiome may contribute to insulin resistance and systemic inflammation in obese rodents: a meta-analysis. Physiol Genomics 2018;50:244–54. https://doi.org/10.1152/physiolgenomics.00114.2017.
[37] Tagliamonte S, Laiola M, Ferracane R, Vitale M, Gallo MA, Meslier V, Pons N, Ercolini D, Vitaglione P. Mediterranean diet consumption affects the endocannabinoid system in overweight and obese subjects: possible links with gut microbiome, insulin resistance and inflammation. Eur J Nutr 2021. https://doi.org/10.1007/s00394-021-02538-8.
[38] Poutahidis T, Kleinewietfeld M, Smillie C, Levkovich T, Perrotta A, Bhela S, Varian BJ, Ibrahim YM, Lakritz JR, Kearney SM, Chatzigiagkos A, Hafler DA, Alm EJ, Erdman SE. Microbial reprogramming inhibits Western diet-associated obesity. PLoS One 2013;8. https://doi.org/10.1371/journal.pone.0068596, e68596.

[39] Erdman SE, Poutahidis T. Probiotic "glow of health": it's more than skin deep. Benefic Microbes 2014;5:109–19. https://doi.org/10.3920/BM2013.0042.
[40] Cani P, Bibiloni R, Knauf C, Waget A, Neyrinck A, Delzenne N, Burcelin R. Changes in gut microbiota control metabolic endotoxemia-induced inflammation in high-fat diet-induced obesity and diabetes in mice. Diabetes 2008;57:1470–81. https://doi.org/10.2337/db07-1403.
[41] Tremaroli V, Bäckhed F. Functional interactions between the gut microbiota and host metabolism. Nature 2012;489:242–9. https://doi.org/10.1038/nature11552.
[42] Nicolucci AC, Hume MP, Martínez I, Mayengbam S, Walter J, Reimer RA. Prebiotics reduce body fat and alter intestinal microbiota in children who are overweight or with obesity. Gastroenterology 2017;153:711–22. https://doi.org/10.1053/j.gastro.2017.05.055.
[43] da Silva Borges D, Fernandes R, Thives Mello A, da Silva Fontoura E, Soares Dos Santos AR, de Moraes S, Trindade EB. Prebiotics may reduce serum concentrations of C-reactive protein and ghrelin in overweight and obese adults: a systematic review and meta-analysis. Nutr Rev 2020;78:235–48. https://doi.org/10.1093/nutrit/nuz045.
[44] Dehghan P, Pourghassem Gargari B, Asghari Jafar-abadi M. Oligofructose-enriched inulin improves some inflammatory markers and metabolic endotoxemia in women with type 2 diabetes mellitus: a randomized controlled clinical trial. Nutrition 2014;30:418–23. https://doi.org/10.1016/j.nut.2013.09.005.
[45] Frost GS, Brynes AE, Dhillo WS, Bloom SR, McBurney MI. The effects of fiber enrichment of pasta and fat content on gastric emptying, GLP-1, glucose, and insulin responses to a meal. Eur J Clin Nutr 2003;57:293–8. https://doi.org/10.1038/sj.ejcn.1601520.
[46] Ivey KL, Hodgson JM, Kerr DA, Lewis JR, Thompson PL, Prince RL. The effects of probiotic bacteria on glycaemic control in overweight men and women: a randomised controlled trial. Eur J Clin Nutr 2014;68:447–52. https://doi.org/10.1038/ejcn.2013.294.
[47] Xia Y, Kelton CML, Guo JJ, Bian B, Heaton PC. Treatment of obesity: pharmacotherapy trends in the United States from 1999 to 2010. Obesity 2015;23:1721–8. https://doi.org/10.1002/oby.21136.
[48] National Institute of Diabetes and Digestive and Kidney Diseases, Prescription medications to treat overweight & obesity | NIDDK [WWW Document], n.d.. National Institute of Diabetes and Digestive and Kidney Diseases. https://www.niddk.nih.gov/health-information/weight-management/prescription-medications-treat-overweight-obesity (accessed 23.08.2021).
[49] Montan PD, Sourlas A, Olivero J, Silverio D, Guzman E, Kosmas CE. Pharmacologic therapy of obesity: mechanisms of action and cardiometabolic effects. Ann Transl Med 2019;7:30. https://doi.org/10.21037/atm.2019.07.27.
[50] Lee Y-S, Jun H-S. Anti-inflammatory effects of GLP-1-based therapies beyond glucose control. Mediators Inflamm 2016;2016:3094642. https://doi.org/10.1155/2016/3094642.
[51] Shiraki A, Oyama J, Komoda H, Asaka M, Komatsu A, Sakuma M, Kodama K, Sakamoto Y, Kotooka N, Hirase T, Node K. The glucagon-like peptide 1 analog liraglutide reduces TNF-α-induced oxidative stress and inflammation in endothelial cells. Atherosclerosis 2012;221:375–82. https://doi.org/10.1016/j.atherosclerosis.2011.12.039.
[52] Liu J, Liu Y, Chen L, Wang Y, Li J. Glucagon-like peptide-1 analog liraglutide protects against diabetic cardiomyopathy by the inhibition of the endoplasmic reticulum stress pathway. J Diabetes Res 2013;2013. https://doi.org/10.1155/2013/630537, 630537.
[53] Newsome P, Francque S, Harrison S, Ratziu V, Van Gaal L, Calanna S, Hansen M, Linder M, Sanyal A. Effect of semaglutide on liver enzymes and markers of inflammation in subjects with type 2 diabetes and/or obesity. Aliment Pharmacol Ther 2019;50:193–203. https://doi.org/10.1111/apt.15316.

[54] Sivalingam S, Larsen EL, van Raalte DH, Muskiet MHA, Smits MM, Tonneijck L, Joles JA, von Scholten BJ, Zobel EH, Persson F, Henriksen T, Diaz LJ, Hansen TW, Poulsen HE, Rossing P. The effect of liraglutide and sitagliptin on oxidative stress in persons with type 2 diabetes. Sci Rep 2021;11:10624. https://doi.org/10.1038/s41598-021-90191-w.

[55] Petersen KE, Rakipovski G, Raun K, Lykkesfeldt J. Does glucagon-like peptide-1 ameliorate oxidative stress in diabetes? Evidence based on experimental and clinical studies. Curr Diabetes Rev 2016;12:331–58. https://doi.org/10.2174/1573399812666150918150608.

[56] Willard FS, Douros JD, Gabe MB, Showalter AD, Wainscott DB, Suter TM, Capozzi ME, van der Velden WJ, Stutsman C, Cardona GR, Urva S, Emmerson PJ, Holst JJ, D'Alessio DA, Coghlan MP, Rosenkilde MM, Campbell JE, Sloop KW. Tirzepatide is an imbalanced and biased dual GIP and GLP-1 receptor agonist. JCI Insight 2020;5. https://doi.org/10.1172/jci.insight.140532, 140532.

[57] Yuan Z, Li D, Feng P, Xue G, Ji C, Li G, Hölscher C. A novel GLP-1/GIP dual agonist is more effective than liraglutide in reducing inflammation and enhancing GDNF release in the MPTP mouse model of Parkinson's disease. Eur J Pharmacol 2017;812:82–90. https://doi.org/10.1016/j.ejphar.2017.06.029.

[58] Pernicova I, Kelly S, Ajodha S, Sahdev A, Bestwick JP, Gabrovska P, Akanle O, Ajjan R, Kola B, Stadler M, Fraser W, Christ-Crain M, Grossman AB, Pitzalis C, Korbonits M. Metformin to reduce metabolic complications and inflammation in patients on systemic glucocorticoid therapy: a randomised, double-blind, placebo-controlled, proof-of-concept, phase 2 trial. Lancet Diabetes Endocrinol 2020;8:278–91. https://doi.org/10.1016/S2213-8587(20)30021-8.

[59] Saisho Y. Metformin and inflammation: its potential beyond glucose-lowering effect. Endocr Metab Immune Disord Drug Targets 2015;15:196–205. https://doi.org/10.2174/1871530315666150316124019.

[60] Dalvi PS, Chalmers JA, Luo V, Han D-Y, Wellhauser L, Liu Y, Tran DQ, Castel J, Luquet S, Wheeler MB, Belsham DD. High fat induces acute and chronic inflammation in the hypothalamus: effect of high-fat diet, palmitate and TNF-α on appetite-regulating NPY neurons. Int J Obes (Lond) 2017;41:149–58. https://doi.org/10.1038/ijo.2016.183.

[61] Phillips CL, Grayson BE. The immune remodel: weight loss-mediated inflammatory changes to obesity. Exp Biol Med (Maywood) 2020;245:109–21. https://doi.org/10.1177/1535370219900185.

[62] Derosa G, Maffioli P, Salvadeo SAT, Ferrari I, Gravina A, Mereu R, D'Angelo A, Fogari E, Palumbo I, Randazzo S, Cicero AFG. Comparison of orlistat treatment and placebo in obese type 2 diabetic patients. Expert Opin Pharmacother 2010;11:1971–82. https://doi.org/10.1517/14656566.2010.493557.

[63] Bougoulia M, Triantos A, Koliakos G. Effect of weight loss with or without orlistat treatment on adipocytokines, inflammation, and oxidative markers in obese women. Hormones (Athens) 2006;5:259–69. https://doi.org/10.14310/horm.2002.11190.

[64] Ali Khan R, Kapur P, Jain A, Farah F, Bhandari U. Effect of orlistat on periostin, adiponectin, inflammatory markers and ultrasound grades of fatty liver in obese NAFLD patients. Ther Clin Risk Manag 2017;13:139–49. https://doi.org/10.2147/TCRM.S124621.

[65] Suleiman JB, Nna VU, Zakaria Z, Othman ZA, Bakar ABA, Mohamed M. Obesity-induced testicular oxidative stress, inflammation and apoptosis: protective and therapeutic effects of orlistat. Reprod Toxicol 2020;95:113–22. https://doi.org/10.1016/j.reprotox.2020.05.009.

[66] Othman ZA, Zakaria Z, Suleiman JB, Ghazali WSW, Mohamed M. Anti-atherogenic effects of orlistat on obesity-induced vascular oxidative stress rat model. Antioxidants (Basel) 2021;10:251. https://doi.org/10.3390/antiox10020251.

[67] Gadde KM, Allison DB, Ryan DH, Peterson CA, Troupin B, Schwiers ML, Day WW. Effects of low-dose, controlled-release, phentermine plus topiramate combination on weight and associated comorbidities in overweight and obese adults (CONQUER): a randomised, placebo-controlled, phase 3 trial. Lancet 2011;377:1341–52. https://doi.org/10.1016/S0140-6736(11)60205-5.

[68] Allison DB, Gadde KM, Garvey WT, Peterson CA, Schwiers ML, Najarian T, Tam PY, Troupin B, Day WW. Controlled-release phentermine/topiramate in severely obese adults: a randomized controlled trial (EQUIP). Obesity (Silver Spring) 2012;20:330–42. https://doi.org/10.1038/oby.2011.330.

[69] Price TO, Farr SA, Niehoff ML, Ercal N, Morley JE, Shah GN. Protective effect of topiramate on hyperglycemia-induced cerebral oxidative stress, pericyte loss and learning behavior in diabetic mice. Int Libr Diabetes Metab 2015;1:6–12.

[70] Brustolim D, Ribeiro-dos-Santos R, Kast RE, Altschuler EL, Soares MBP. A new chapter opens in anti-inflammatory treatments: the antidepressant bupropion lowers production of tumor necrosis factor-alpha and interferon-gamma in mice. Int Immunopharmacol 2006;6:903–7. https://doi.org/10.1016/j.intimp.2005.12.007.

[71] Ahmed M, El-Bakly WM, Zaki AM, abd Alzez LF, El Serafi O. Bupropion effects on high-fat diet-induced steatohepatitis and endothelial dysfunction in rats: role of tumour necrosis factor-alpha. J Pharm Pharmacol 2014;66:793–801. https://doi.org/10.1111/jphp.12213.

[72] Wang X, Sun Z-J, Wu J-L, Quan W-Q, Xiao W-D, Chew H, Jiang C-M, Li D. Naloxone attenuates ischemic brain injury in rats through suppressing the NIK/IKKα/NF-κB and neuronal apoptotic pathways. Acta Pharmacol Sin 2019;40:170–9. https://doi.org/10.1038/s41401-018-0053-3.

[73] Anttila JE, Albert K, Wires ES, Mätlik K, Loram LC, Watkins LR, Rice KC, Wang Y, Harvey BK, Airavaara M. Post-stroke intranasal (+)-naloxone delivery reduces microglial activation and improves behavioral recovery from ischemic injury. eNeuro 2018;5. https://doi.org/10.1523/ENEURO.0395-17.2018. ENEURO.0395-17.2018.

[74] Guedes MR, Fittipaldi-Fernandez RJ, Diestel CF, Klein MRST. Impact of intragastric balloon treatment on adipokines, cytokines, and metabolic profile in obese individuals. Obes Surg 2019;29:2600–8. https://doi.org/10.1007/s11695-019-03891-8.

[75] Albuquerque A, Sarmento J, Azevedo R, et al. Intra-gastric balloon leads to a proportional decrease between body mass index and serum C-reactive protein levels. J Gastroenterol Hepatol 2013;495.

[76] Madeira E, Madeira M, Guedes E, et al. Impact of weight loss with intragastric balloon on bone density and microstructure in obese adults. J Clin Densitom 2019;22(2):279–86. https://doi.org/10.1016/j.jocd.2017.12.002.

[77] Nyström M, Machytka E, Norén E, Testoni PA, Janssen I, Turró Homedes J, Espinos Perez JC, Turro Arau R. Aspiration therapy as a tool to treat obesity: 1- to 4-year results in a 201-patient multi-center post-market European registry study. Obes Surg 2018;28:1860–8. https://doi.org/10.1007/s11695-017-3096-5.

[78] Thompson CC, Abu Dayyeh BK, Kushner R, Sullivan S, Schorr AB, Amaro A, Apovian CM, Fullum T, Zarrinpar A, Jensen MD, Stein AC, Edmundowicz S, Kahaleh M, Ryou M, Bohning JM, Ginsberg G, Huang C, Tran DD, Glaser JP, Martin JA, Jaffe DL, Farraye FA, Ho SB, Kumar N, Harakal D, Young M, Thomas CE, Shukla AP, Ryan MB, Haas M, Goldsmith H, McCrea J, Aronne LJ. Percutaneous gastrostomy device for the treatment of class II and class III obesity: results of a randomized controlled trial. Am J Gastroenterol 2017;112:447–57. https://doi.org/10.1038/ajg.2016.500.

[79] Jirapinyo P, de Moura DTH, Horton LC, Thompson CC. Effect of aspiration therapy on obesity-related comorbidities: systematic review and meta-analysis. Clin Endocrinol 2020;53:686–97. https://doi.org/10.5946/ce.2019.181.

[80] Sharaiha RZ, Hajifathalian K, Kumar R, Saunders K, Mehta A, Ang B, Skaf D, Shah S, Herr A, Igel L, Dawod Q, Dawod E, Sampath K, Carr-Locke D, Brown R, Cohen D, Dannenberg AJ, Mahadev S, Shukla A, Aronne LJ. Five-year outcomes of

endoscopic sleeve gastroplasty for the treatment of obesity. Clin Gastroenterol Hepatol 2021;19:1051–1057.e2. https://doi.org/10.1016/j.cgh.2020.09.055.
[81] The National Institutes of Health (NIH) Consensus development program: gastrointestinal surgery for severe obesity [WWW Document], n.d.. https://consensus.nih.gov/1991/1991GISurgeryObesity084html.htm (accessed 08.08.2021).
[82] American Diabetes Association. 7. Obesity management for the treatment of type 2 diabetes: *Standards of medical care in diabetes—2018*. Diabetes Care 2018;41:S65. https://doi.org/10.2337/dc18-S007.
[83] Anhê FF, Varin TV, Schertzer JD, Marette A. The gut microbiota as a mediator of metabolic benefits after bariatric surgery. Can J Diabetes 2017;41:439–47. https://doi.org/10.1016/j.jcjd.2017.02.002.
[84] Chiappetta S, Schaack HM, Wölnerhannsen B, Stier C, Squillante S, Weiner RA. The impact of obesity and metabolic surgery on chronic inflammation. Obes Surg 2018;28:3028–40. https://doi.org/10.1007/s11695-018-3320-y.
[85] Billeter AT, Vittas S, Israel B, Scheurlen KM, Hidmark A, Fleming TH, Kopf S, Büchler MW, Müller-Stich BP. Gastric bypass simultaneously improves adipose tissue function and insulin-dependent type 2 diabetes mellitus. Langenbecks Arch Surg 2017;402:901–10. https://doi.org/10.1007/s00423-017-1601-x.
[86] Butner KL, Nickols-Richardson SM, Clark SF, Ramp WK, Herbert WG. A review of weight loss following Roux-en-Y gastric bypass vs restrictive bariatric surgery: impact on adiponectin and insulin. Obes Surg 2010;20:559–68. https://doi.org/10.1007/s11695-010-0089-z.
[87] Biobaku F, Ghanim H, Monte SV, Caruana JA, Dandona P. Bariatric surgery: remission of inflammation, cardiometabolic benefits, and common adverse effects. J Endocr Soc 2020;4:bvaa049. https://doi.org/10.1210/jendso/bvaa049.
[88] Holdstock C, Lind L, Engstrom BE, Ohrvall M, Sundbom M, Larsson A, Karlsson FA. CRP reduction following gastric bypass surgery is most pronounced in insulin-sensitive subjects. Int J Obes (Lond) 2005;29:1275–80. https://doi.org/10.1038/sj.ijo.0803000.
[89] Sala P, de Miranda Torrinhas RSM, Fonseca DC, Machado NM, Singer J, Singer P, Ravacci GR, Belarmino G, Ferreira BAM, Marques M, Ishida RK, Guarda IFMS, de Moura EGH, Sakai P, Santo MA, Sunaga DY, Heymsfield SB, Bezerra DPDS, Corrêa-Giannella ML, Waitzberg DL. Intestinal expression of toll-like receptor gene changes early after gastric bypass surgery and association with type 2 diabetes remission. Nutrition 2020;79–80. https://doi.org/10.1016/j.nut.2020.110885, 110885.
[90] Liou AP, Paziuk M, Luevano J-M, Machineni S, Turnbaugh PJ, Kaplan LM. Conserved shifts in the gut microbiota due to gastric bypass reduce host weight and adiposity. Sci Transl Med 2013;5:178ra41. https://doi.org/10.1126/scitranslmed.3005687.
[91] Furet J-P, Kong L-C, Tap J, Poitou C, Basdevant A, Bouillot J-L, Mariat D, Corthier G, Doré J, Henegar C, Rizkalla S, Clément K. Differential adaptation of human gut microbiota to bariatric surgery-induced weight loss: links with metabolic and low-grade inflammation markers. Diabetes 2010;59:3049–57. https://doi.org/10.2337/db10-0253.
[92] Kim YJ, Womble JT, Gunsch CK, Ingram JL. The gut/lung microbiome axis in obesity, asthma, and bariatric surgery: a literature review. Obesity (Silver Spring) 2021;29:636–44. https://doi.org/10.1002/oby.23107.
[93] Shen N, Caixàs A, Ahlers M, Patel K, Gao Z, Dutia R, Blaser MJ, Clemente JC, Laferrère B. Longitudinal changes of microbiome composition and microbial metabolomics after surgical weight loss in individuals with obesity. Surg Obes Relat Dis 2019;15:1367–73. https://doi.org/10.1016/j.soard.2019.05.038.
[94] Balistreri CR, Caruso C, Candore G. The role of adipose tissue and adipokines in obesity-related inflammatory diseases. Mediators Inflamm 2010;2010. https://doi.org/10.1155/2010/802078, 802078.

[95] Goktas Z, Moustaid-Moussa N, Shen C-L, Boylan M, Mo H, Wang S. Effects of bariatric surgery on adipokine-induced inflammation and insulin resistance. Front Endocrinol 2013;4:69. https://doi.org/10.3389/fendo.2013.00069.
[96] Hankir MK, Rullmann M, Seyfried F, Preusser S, Poppitz S, Heba S, Gousias K, Hoyer J, Schütz T, Dietrich A, Müller K, Pleger B. Roux-en-Y gastric bypass surgery progressively alters radiologic measures of hypothalamic inflammation in obese patients. JCI Insight 2019;4. https://doi.org/10.1172/jci.insight.131329, 131329.
[97] Kelly AS, Ryder JR, Marlatt KL, Rudser KD, Jenkins T, Inge TH. Changes in inflammation, oxidative stress and adipokines following bariatric surgery among adolescents with severe obesity. Int J Obes (Lond) 2016;40:275–80. https://doi.org/10.1038/ijo.2015.174.
[98] Subramaniam R, Aliakbarian H, Bhutta HY, Harris DA, Tavakkoli A, Sheu EG. Sleeve gastrectomy and Roux-en-Y gastric bypass attenuate pro-inflammatory small intestinal cytokine signatures. Obes Surg 2019;29:3824–32. https://doi.org/10.1007/s11695-019-04059-0.
[99] Pucci A, Batterham RL. Mechanisms underlying the weight loss effects of RYGB and SG: similar, yet different. J Endocrinol Invest 2019;42:117–28. https://doi.org/10.1007/s40618-018-0892-2.
[100] Aron-Wisnewsky J, Prifti E, Belda E, Ichou F, Kayser BD, Dao MC, Verger EO, Hedjazi L, Bouillot J-L, Chevallier J-M, Pons N, Le Chatelier E, Levenez F, Ehrlich SD, Dore J, Zucker J-D, Clément K. Major microbiota dysbiosis in severe obesity: fate after bariatric surgery. Gut 2019;68:70–82. https://doi.org/10.1136/gutjnl-2018-316103.
[101] Hafida S, Mirshahi T, Nikolajczyk BS. The impact of bariatric surgery on inflammation: quenching the fire of obesity? Curr Opin Endocrinol Diabetes Obes 2016;23:373–8. https://doi.org/10.1097/MED.0000000000000277.
[102] Johansson H-E, Haenni A, Zethelius B. Platelet counts and liver enzymes after bariatric surgery. J Obes 2013;2013. https://doi.org/10.1155/2013/567984, 567984.
[103] Arble DM, Evers SS, Bozadjieva N, Frikke-Schmidt H, Myronovych A, Lewis A, Toure MH, Seeley RJ. Metabolic comparison of one-anastomosis gastric bypass, single-anastomosis duodenal-switch, Roux-en-Y gastric bypass, and vertical sleeve gastrectomy in rat. Surg Obes Relat Dis 2018;14:1857–67. https://doi.org/10.1016/j.soard.2018.08.019.
[104] Anon. Clinical guidelines on the identification, evaluation, and treatment of overweight and obesity in adults—the evidence report. national institutes of health. Obes Res 1998;6 Suppl. 2:51S–209S.
[105] Lyznicki JM, Young DC, Riggs JA, Davis RM, Council on Scientific Affairs, American Medical Association. Obesity: assessment and management in primary care. Am Fam Physician 2001;63:2185–96.
[106] Lee A, Jeon KJ, Kim MS, Kim H-K, Han SN. Modest weight loss through a 12-week weight management program with behavioral modification seems to attenuate inflammatory responses in young obese Koreans. Nutr Res 2015;35:301–8. https://doi.org/10.1016/j.nutres.2015.02.004.

CHAPTER 16

New therapeutic strategies in the management of obesity-modulated inflammation

Ronald Tyszkowski[a] and Raman Mehrzad[b]
[a]Private Practice, Allied Health, Women and Infants Hospital, Providence, RI, United States
[b]Division of Plastic and Reconstructive Surgery, Rhode Island Hospital, The Warren Alpert School of Brown University, Providence, RI, United States

The current approach to management of obesity is not working. The data are overwhelming that the incidence of obesity will continue to climb and result in massive financial, social, and health costs. So where does that leave us as practitioners? How do we rethink the strategies so ingrained in our practice and society? Clinical research into the origins and perpetuating factors of obesity and obesity-related inflammation is significant and continues to grow. What it shows us is the unbelievably complex web of physiological changes beyond simple weight gain these conditions produce. Additionally, the roots of obesity can even precede poor lifestyle choices. Vulnerabilities to epigenetic factors can be in place before birth. A concerted effort to bring the information gleaned in the laboratory to the battleground of the clinician's office in the form of effective and current treatment strategies is necessary to have any chance of stemming the tide of the obesity pandemic.

Staging obesity-related inflammation

Physiologic changes due to obesity go far beyond the morphologic. Research continues to uncover myriad alterations in cellular function, not the least of which is the inflammatory state. This concurrent state heightens the urgency of an adequate management strategy to head off a slow decline into chronic disease in the obese patient. However, it can also give us clues to the same strategy. In many cases, the alterations in cellular function can be measured, particularly those associated with inflammation. In this way, the patient may be "staged," and management of associated risk factors can be undertaken. Since obesity can have a synergistic relationship with inflammation, this treatment directed toward specific anti-inflammatory measures

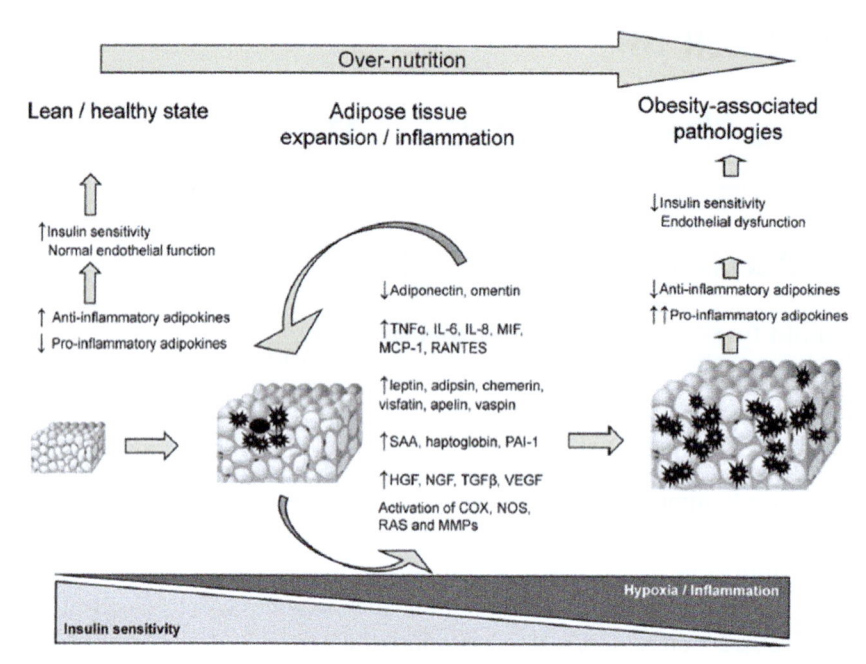

Fig. 1 A continuum of obesity-related physiological stages [1]. Patients may be able to be placed on the continuum based upon testable inflammatory biomarkers and more specific and effective treatment strategies may result.

in addition to recommendations toward improving BMI may improve the chances of success. Fig. 1 shows how the degree and/or duration of obesity in the patient can indicate the amount of concomitant predisease and outright pathology associated with it.

A renewed approach that takes into account increased BMI and subsequent increased inflammatory markers may give the practitioner insights into the level of pathology and a more comprehensive approach to treatment.

Management of obesity-related inflammation presents many challenges. Prime among them are the complex biochemical and pathophysiological changes that can occur in response to the synergistic relationship between the obese and inflammatory states, i.e., they can work to perpetuate each other. For this reason, addressing one without the other can be a recipe for failure. Classical management strategies for the obese patients, when they are actually undertaken, tend to minimize or ignore altogether these biochemical and pathophysiological factors.

Newer approaches, in an attempt to reverse decades of obesity mitigation failures, seek to incorporate the evaluation of glucose-insulin homeostasis

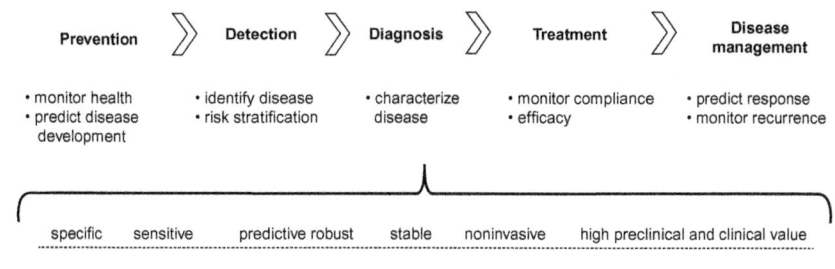

```
  Prevention    >  Detection    >  Diagnosis    >  Treatment    >  Disease
                                                                   management

• monitor health    • identify disease   • characterize    • monitor compliance   • predict response
• predict disease   • risk stratification  disease         • efficacy             • monitor recurrence
  development
```

specific   sensitive   predictive robust   stable   noninvasive   high preclinical and clinical value

Biomarker requirements

Fig. 2 Potential uses and essential features of biomarkers in preclinical and clinical settings [2]. Biomarkers may be helpful at the different stages of obesity including what we may now consider to be a predisease state.

biomarkers, adipose tissue biomarkers, inflammation biomarkers, and omics-based biomarkers. These biomarkers can help to identify those at risk for disease, to monitor disease progression and prognosis, and to target intervention that allows for more personalized treatment options. [2]. Patients can then be "staged" as to relative risk for additional chronic disease beyond obesity based upon more than BMI and waist circumference [2] (Fig. 2).

Glucose-insulin homeostasis biomarkers

The correlation between obesity and elevated insulin levels is indisputable. However, the initiating factor remains unclear [3]. Does hyperinsulinemia precede insulin resistance, defined as a decrease in a target cell's response to insulin, or occur as a result of it [2]? Research into the management of type 2 diabetes and other metabolic sequelae will ultimately answer that question. Regardless, evidence suggests a connection with sustained higher insulin levels and risk of various diseases. Thus, it has value as an indicator and potential stage definer of the deleterious effects of obesity and obesity-related inflammation.

Insulin and proinsulin

Insulin resistance and hyperinsulinemia have been studied extensively as they relate to chronic disease. Increased insulin and the precursor molecule, proinsulin, have been suggested as a link between obesity and type 2 diabetes and between cardiovascular diseases and cancer [4]. Recent meta-analyses have shown increased insulin levels being associated with higher incidences of hypertension and coronary heart disease [5].

C-peptides

C-Peptide is released in equal amounts to insulin when proinsulin is cleaved during insulin synthesis. Increased levels have been shown to be reliable predictors of all mortality in nondiabetic adults [6,7].

Adipose tissue biomarkers

As described in detail in the chapter *Obesity and Inflammation*, morphologic changes to adipose tissue in response to excess calories and subsequent energy imbalances result in the secretion of adipokines and cytokines. These substances have a variety of autocrine, paracrine, and endocrine effects [8], which can contribute to "the pathogenesis of obesity associated metabolic and cardiovascular complications" [9].

Adiponectin

Adiponectin is an extremely common circulating peptide [10] associated with beneficial insulin sensitizing, anti-inflammatory, antiatherogenic, and cardioprotective properties [11]. Decreased serum concentration is noted in obesity and obesity-linked diseases [12].

Resistin

Resistin is a polypeptide that induces low-grade inflammation [13]. Increased serum resistin levels are associated with increased insulin levels in relation to insulin resistance [14], increased severity of cardiovascular diseases [15], and all-cause mortality in patients with type 2 diabetes [16].

Inflammatory biomarkers
C-reactive protein

C-reactive protein continues to be used as a biomarker for systemic inflammation and consequently a risk factor for cardiovascular disease. However, recent evidence shows that this relationship is unclear [17], and actual risk is determined by conventional risk factors and other inflammatory biomarkers.

Cytokines

Secretion of cytokines in adipose cell composition remodeling in obesity can disrupt the balance between proinflammatory and anti-inflammatory effects [18], particularly in the promotion of insulin resistance. Laboratory analysis of cytokines remains an evolving technology, which will play a more significant role in the future [2].

Omic-based biomarkers

Omics is defined as the study of related sets of biological molecules in a comprehensive fashion [19]. Single biomarkers can ultimately be difficult to quantify, as they exist within a system in which multiple pathways interact in a complex manner [2]. Identification of novel omic-based biomarkers, in which the role of the biomarker is interpreted with respect to its role within the -omic system, holds promise for future clinical use. Omics platforms can include the following:
- *Genomics*: the branch of molecular biology concerned with the structure, function, evolution, and mapping of genomes
- *Transcriptomics*: the study of all messenger RNA molecules expressed from the genes of an organism
- *Metabolomics*: the scientific study of chemical processes involving metabolites, the small molecule substrates, intermediates, and products of cell metabolism
- *Proteomics*: the study of the entire complement of proteins that is or can be expressed by a cell, tissue, or organism
- *Lipidomics*: the study of all lipids in the cell

Omics-based biomarkers hold much promise, and as research into their application continues, they will be able to be applied in clinical situations.

Improvements in our ability to detect and quantify inflammatory biomarkers in the obese patient will allow for a better understanding of concomitant pathology and risk of future chronic disease.

The microbiome and obesity

Gut Microbiota is considered as an assortment of microorganisms that inhabit the gastrointestinal tract [20]. Human microbiota is mainly composed of five phyla of bacteria: Bacteroidetes, Firmicutes, Actinobacteria, Protobacteria, and Verrucomicrobia [21]. Composition of the gut microbiota is altered in the obese patient. A decreased richness [22] of microorganisms in the gut has been correlated to incidence of overall adiposity, insulin resistance, and dyslipidemia (Fig. 3).

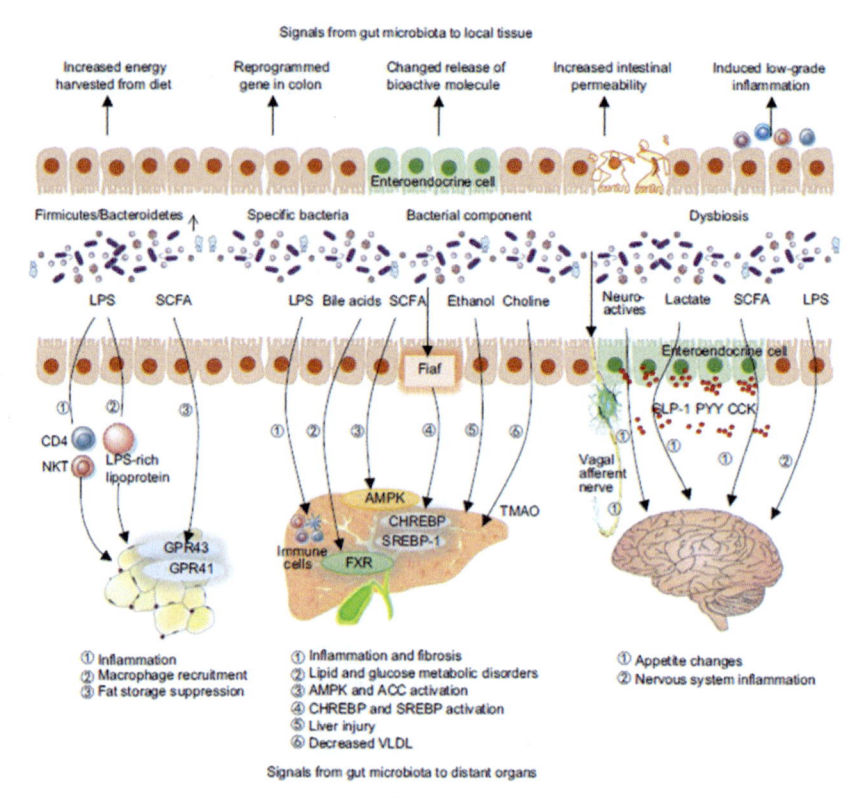

Fig. 3 This drawing shows the many effects that the altered microbiome can have on human physiology [23]. Gut microbiota communicate with adipose tissue, the liver, and the brain through lipopolysaccharides, short-chain fatty acids, and other mediators.

Gut microbiota effects these changes via a multitude of alterations to physiology. In local tissues, obesity-associated gut microbiota have an increased capacity to:
- harvest energy from the diet,
- stimulate gene reprogramming in the colon,
- change polypeptide hormones and other bioactive molecules released by enterochromaffin cells,
- decrease the intestinal barrier
- disturb immune homeostasis [23]

The decrease of the intestinal barrier can progress to a syndrome known as "leaky gut." "Leaky gut" is a euphemism for intestinal barrier dysfunction or increased intestinal permeability and its resulting sequelae. Non-GI disease and its relationship to "leaky gut" are an evolving area of research

[24]. Hypotheses contend that intestinal barrier dysfunction can result in substances leaking into the body, which can alter physiology, producing multiple predisease states including that of obesity. The introduction of bacteriogenic lipopolysaccharides (LPSs) and short-chain fatty acids (SCFAs) through the intestinal barrier can induce low-grade inflammation and exaggerated immune responses.

Gut microbiota also can directly affect adipose tissue by participating in the regulation of adipogenesis. SCFAs, from the microbiota, participate in insulin-mediated fat accumulation in adipocytes via activation of their receptors GPR43 and GPR41, which can inhibit lipolysis and encourage adipocyte differentiation [23].

In the liver, microbiota-derived LPS and other compounds that have exited the dysfunctional intestinal barrier can promote inflammation by stimulating immune cells and consequently playing a role in the pathophysiology of nonalcoholic fatty liver disease [23].

Promoting a healthy microbiota in obese patients (and correcting intestinal barrier dysfunction) may have important effects in improved BMI as well as decreased systemic inflammation and should continue to be studied as a viable clinical intervention.

Alternative treatments for obesity

Classical treatments of obesity based on physical activity and decreased caloric intake are simply not enough. Approximately ⅔ of people who lose weight will regain it within a year, and almost all of them within 5 years. [25]. A fundamentally different approach to the problem is not just indicated, but necessary to avoid catastrophe.

Treating the individual

Each individual patient brings a unique set of causative factors to their obesity diagnosis such as their unique physiology, genetic factors, medical history, and even socioeconomic stressors (Fig. 4). As such, cookie-cutter approaches may be extremely difficult to implement depending on the patient. Low-income patients will have a different amount of access to high-quality food and consistent, effective exercise as compared with middle- and high-income patients. In fact, the number of pertinent variables can be exceedingly high and a challenge for the busy practitioner to manage in what typically is a relatively brief in-office encounter.

```
┌─────────────────────────────────────────┐
│   Assess for root causes of weight gain │
└─────────────────────────────────────────┘
```

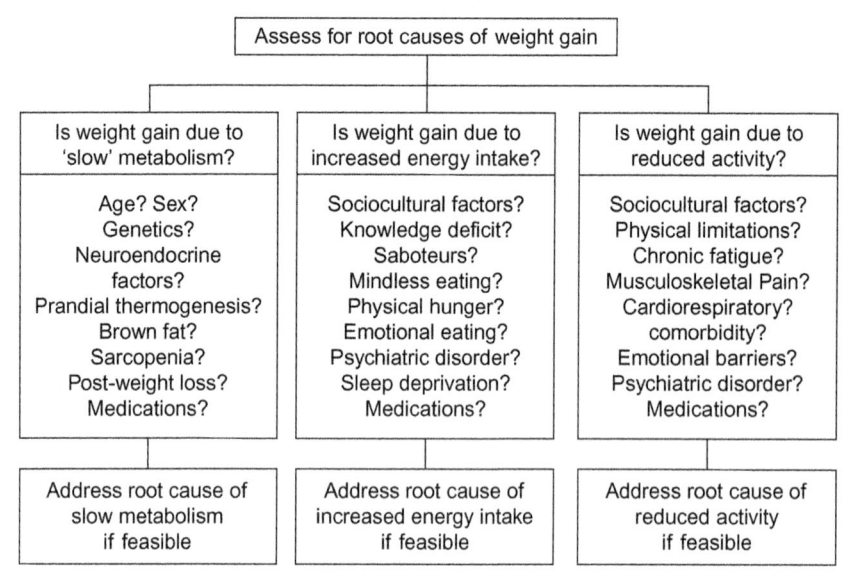

Is weight gain due to 'slow' metabolism?	Is weight gain due to increased energy intake?	Is weight gain due to reduced activity?
Age? Sex? Genetics? Neuroendocrine factors? Prandial thermogenesis? Brown fat? Sarcopenia? Post-weight loss? Medications?	Sociocultural factors? Knowledge deficit? Saboteurs? Mindless eating? Physical hunger? Emotional eating? Psychiatric disorder? Sleep deprivation? Medications?	Sociocultural factors? Physical limitations? Chronic fatigue? Musculoskeletal Pain? Cardiorespiratory? comorbidity? Emotional barriers? Psychiatric disorder? Medications?
Address root cause of slow metabolism if feasible	Address root cause of increased energy intake if feasible	Address root cause of reduced activity if feasible

Fig. 4 An algorithmic approach to determining some of root causes of obesity in the individual patient. The many different contributing factors can be significant [25].

Epigenetic factors in the development of obesity

Epigenetics and its role in the development of pathology are at the forefront of functional medicine and its approach to management and prevention. The overwhelming incidence of obesity has driven scientists to look carefully for genetic predisposition as well as genetic vulnerabilities to environmental factors, which may be playing a role in this pandemic.

Epigenetic changes to DNA affect the relative state of activity of a given gene. Contrary to true genetic modification or mutation, the epigenetic effect is reversible. The best understood epigenetic change is the addition of a methyl group to DNA (methylation). "Importantly, although the DNA sequence of genes in an individual (the genome) is largely stable, the epigenome has the potential to be reversibly modified by exposure to a range of nutritional and environmental factors [26]."

Studies have shown that the epigenetic factor of poor nutrition during development, as a result of either an excess or deficient maternal caloric or micronutrient intake, is associated with an increased risk of a range of chronic diseases, including obesity, type 2 diabetes, and cardiovascular disease in later life [27].

Extending the treatment window for obesity from reactive to proactive, with the recognition that lifestyle factors starting in the prenatal stage influence expression of genes much later in life, is clearly an important step in the necessary evolution of care.

Artificial intelligence and management of obesity

Recent studies have shown that Artificial Intelligence (AI) may have a dramatic effect on the evolution in the management and prevention of obesity. Energy balance or amount of calories ingested as compared with amount of calories expended is a significant factor in the etiology of obesity. There are a number of measurable factors that can affect this balance that are specific to the individual, e.g., calorie content of specific foods, health status, and level of physical activity. Sefa-Yeboah et al. [28] proposed a web and/or mobile-based application that uses an algorithm designed to take these factors into account for the individual to help them make real-time eating decisions. Additionally, it can track progress, in order to maintain health as weight loss occurs. In another study by Halberg et al. [29], a novel model of treatment for type 2 diabetes was investigated using a technology-based intervention. Their Continuous Care Intervention (CCI), in which diabetic patients were continuously monitored and instructed relative to medication and diet, produced profound changes in HbA1c, use of medication, and body weight in a relatively short period of time with sustainable changes out to at least a year.

This is just one example of how next-generation computing solutions may be able to aid physicians in the management of obesity. The pathways to obesity consist of a multitude of poor decisions regarding energy balance, which in turn spawn other related changes similar to a snowball rolling down a hill. Machine learning can eventually be directed to process the massive number of variables at any given time that can promote or reverse obesity and obesity-related inflammation in real time to direct the individual patient to better choices. As mentioned in the previous section, the personal genome of the individual and its epigenetic status may also be eventually factored into real-time AI decision guiding.

The physician or healthcare provider spends only a fraction of crucial decision-making time with the patient, so the number of decisions they can affect is minimal. Adding in an intelligent program to aid in restoring and maintaining proper energy balance is an exciting application of AI and an exciting new approach in treating obesity.

Botanicals in the treatment of obesity and obesity-related inflammation

The use of botanical agents in the treatment of pathology spans thousands of years and hundreds of civilizations. Continued modern research shows that many traditional botanical agents have high efficacy and excellent safety in the treatment of obesity and obesity-related inflammation.

Curcumin

Curcumin is a yellow [30] pigment derived from the spice turmeric. It has been used as a treatment for obesity and obesity-related metabolic diseases.

Curcumin directly interacts with adipocytes, pancreatic cells, hepatic stellate cells, macrophages, and muscle cells where it can suppress proinflammatory transcription factors, leading to the downregulation of adipokines, including tumor necrosis factor, interleukin-6, resistin, leptin, and monocyte chemotactic protein-1 [30]. It an also aid in the upregulation of adiponectin. Adiponectin is a protein that has regulatory effects on homeostasis, glucose and lipid metabolism, and anti-inflammatory action. It is produced exclusively in the adipose tissue [31]. Additionally, it results in overall impaired adipogenesis [32].

These curcumin-induced alterations can reverse insulin resistance, hyperglycemia, hyperlipidemia, and other symptoms linked to obesity [30]. Other structurally similar botanical agents, specifically those derived from red chili, cinnamon, cloves, black pepper, and ginger, also exhibit effects against obesity and insulin resistance.

Berberine

Berberine, a naturally occurring alkaloid, is found in certain species of flowering plants such as *Berberidaccae, Coptis rhizomes,* and *Hydrastis Canadensis.* Clinical research and animal studies have shown that [33,34] berberine can affect glucose, lipid metabolism and attenuate insulin resistance [35].

Studies have shown that Berberine can act as a preventative agent against obesity via the modulation of gut microbiota, gene regulation, intestinal permeability, and hepatic gluconeogenesis [33–35].

Safe and effective pharmacological agents for the management of obesity and obesity related inflammation are in high demand. The physiological effects of botanical agents as well as their relative safety make them worthy candidates for continued study, and practitioners should educate themselves regarding their clinical applications.

Sleep and obesity

Multiple studies have linked alterations in sleep quality and duration to an increased incidence of obesity and obesity-related inflammation.

The risk of obesity has been shown to be greater in short sleepers (generally those reporting sleeping <7 h/night) than normal sleepers (those reporting sleeping 7–8 h/night) and that there is a greater prevalence of obesity among short than normal sleepers [36]. Shorter duration of sleep is also related to improper energy balance as it may result in consumption in greater number of calories and often poorer quality of food [37]. This sleep–obesity relationship may have consequences for obesity treatments, as it appears that short sleepers have reduced ability to lose weight [36].

Morphologic changes associated with obesity can contribute to a high incidence of obstructive sleep apnea (OSA) [38]. OSA, in turn, can result in an increase in inflammatory markers in affected patients [39].

Fig. 5 shows the positive feedback loop of decreased body weight and increased sleep duration. As weight is lost, sleep quality and duration improve. As sleep quality and duration improve, more body weight is lost [36]. Unfortunately, as is the case with obesity and inflammation, obesity and dysfunctional sleep also synergistically interact to worsen the clinical status of the patient. For this reason, obesity and obesity-related inflammation

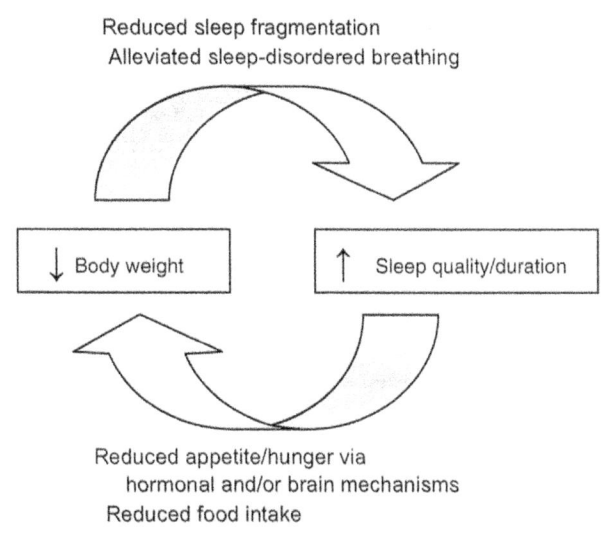

Fig. 5 The drawing illustrates the positive feedback loop of decreased body weight and increased sleep duration [36].

targeted treatment plans should include evaluation of sleep status and a plan to address any dysfunction in order to maximize effectiveness and improve chances of success.

Sleep medicine is an important addition to the management of the obese patient and should be included in any multidisciplinary approach.

References

[1] Karastergiou K, Mohamed-Ali V. The autocrine and paracrine roles of adipokines. Mol Cell Endocrinol 2010;318(1–2):69–78.
[2] Aleksandrova K, Mozaffarian D, Pischon T. Addressing the perfect storm: biomarkers in obesity and pathophysiology of cardiometabolic risk. Clin Chem 2018;64(1):142–53.
[3] Czech MP. Insulin action and resistance in obesity and type 2 diabetes. Nat Med 2017;23(7):804–14.
[4] Aleksandrova K, et al. Adiposity, mediating biomarkers and risk of colon cancer in the European prospective investigation into cancer and nutrition study. Int J Cancer 2014;134(3):612–21.
[5] Xun P, et al. Fasting insulin concentrations and incidence of hypertension, stroke, and coronary heart disease: a meta-analysis of prospective cohort studies. Am J Clin Nutr 2013;98(6):1543–54.
[6] Patel N, et al. Fasting serum C-peptide levels predict cardiovascular and overall death in nondiabetic adults. J Am Heart Assoc 2012;1(6), e003152.
[7] Min J-y, Min K-b. Serum C-peptide levels and risk of death among adults without diabetes mellitus. CMAJ 2013;185(9):E402–8.
[8] Heymsfield SB, Wadden TA. Mechanisms, pathophysiology, and management of obesity. N Engl J Med 2017;376(3):254–66.
[9] Shibata R, et al. The role of adipokines in cardiovascular disease. J Cardiol 2017;70(4):329–34.
[10] Scherer PE, et al. A novel serum protein similar to C1q, produced exclusively in adipocytes. J Biol Chem 1995;270(45):26746–9.
[11] Turer AT, Scherer PE. Adiponectin: mechanistic insights and clinical implications. Diabetologia 2012;55(9):2319–26.
[12] Schöndorf T, et al. Biological background and role of adiponectin as marker for insulin resistance and cardiovascular risk. Clin Lab 2005;51(9–10):489–94.
[13] Patel SD, et al. Disulfide-dependent multimeric assembly of resistin family hormones. Science 2004;304(5674):1154–8.
[14] Park HK, Ahima RS. Resistin in rodents and humans. Diabetes Metab J 2013;37(6):404–14.
[15] Zhang J-Z, et al. Increased serum resistin level is associated with coronary heart disease. Oncotarget 2017;8(30):50148.
[16] Fontana A, et al. Association between resistin levels and all-cause and cardiovascular mortality: a new study and a systematic review and meta-analysis. PLoS One 2015;10(3), e0120419.
[17] Emerging Risk Factors Collaboration. C-reactive protein concentration and risk of coronary heart disease, stroke, and mortality: an individual participant meta-analysis. Lancet 2010;375(9709):132–40.
[18] Makki K, Froguel P, Wolowczuk I. Adipose tissue in obesity-related inflammation and insulin resistance: cells, cytokines, and chemokines. Int Sch Res Notices 2013;2013.
[19] Fiocchi C. Integrating omics: the future of IBD? Dig Dis 2014;32(Suppl. 1):96–102.

[20] Castaner O, et al. The gut microbiome profile in obesity: a systematic review. Int J Endocrinol 2018;2018.
[21] Qin J, et al. A human gut microbial gene catalogue established by metagenomic sequencing. Nature 2010;464(7285):59–65.
[22] Le Chatelier E, Nielsen T, Qin J, Prifti E, Hildebrand F, Falony G, Almeida M, Arumugam M, Batto JM, Kennedy S, et al. Richness of human gut microbiome correlates with metabolic markers. Nature 2013;500:541–6.
[23] Sun L, et al. Insights into the role of gut microbiota in obesity: pathogenesis, mechanisms, and therapeutic perspectives. Protein Cell 2018;9(5):397–403.
[24] Camilleri M. Leaky gut: mechanisms, measurement and clinical implications in humans. Gut 2019;68(8):1516–26.
[25] Sharma AM, Padwal R. Obesity is a sign—over-eating is a symptom: an aetiological framework for the assessment and management of obesity. Obes Rev 2010;11(5):362–70.
[26] Waterland RA, Michels KB. Epigenetic epidemiology of the developmental origins hypothesis. Annu Rev Nutr 2007;27:363–88.
[27] Van Dijk SJ, et al. Epigenetics and human obesity. Int J Obes (Lond) 2015;39(1):85–97.
[28] Sefa-Yeboah SM, et al. Development of a mobile application platform for self-management of obesity using artificial intelligence techniques. Int J Telemed Appl 2021;2021.
[29] Hallberg SJ, et al. Effectiveness and safety of a novel care model for the management of type 2 diabetes at 1 year: an open-label, non-randomized, controlled study. Diabetes Ther 2018;9(2):583–612.
[30] Aggarwal BB. Targeting inflammation-induced obesity and metabolic diseases by curcumin and other nutraceuticals. Annu Rev Nutr 2010;30:173–99.
[31] Kadowaki T, Yamauchi T. Adiponectin and adiponectin receptors. Endocr Rev 2005;26(3):439–51.
[32] Bradford PG. Curcumin and obesity. Biofactors 2013;39(1):78–87.
[33] Zhang W-L, Zhu L, Jiang J-G. Active ingredients from natural botanicals in the treatment of obesity. Obes Rev 2014;15(12):957–67.
[34] Zhang Y, et al. Treatment of type 2 diabetes and dyslipidemia with the natural plant alkaloid berberine. J Clin Endocrinol Metab 2008;93(7):2559–65.
[35] Ilyas Z, et al. The effect of berberine on weight loss in order to prevent obesity: a systematic review. Biomed Pharmacother 2020;127, 110137.
[36] St-Onge M-P, Shechter A. Sleep disturbances, body fat distribution, food intake and/or energy expenditure: pathophysiological aspects. Horm Mol Biol Clin Invest 2014;17(1):29–37.
[37] Markwald RR, et al. Impact of insufficient sleep on total daily energy expenditure, food intake, and weight gain. Proc Natl Acad Sci 2013;110(14):5695–700.
[38] Schwartz AR, et al. Obesity and obstructive sleep apnea: pathogenic mechanisms and therapeutic approaches. Proc Am Thorac Soc 2008;5(2):185–92.
[39] Nadeem R, et al. Serum inflammatory markers in obstructive sleep apnea: a meta-analysis. J Clin Sleep Med 2013;9(10):1003–12.

Index

Note: Page numbers followed by *f* indicate figures and *t* indicate tables.

A

Abdominal aortic aneurysms (AAA), 124–125
Activating transcription factor 6 (ATF-6), 190
Adipocytes, 190
Adipokines origins, effects, 72–73
Adiponectin, 74
Adipose tissue biomarkers, 266
   adiponectin, 266
   resistin, 266
Adipose tissue changes, 72
Adjustable gastric banding/lap banding, 249
Advanced-glycation end-products (AGEs), 85–86
AI. *See* Artificial intelligence (AI)
Aneurysmal disease, 124–126
Antiinflammatory diet, 222–224
   benefits, 224–227
   weight loss, 224
Antiinflammatory intervention, aging-related illnesses, 92–93
   mediators, aging, longevity, 92–93
   targeting inflammation, 93
Aortic stenosis, 123–124
Arrhythmias, 122–123
AspireAssit, 248
Aspirin triggered lipoxin (ATL), 183
Atherosclerosis, coronary artery disease, 119–120

B

Bariatric interventions, 248–252
   bariatric surgery, 248–252
      other procedures, 252
      Roux-en-y gastric bypass (RYGB), 250–251
      sleeve gastrectomy, 251
   endoscopic/surgical, 248
Behavioral weight management strategies, 233–237
   diet, 233–236, 234*t*
   exercise, 236–237
Biliopancreatic diversion with duodenal switch (BPD/DS), 249

Blood pressure (BP), 224
Body mass index (BMI), 102, 194–196, 213
BPD/DS. *See* Biliopancreatic diversion with duodenal switch (BPD/DS)
British Regional Heart Study, 194

C

Carbohydrate insulin model, 217–218
Cardiovascular Health Study (CHS), 194
Cardiovascular Risk factors in Patients with Diabetes—a Prospective study in Primary care (CARDIPP), 196
CBC. *See* Complete blood count (CBC)
CCI. *See* Continuous Care Intervention (CCI)
Central nervous system (CNS), 105, 131
Central nervous system (CNS) disorders, obesity, 132–144
   autoimmune, 138–141
   cognition, 141–144
   idiopathic intracranial hypertension, 132–136
   stroke, 136–138
Chemo-attracting adipokines, 131–132, 133*f*
Chronic low-grade inflammation, 202–203
CHS. *See* Cardiovascular Health Study (CHS)
c-Jun N-terminal kinase (JNK), 190
Clonal hematopoiesis of indeterminate potential (CHIP), 91
CoLaus study, 194
Complete blood count (CBC), 253
Continuous Care Intervention (CCI), 271
Cooperative Lifestyle Intervention Program, 202–203
COVID-19, 107–108
C-reactive protein (CRP), 105, 234–235
Cytokines/adipokines, 213–214

D

Damage associated molecular patterns (DAMPs), 85–86
Dietary inflammation index (DII), 223, 235–236
Dietary intervention randomized control trial (DIRECT), 233–234

Dietary recommendations, inflammation, 226f, 227
DII. See Dietary inflammation index (DII)
DIRECT. See Dietary intervention randomized control trial (DIRECT)
Docosahexaenoic acid (DHA), 182, 219–220

E

Eicosapentaenoic acid (EPA), 182, 219–220
Endoscopic sleeve gastroplasty, 248
Endothelial, microvascular dysfunction, 76–77
Endothelin nitrous oxide synthase (eNOS), 137
Epidemiology, 6–7f, 7, 101–102
  BMI, obesity, 102
Erythrocyte sedimentation rate (ESR), 105
Exercise, 194
Extracellular matrix (ECM), 105

F

Fast-food diet, 235–236
Fecal transformation, 241–242
Fibroblast growth factor (FGF) 2, 193
Free fatty acids (FFAs), 106–107

G

Gastroesophageal reflux disease (GERD), 108
Glucagon-like peptide-1 receptor agonists (GLP1-RAs), 242–243
Glucose-insulin homeostasis biomarkers, 265–266
  C-peptides, 266
  insulin, proinsulin, 265
Gut microbiota, 267

H

HDL. See High-density lipoprotein (HDL)
Health, Aging, and Body Composition (Health ABC) study, 196–197
Heart and soul study, 194
Heart failure, 120–122
High-carbohydrate diets, 217
High-density lipoprotein (HDL), 220–221
High-fiber DASH diet, 224
High-intensity exercise training (HIIT), 193
High-intensity training (HIT), 237
High-sensitivity C-reactive protein (hsCRP), 215

HIIT. See High-intensity exercise training (HIIT)
HIT. See High-intensity training (HIT)
Human cytomegalovirus (HCMV), 84
Human microbiota, 267
Hyperinsulinemia, 265
Hypertrophic adipocytes, 219
Hypoxia-induced factor 1α (HIF-1α), 192–193

I

IBD. See Inflammatory bowel disease (IBD)
IBS. See Irritable bowel syndrome (IBS)
IMIAS. See International Mobility in Aging Study (IMIAS)
InCHIANTI study, 194
Indonesian family life survey, 194
Inflammation, 1, 19–20, 190
  aging, 83–87
    cell debris, 85–86
    cell senescence, 86–87
    gut dysbiosis, 84–85
    immunosenescence, 83–84
  allostasis, allostatic load, 20, 20–21f
  associated foods, 235–236
  chronic infections, 26
  chronic stress, 25
  consequences, 49–51, 50–52f
    mechanism, 53–55
    obesity-induced chronic inflammation, 65–67, 66f
    cardiovascular diseases, 55–56, 56f
    central nervous system, 63–65, 65f
    endocrine diseases, 57–59, 58f
    gastrointestinal diseases, 59–62, 59f, 61f
    musculoskeletal diseases, 62–63, 63f
  diet, 24–25
  disturbed sleep, 25–26, 26f
  dysbiosis, 22–24, 24f
  obesity, 20–22, 87–88
    adipocyte senescence, 87–88
    metabolic inflammation, 87
  obesity, aging, 88–92
    Alzheimer's disease, 91–92
    atherosclerosis, 89–91
    immunocompromise, 88
    insulin resistance, 89
  physical activity, 22, 23f

triggers, 20, 21f
xenobiotics, 26–28, 27f
Inflammation resolution, 175, 176f
  apoptotic cells, clearance, 180–181
    therapeutic applications, 180–181, 180f
  cyclopentenone prostaglandins (CyPGs), 176–177, 177–178f
    therapeutic applications, 177, 179f
  lipid mediators, 182, 182–183f
  lipoxins, 183, 184f
    therapeutic applications, 183
  maresins, 185
    therapeutic applications, 185
  microRNAs (miRNAs), 181–182
    therapeutic applications, 182
  protectins (PDs), 185–186
    therapeutic applications, 186
  resolvins, 183–185, 184f
Inflammatory biomarkers, 266–267
  C-reactive protein, 266
  cytokines, 266–267
Inflammatory bowel disease (IBD), 226–227
Inflammatory components, 196–197
Inflammatory diets, 235–236
Inhibitor of κ kinase (IKK), 190
Inositol-requiringenzyme 1 (IRE-1), 190
Insulin resistance, 75–76, 193, 265
Intercellular adhesion molecule-1 (ICAM-1), 253
Interferon gamma (IFN-γ)), 238
Interleukin 6, 73–74
Intermittent fasting diet, 225
International Mobility in Aging Study(IMIAS), 194
Interventions, GI diseases, 112–113
  management, 113
  prevention, 113
Intragastric balloon (IGB), 248
Irritable bowel disease (IBD), 111–112
Irritable bowel syndrome (IBS), 226–227

K
Ketogenic diet, 225

L
LDL. See Low-density lipoprotein (LDL)
Leaky gut syndrome, 268–269
Leptin resistance, 214–215

Lipid mediator class switch, 175
Lipopolysaccharides (LPSs), 106, 268–269
LIT. See Low-intensity training (LIT)
Low-carbohydrate diets, 217
Low-density lipoprotein (LDL), 90, 220–221
Low-fat diet, 224
Low-intensity training (LIT), 237

M
MacArthur studies of aging, 194
Macrobiotic diet, 254
Macrophages, 191–192
Mediterranean diet, 224–225
Med Weight Registry study, 204–205
MESA. See Multi-Ethnic Study of Atherosclerosis (MESA)
Messenger RNA (mRNA), 181
Metabolic surgery, 248–249
Metformin, 243
Michael addition reaction, 177
Microbiome, 237–242
  prebiotics, 240–241
  probiotics, 238–240
  synbiotics, 241–242
MicroRNA, 76
Middle cerebral arteries (MCAs), 136–137
Mineralocorticoid receptors (MRs), 134–135
Multi-Ethnic Study of Atherosclerosis (MESA), 194
Multiple sclerosis (MS), 132

N
Naltrexone, 245
National Health and Nutrition Examination Survey, 213
New England Journal of Medicine, 233–234
Nonalcoholic fatty liver disease (NAFLD), 108
Nonrandomized clinically controlled trials, 201–202
Nonsteroidal antiinflammatory drugs (NSAIDs), 183
Nuclear factor kB (NFkB), 190

O
OAGB. See One anastomosis gastric bypass (OAGB)
Obese (ob) gene, 193

Obese patients, inflammation
  standardized evaluation, 252–253
  weight management, stepwise approach, 253–255
Obesity, 1, 189
  alternative treatments, 269–271
    epigenetic factors, 270–271
    unique causative factors, 269, 270f
  artificial intelligence (AI), 271
  disease, 5–6
  etiology, genetics, 104–105
  gastrointestinal diseases, 108–112, 109t
    hepatobiliary, 111
    small intestine, colon, 111–112
    upper GI tract, 110
  incidence, certain groups, 83–84
    pediatric populations, 102–103
    socioeconomic, racial, equitable healthcare, 103–104
  inflammation, 71–72, 105–108
    acute disease processes, 107–108
    cancer, 77–79, 78f
    chronic diseases processes, 108
    pathogenesis, 105–107
  inflammatory pathway, 213
    diet, 216
    epidemic, 213, 214t
    essential fatty acids, 219–220
    high fat, 219
    inflammation markers, 215–216
    leptin, 214–215
    pathophysiology, 213–214
    saturated, unsaturated fatty acids, 220–221, 220f
    sugar, 216–218
    trans fatty acids, 221, 222f
  microbiome, 267–269, 268f
  paradox, 126
  relative muscle weakness, 153–156
    clinical consequences, 155
    mechanisms, 154
    prevention, treatment, 155–156
  sleep, 273–274, 273f
Obesity, pandemic
  behavioral factors, 10–12, 11–13f
  disease, 13
    cancer, 14
    type 2 diabetes, 13–14
    failures, management, 14–16
      poor training, 14–15
      practitioner bias, 15–16
  global impact, 7–8
    worldwide, 7–8, 8–9f
  increased incidence, 8, 10f
  origins, 8
  sociodemographic factors, 8–10
Obesity-related inflammation
  botanicals, 272
    berberine, 272
    curcumin, 272
  physical activity, 190–203, 191–192f
    interventional studies, 199–203, 200t
    observational studies/data, 194–199, 195t
    weight loss, maintenance, 203–205
  staging, 263–265, 264–265f
Obstructive sleep apnea (OSA), 273
Okinawa diet, 222
Omega 3 polyunsaturated fatty acid (n-3 PUFA), 219
Omega 6 poly unsaturated fatty acid (n-6 PUFA), 219
Omic-based biomarkers, 267
Omics, 267
One anastomosis gastric bypass (OAGB), 249
OSA. *See* Obstructive sleep apnea (OSA)

P

Pathophysiology obesity
  adipose tissue structure, 31–32
  endocrine action, obese state, 37–39
    adiponectin, 38–39
    leptin, 37–38
    microRNAs (miRNAs), 39
  metabolic syndrome, treatment, 39–41
    harnessing brown adipose tissue, 40
    resolving endocrine dysfunction, 41
    resolving inflammation, 40–41
    restoring energy balance, 40
  phenotype, 32–37
    brown adipose tissue loss, 36–37
    chronic inflammation, 35
    ectopic fat deposition, 33–35
    insulin resistance, 36
Pattern recognition receptors (PRRs), 85–86
Pharmacotherapy, 242

Physical fitness, 193
Physical inactivity/sedentary behavior physiology, 193
PKR-like eukaryotic initiation factor 2 α kinase (PERK), 190
Plant-based diet, 223
Plant-rich diet, 238
Poly-morphonuclear monocytes (PMNs), 175
Polyunsaturated fatty acid (PUFA), 222–223
Precursor miRNA (pre-miRNA), 181
Primary miRNA (pri-miRNA), 181
Proinflammatory diet, 223
Promotion inflammation, 74–75, 75f
Pro-resolving lipid mediators (SPMs), 175
Pro-resolving macrophages, 175
Protein kinase R, 190
PRRs. See Pattern recognition receptors (PRRs)
PUFA. See Polyunsaturated fatty acid (PUFA)

R
Randomized control trials (RCTs), 201, 235
Reactive oxygen species (ROS), 85–86
Regulatory T cells (Treg), 238
Residual basal metabolic rate (RMR), 236
Resistin, 213–214
Ribonucleic acids (RNAs), 181
RNA-induced silencing complex (RISC), 181
Roux-en-Y gastric bypass (RYGB), 249

S
Sarcopenic obesity, 156–167
  clinical consequences, 165–166
    coexisting conditions, 166
      sarcopenic obesity, cancer, 165–166
      sarcopenic obesity, frailty, 165
  definitions, 156–157
  mechanisms, 158–165
    adipokines, 160–161
    hormones, 164–165
    myokines, 161–164, 163f
    proinflammatory cytokines, 160
    reduced physical activity, 158–160, 159f

prevalence, 157–158
treatment, 166–167
Sears, Barry, 222
Semaglutide, 243
Senescence-associated secretory phenotype (SASP), 86–87
Short-chain fatty acids (SCFAs), 85, 238, 268–269
Single Anastomosis Duodeno-Ileal bypass (SADI), 249
Sleeve gastrectomy (SG), 249
SPMs. See Pro-resolving lipid mediators (SPMs)
Swedish Obese Subjects trial, 248–249

T
T helper (Th) cells, 238
Third National Health and Nutrition Examination Survey (NHANES III), 194
Tirzepatide, 243
TNF receptor-associated factor 2 (TRAF2), 190
Toll-like receptor (TLR), 240
Trans-activation response RNA-binding protein (TRBP), 181
Tumor necrosis factor-alpha (TNF-α), 73, 235–236

U
Unfolded protein response (UPR), 190

V
Vascular cell adhesion molecule-1 (V-CAM-1), 253
Vascular endothelial growth factor (VEGF), 193
Visceral fat, 219

W
Weight loss medications, 242–245, 246–247t
Western diet, 223
White adipose tissue (WAT), 190
World Health Organization (WHO), 5

Z
Zone diet, 222

CPI Antony Rowe
Eastbourne, UK
December 19, 2022